Technological Change in Modern Surgery

Rochester Studies in Medical History

Senior Editor: Theodore M. Brown
Professor of History and Preventive Medicine
University of Rochester

Additional Titles of Interest

Female Circumcision and Clitoridectomy in the United States: A History of a Medical Treatment
Sarah B. Rodriguez

The Spanish Influenza Pandemic of 1918–1919: Perspectives from the Iberian Peninsula and the Americas
Edited by María-Isabel Porras-Gallo and Ryan A. Davis

Infections, Chronic Disease, and the Epidemiological Transition: A New Perspective
Alexander Mercer

Save the Babies: American Public Health Reform and the Prevention of Infant Mortality, 1850–1929
Richard A. Meckel

Intrusive Interventions: Public Health, Domestic Space, and Infectious Disease Surveillance in England, 1840–1914
Graham Mooney

The Antivaccine Heresy: "Jacobson v. Massachusetts" and the Troubled History of Compulsory Vaccination in the United States
Karen L. Walloch

Healthy Boundaries: Property, Law, and Public Health in England and Wales, 1815–1872
James G. Hanley

Psychiatry and Racial Liberalism in Harlem, 1936–1968
Dennis A. Doyle

Childbirth, Maternity, and Medical Pluralism in French Colonial Vietnam, 1880–1945
Thuy Linh Nguyen

Setting Nutritional Standards: Theory, Policies, Practices
Edited by Elizabeth Neswald, David F. Smith, and Ulrike Thoms

A complete list of titles in the Rochester Studies in Medical History series may be found on our website, www.urpress.com.

Technological Change in Modern Surgery

Historical Perspectives on Innovation

EDITED BY THOMAS SCHLICH
AND CHRISTOPHER CRENNER

UNIVERSITY OF ROCHESTER PRESS

The University of Rochester Press gratefully acknowledges generous support from the James McGill Chair program of McGill University and the Kansas University Endowment Association.

First published 2017

University of Rochester Press
668 Mt. Hope Avenue, Rochester, NY 14620, USA
www.urpress.com
and Boydell & Brewer Limited
PO Box 9, Woodbridge, Suffolk IP12 3DF, UK
www.boydellandbrewer.com

ISBN-13: 978-1-58046-594-6
ISSN: 1526-2715

Library of Congress Cataloging-in-Publication Data

Names: Schlich, Thomas, editor. | Crenner, Christopher, 1961– editor.
Title: Technological change in modern surgery : historical perspectives on innovation / edited by Thomas Schlich and Christopher Crenner.
Other titles: Rochester studies in medical history ; v. 39. 1526-2715
Description: Rochester, NY : University of Rochester Press, 2017. | Series: Rochester studies in medical history, ISSN 1526-2715 ; vol. 39 | Includes bibliographical references and index.
Identifiers: LCCN 2017008053 | ISBN 9781580465946 (hardcover : alk. paper) Subjects: | MESH: Specialties, Surgical—history | Surgical Procedures, Operative—trends | Inventions—history | History, Modern 1601–
Classification: LCC RD32 | NLM WO 11.1 | DDC 617—dc23 LC record available at https://lccn.loc.gov/2017008053

This publication is printed on acid-free paper.
Printed in the United States of America.

We would like to dedicate this book to
Dr. Marc Asher for his inspiration and support.

Contents

Chapter One

Technological Change in Surgery

An Introductory Essay

THOMAS SCHLICH AND CHRISTOPHER CRENNER

Surgery over the last two hundred years has gone through enormous technological transformations and continues to be a hotbed of technical innovation, as recent developments in transplantation, osteosynthesis, minimally invasive surgery, artificial organs, and implanted assistive devices testify. Surgery is thus an ideal field for examining the processes of technological change in medicine. It is also a field that has some specific and distinct features, which makes it particularly interesting for investigating technological change: Within medicine, surgery is most closely associated with bodily practices. Surgery is performed on the living body of the patient, which becomes the material of the surgeon's craft. It is further linked to the manual skills and the immediate physical presence of the surgeon. All of this makes it a practice with high and highly visible stakes for all involved, especially in the implementation of new technologies.

Surgery itself can be described as a technology. Under the comprehensive definition proposed by scholars in science and technology studies, the word "technology" has three layers of meaning.[1] First, there is the physical level. In surgery, this involves the instruments, the operating room, and so on. Second, technology can be seen as an activity, as a means to accomplish a specific goal. This refers to what the surgeon does in the operative procedure. Finally, technology is what people know: having instruments and starting to use them on bodies was not enough for successful surgery; surgeons also had to know how to apply the tools and the techniques within their sphere of activity. A surgical technology cannot be spread without the relevant knowledge, know-how, and practical skills. In surgery, the provider-user relationship is also unusually complex. The primary user of surgical technology is the surgeon, but the surgeon applies the technology to another participant in the setting, a patient, who thus becomes in a way the end-user of surgical technology and, in certain instances, an active participant in the employment of new tools and techniques.

Innovation

For explaining change in medicine, historians have traditionally focused on the point of discovery of a new principle or the invention of a new technique. The truth of the discovered principle and the usefulness of the invention itself were seen as the reason for change.[2] But, as more recent historical studies have shown, even superior techniques do not inevitably spread. To understand the successful adoption of a surgical technology one has to explain the wider conditions of its success. Among these conditions, the technology itself is just one element. It must be examined in the context of the prevailing social, political, and economic conditions, as well as the work that historical actors put into making the new technique effective, useful, and practicable.[3]

In the last couple of decades many historical studies have used the conceptual framework of "innovation" in order to follow this more comprehensive approach in explaining change in medicine.[4] They have broadened their perspective to look at the complex processes of the introduction of novel techniques into specific social or economic contexts and looked beyond the simple development of a new technique to examine how it was used, regulated, and controlled, what skills and resources were needed to make it work, and what meaning it was given.

The concept of "innovation" became particularly popular in the history of medicine in the early 1990s. At a time when change in medicine was perceived as a "mixed blessing and evaluations of modern medicine oscillate[d] between eloquent praise and sharp criticism,"[5] using the concept of innovation was an attempt to overcome naïve and teleologically charged ideas of "progress" and "advance." "It suits our time," John Pickstone wrote in 1992, and explained that "as public programs recede before the protagonists of market mechanisms, so new technology comes to be identified with new products for markets, rather than with grand designs for the better provision of energy, food or welfare."[6] The innovation framework thus corresponded to a view of medicine as a market rather than a humanitarian enterprise. New technologies did not automatically denote successful or failed progress. They were now "innovations," which were either successful or not in the medical and societal marketplace. Thus innovation still denoted progress, but progress defined in market terms.

By 1999 Jennifer Stanton was able to refer to a "new school" of historians, "which treats medical technology as another element in the social, political, and economic history of medicine relating it to professionalization, changing notions about disease, and the organization of medical care."[7] Numerous case studies now demonstrated "an awareness that medical technologies fit into the power structures of medicine and wider society," and that "their images, uses, successes and failures have to be seen in that light."[8] In this way, the historical study of innovation provided "a privileged site of investigation of the multiple dimensions of medicine," as Ilana Löwy has phrased it. It helped to better understand the "close links between different aspects of medicine as a body of knowledge, laboratory and bedside practice, and social institution."[9] History of this kind was potentially fruitful for understanding present conditions and future developments.[10]

The innovation framework with its broader view of change beyond discovery or invention came with a model of a "staged career." This model encompassed the introduction of new technologies into social and economic contexts as well as their subsequent "diffusion" when the innovation became more widely adopted.[11] The approach was applicable to surgical operations too, so that, as Sally Wilde describes it, operations were seen to "have careers, and the processes through which they are developed have many parallels to the processes through which other technological innovations are developed."[12]

However, more recently, the use of the innovation framework has been viewed more critically. Sally Frampton has argued that the staged career model only works well if technologies remain identical over time. This can be problematic when we investigate surgery, since surgical interventions are unstable entities to start with. "Meanings of different operations," she points out, "shift continually, no matter how long and established their history. A tonsillectomy is performed and experienced quite differently today than from how it was in the 1920s." In the end, "labels such as 'ovariotomy,' helped to make sense of surgical innovation, to give a firm, single identity and status to the operation," but, "underneath that label, . . . there often struggled multiple identities and meanings, over which were layered differing representations."[13] It is thus questionable how useful the staged career model is, with its distinction between innovation, invention, and diffusion, in a situation where "both the context and the technology of a surgical innovation are liable to change."[14]

The whole notion of a linear development of surgical innovation has to be viewed critically. It risks making the acceptance of new techniques look inevitable, and oversimplifies its often complex and convoluted character. It is rare, for example, that the idea of a new procedure leads directly to its use. Normally the "relationship between theory and practice in the construction of a 'new' operation" is "complex and circular."[15] In many cases, there is no clear direction of innovation pointing from scientific theory to surgical practice. In the introduction of antisepsis and asepsis, for example, scientific research in the laboratory and surgical practices stood in complicated mutual relationships.[16] The same is true for organ transplantation where the emergence of the concept of "organ replacement" went hand in hand with the development of the surgical practice of transplantation.[17] Moreover, many innovations in surgery were first used in practice and only later justified by scientific research, for example, osteosynthesis (the operative treatment of broken bones by metal implants, such as plates and screws).[18]

Instead of a linear development, one can think of the rise of modern surgery as the emergence of a network of various and heterogeneous control technologies.[19] The network metaphor is also being used in science and technology studies for comprehensive explanatory accounts of transformations, so that innovators can be characterized as "network builders,"[20] as John Law has called it. In surgery, the introduction of, for example, a technology like osteosynthesis can be analyzed as "the building of a complex network of specific practices, actors and objects linked to different localities."[21]

Newness

Innovation studies focus on the new. They are, as Stanton states, "about change and the excitement of new developments," reflecting the "fascination in the media, among the public, and in museums and popular literature" about "medical 'breakthrough.'"[22] In the past decades, innovation with its claim to newness has become a buzzword for business and organizations of all kinds, including health care, where it has been a common strategy to try and optimize medical services by "the creation and diffusion of new products and processes."[23] Since the 1990s, the concept of innovation has been escalated into its maximum version—"disruptive innovation." Disruptive innovation is being recommended as the only way to survive in a world in which the old recipes for economic success no longer work.[24] In a dog-eat-dog world of neoliberalism the choice is between being either an agent of disruption or a victim of it.[25] The history of minimally invasive surgery (keyhole surgery) has been told as a story of disruptive innovation. In this narrative, general surgeons nearly missed the boat on introducing the new disruptive technology, losing their market to internist and radiologists.[26]

To be sure, for the historical actors in their time period, it was often important to claim novelty for the techniques they proposed. In science and medicine, credit, priority, and intellectual property have always been closely linked up to originality.[27] However, historians cannot simply accept such claims at face value: "what constitutes an innovation was very much a matter of perspective, and often a matter of conflicting perspectives," Löwy wrote in 1992,[28] and as Frampton has found for ovariotomy, fundamentally, "the 'new' is very much a representation," it is "fixed to a specific time period." Ovariotomy could be presented as new or as old, according to the needs of the historical actors in particular contexts. "Thus," she concludes, "notions of 'newness' are to be seen as constructed rather than necessarily pertaining to a linear temporality."[29] This is a position that makes it possible for the historian to escape the conscription into the retrospective adjudication of priority claims.[30]

Going beyond the awareness of the historically constructed nature of novelty, other authors have criticized the exclusive interest in the new in an "innovation-centric history." In his monograph *The Shock of the Old*, the historian of science and technology David Edgerton observes a widespread assumption "that the new is much superior to older methods."[31] In reality, he argues, this judgment is often not well-founded. It is a widespread but often erroneous belief "that the new would be better in the longer run"[32]—a belief that can even become a self-fulfilling prophecy. As he further points out, the unreflecting assumption of the superiority of the new has a significant historiographical corollary. If we accept it, we need to explain why some historical actors did not take on the new, why they put up "resistance," as it is called. "Resistance to new technology" becomes a puzzle to be solved with the help of psychological and sociological factors.[33] Often individual attitudes and emotional influences are used for this purpose—conservativism, jealousy, or worse, stupidity and ignorance.

However, "the idea of 'resistance' only makes sense if there are no alternatives."[34] Unfortunately, many historical accounts of technologies are indeed implicitly based on the "hidden counterfactual assumption" that the uptake and use of a technology shows "that there was no alternative" at the time.[35] But this is not the case: There "usually have been comparable alternatives" to new technologies: there were computing machines before electronic computers, there were multiple means of transporting people when the railway came up, the Internet is not the only way of communicating over long distances.[36] It is often difficult for historians to identify such alternatives, since they sometimes become almost invisible in retrospect.[37] But at closer examination we can see "alternatives . . . for almost any major modern invention." Veritable "clusters of related innovations" can be found, which are "waiting to be selected" and which "exist to fulfill virtually any of our wants, needs or whims."[38] In general, "societies have long thrown up many more innovations than have actually been used, or probably could be used." This means that, in fact, the majority of technologies had to be "resisted."[39] Resisting the introduction of new technologies is thus nothing unusual, that is, in special need of explanation.[40] "In a world where individuals or societies simply could not accept every innovation on offer, resistance is required.

In choosing one technology, society [is] necessarily resisting *many* 'old' and 'new' alternative technologies"[41]

Acceptance and Rejection

Despite the problems with such a simplistic concept, studies on innovation in medicine are usually couched in terms of diffusion versus resistance, success versus failure. They are structured around this distinction in order to explain "how and why changes have spread" and how they will spread in the future.[42] In the history of surgery historians apply the same dichotomy and examine how "new operations were invented and either flourished and developed or declined into oblivion."[43] But this dichotomy restricts analysis. It cannot account for more complex developments, which emerge when the identity of the interventions changes over time, but also when, for example, the indication for a particular surgical intervention varies.[44] Some operations, such as tonsillectomy, seem to have been relatively stable and widespread over time. So one could call them successful. Others have gone through a period of popularity and then disappeared. Examples are ovariotomy for treating "insanity" in women (Battey's operation) and nephropexy to fix "floating kidneys." These are the "failures."[45]

In the case of ovariotomy most of the time both acceptance and rejection were present, which was further complicated by a changing and inconsistent nomenclature. In the end, the question of whether ovariotomy was accepted or rejected revolves around the meaning that was given to the operation at a certain point in time.[46] Frampton also points to the example of nephropexy, which shows how, with time, these meanings can change. Nephropexy, once ridiculed by much of the surgical profession, is in use again today, but it is framed by an entirely different medico-cultural context.[47] To some degree these operations are not even identical in the different contexts. In any case, "such occurrences speak to the continual negotiation between surgical nomenclature and the meaning of operations, which complicates notions of success or failure."[48]

Many surgical examples show the precariousness of the categories of "success" and "failure." Organ transplantation, for example, first introduced in the 1880s, was abandoned in the 1920s because transplants between different individuals hit an obstacle that turned out to be insurmountable for the time being. The method was taken up again only in 1945, but transplant rejection remained an irresolvable problem until the 1960s. Transplants only became a viable technology when pharmaceuticals were introduced that prevented the recipient's immune system from attacking the transplanted organ.[49] As a result of this, the early period of transplantation, between 1880 and 1920, is today seen as a time of pioneering innovation. But it's easy to see that transplants could have easily gone down in history as a bizarre aberration.

Interestingly, the construction of a historical narrative is already part of the innovation process. It helps to define a particular procedure as an innovation and gives relevance to it. This is true for ovariotomy[50] as much as it is true for transplant surgery. Frequently, the narrative is extended into the earlier past, or a fictitious version of it. Some transplant surgeons went to the extreme of reinterpreting all kinds of cultural material from the past as being evidence of the idea of "organ transplantation." Ganesha, the Indian god of wisdom who has the head of an elephant, as well as ancient Greek chimeras and other mythological figures, ended up as examples of early transplantation, or at least the existence of the idea of transplantation.[51] Even more recent accounts of the history of organ transplants cast the Saints Cosmas and Damian as predecessors of modern transplant surgeons because, according to the medieval *legenda aurea*, one of the miracles the saintly brothers worked was replacing the "bad" leg of a worshipper in his dream with the leg of recently deceased moor, which they took from the graveyard.[52] The creation of predecessors and pioneers can even be understood as a narrative effect of the structure of the normal scientific paper with its reference to past work on the topic, which is then enhanced in some of the historical papers written by doctors and scientists.[53]

The status of supposed predecessor techniques varies according to the context in which the narrative is being written. For example, operative fracture care with screws, wire, and plates was tried out by several surgeons in the nineteenth and twentieth centuries.[54] For a long time, however, such attempts remained isolated and nonoperative treatment with plaster casts or traction was the standard of care. Within this context, the early attempts at osteosynthesis looked like an item on the list of bizarre alternative innovations, together with other abandoned approaches such as Just Lucas-Championnière's massage treatment. However, in the 1960s an organization of Swiss surgeons (the AO/ASIF) organized and standardized operative fracture care in a way that made it applicable on a large scale. Once this technology was established, the earlier work was reinterpreted as pioneer work for an ultimately successful innovation. What needed to be explained now was how surgeons could ever have been critical of osteosynthesis and "resist" innovation. We can see how there is a constant reevaluation of the past in light of the present. This fluidity of the past renders judgments and categorization fragile and susceptible to being overturned and even ridiculed in the future. Today's innovators can easily be tomorrow's cranks.

It is therefore worthwhile for historians to step out of the normatively loaded terminology of acceptance and rejection, success and failure. A good way of doing this is to widen the focus by giving more room to alternatives and examining the landscape of technologies that were both in use and coming into use in a certain time period or context.

Alternatives

Looking for alternatives is not new. There has been a long-standing interest on part of some historians of technology in alternatives, in "paths not taken."[55] However, the problem is not just the neglect of alternatives. Even if the existence of alternatives is being acknowledged, there is often an assumption that there was no *comparable* alternative, in other words it is assumed that, as Edgerton explains, "the newest was radically more effective, efficient, powerful and generally better than what it superseded." "But," he continues, "to become widely used, a thing does not have to be massively better than what preceded it; it needs only to be *marginally* better than alternatives (assuming for the moment that better technologies will replace worse ones)."[56] We can go even further. If we consider existing alternatives in the history of technological transformation in a serious way, Edgerton argues, we can also see that new technologies were not necessarily superior to the old ones at all. Studies into the choice of technology have shown not only "that alternatives often exist" but also "that the fact that one technology supersedes another is not even evidence of superiority at all, since other factors are involved." If we take the increase of general welfare as the equivalent of superiority, we can see that some new technologies actually reduced welfare, compared with the best alternative. Edgerton mentions nuclear power as an example. This example also points to the fact that "societies can get locked into technologies which are worse than real alternatives."[57]

It is true that, for understanding how medicine became what it is today, one has to look at success stories, for example, transplants and operative fracture treatment, which have both become common procedures. Because they were successful, these innovations were able to shape medical practice. As historians, however, we also want to understand the conditions that made these technologies successful, and a crucial element among these conditions are the other technologies that were around or arose at the time when a new technology was introduced.

Historians need to examine the negotiations about new surgical interventions and techniques in a context where the innovation is being compared with other options for addressing the same problem, either old or new, either operative or nonoperative.[58] However, "because the world changes in so many ways," it can be very difficult to understand the rationale of such comparisons retrospectively.[59] But without looking at alternatives, we risk fundamentally misinterpreting the processes of transformation in surgery, for example, by attributing irrationality to historical actors who were following alternative trajectories. Taking alternatives into account, we can write history without blaming historical actors of conservativism, blindness, or stubbornness—an attitude that can also be useful for understanding such processes in the present time.

If we take, for example, the introduction of rubber gloves into surgical practice, many historical accounts show deep impatience with past surgeons' hesitation to adopt surgical gloves. They find it "curious that it took lively minds so long to come around with the notion of an impermeable glove in surgery," and "even more curious that, when the proposal was finally made in the eighteen-nineties, it required more than a decade of passionate argument before final universal acceptance could be achieved," the explanation being that "the human mind does not always dart straight to the obvious."[60] A closer investigation of the discussions at the time shows that many surgeons were skeptical about gloves for good reasons. They hesitated exchanging the manual dexterity of their uncovered hands against an unclear benefit in infection control.[61] We don't need deviance of the mind as an explanation. Another example of this is the story of the first introduction of rubber gloves into the operating room. This happened in 1889 at the Johns Hopkins Department of Surgery headed by William Halsted. As Halsted recalled later, the nurse in charge of his operating room "complained that the solution of mercuric chloride [the antiseptic substance that he used at the time] produced a dermatitis of her arms and hands." As the surgeon wanted to keep this "unusually efficient woman" in his OR, he "one day in New York requested the Goodyear Rubber Company to make as an experiment two pair of thin rubber gloves with gauntlets."[62] The fact that this nurse was Halsted's future wife makes for a popular story among the anecdotes of medical history. But the story also has less sanguine part: For a long time it was only the nurses who used the gloves. It took seven years until the operating surgeons wore them on a routine basis.[63] This "delay" has been a puzzle for historians of medicine. Even Halsted himself wondered in retrospect how he "could have been so blind as not to have perceived the necessity for wearing them invariably at the operating table."[64]

Carelessness is a very improbable explanation, since Halsted was known for his extreme fastidiousness in all things that had to do with asepsis.[65] There is another explanation for the fact that gloves were not his main concern at that time, and that is that he was busy working at a different strategy of preventing wound infection. Interestingly, Halsted had developed his alternative strategy because of his interest in bacteriology. He had used bacteriological methods to test Joseph Lister's system of antisepsis, and he found that it was not possible to eliminate all bacteria in the wound with antiseptics. As a reaction, Halsted tried to figure out some other way of preventing wound infection. He aimed at creating conditions in the patient's wound and tissues that would prevent bacteria that were in the wound from causing a wound infection. In one experiment, for example, he introduced bacteria into the peritoneal cavity of dogs and noticed that no harm occurred "as long he carefully avoided any mechanical injury to the tissues." However, if he bruised the tissue or cut off some small part of it from its blood supply, "a single bacterium . . . was able to multiply and cause a fatal peritonitis."[66] As a consequence, Halsted put his focus on his careful and gentle operating technique. He wrote in 1891 that "the obstruction to the circulation produced by sutures and ligatures is often the immediate cause of suppuration in infected wounds."[67] As Halsted's first biographer William MacCallum put it, Halsted's procedures were "of mathematical precision, with healing almost as precisely ensured."[68] Thus much of Halsted's infection prophylaxis was embodied in his surgical technique rather than in preventing contamination from outside. For this reason gloves were not high on his agenda.

This example shows how the conventionally narrow focus on a single surgical technology and its acceptance or rejection, in this case the gloves, can lead to the serious misinterpretation of events and developments. Moreover, Halsted's careful operating style was not the only alternative to the use of surgical gloves. There was, for example, a whole range of different techniques of hand disinfection in use. Another strategy consisted in keeping one's hands clean between operations and abstaining from handling infectious material, even when not on the job—an approach that among some authors amounted to a whole regime of living.[69] Separation between septic and aseptic cases, rooms and operators, was another common strategy.[70] Other surgeons developed no-touch techniques for their operations. William Arbuthnot Lane designed a particular set of instruments that had long handles to use for operative fracture treatment—a method that has mockingly been called "the knife and fork method of operating."[71] But the no-touch approach was used in various contexts later on too. Still another strategy consisted in coating the surgeon's hands with a layer of some substance in order to prevent contamination of the wound without limiting manual dexterity.[72] For this purpose surgeons tried paraffin,[73] or a special wax paste as an aseptic "microscopic glove," which was to be "impermeable for water, blood juices, and bacteria."[74] None of these methods was taken up on a large scale, mainly, it seems, because the coatings were not durable enough to last through a surgical intervention. The theme, however, persisted. In 1943 three researchers at the University of Chicago reported their observation that "cationic detergents deposit an invisible, non-perceptible film on the hands which retains bacteria under it," and which was supposedly quite durable and had considerable "bactericidal power."[75] Still another approach to dealing with wound infection was systemic and took vaccination as its model. Various surgeons tried to create either specific immunity against wound infection or to boost the body's immune defense more generally before surgical operations. Johannes Mikulicz, for example, a leading surgeon of his time who, among other things, added the face mask to the surgical equipment, submitted his patients to preoperative injection of nucleic acid in order to increase their white blood cell count and thus strengthen their immune defense.[76] Such attempts were similar to antibiotic prophylaxis as it was introduced a couple of decades later.

The negligence of alternatives and its consequences is very well visible in the traditional historiography of the introduction of antisepsis. For a long time, the history of antisepsis has been told as a story of innovative spirit versus conservative stubbornness. Surgeons who accepted Lister's antisepsis were seen as avant-garde. Those who didn't were thought to be resistant to innovation. The story was teleological. It assumed that the adoption of antisepsis was the quasi-natural outcome of history. In the past two decades new historical work has resulted in a different perspective: Historians have shown that a lot of surgeons were not particularly interested in Lister's ideas and practices at the time—*not* because they were conservative or stubborn, but because they were busy developing their *own* innovations. They were finding other ways and strategies of preventing wound disease. There was, for example, a group of doctors, scientists, and administrators in Lister's time who, as Michael Worboys writes, "transferred the rhetoric and prescriptions of the sanitary movement from the urban environment . . . to urban hospitals and their patients."[77] For the proponents of sanitation, Lister's focus on applying one chemical substance was a distraction from what really needed to be done, namely, reforming the hospitals.[78] Seen from that perspective, antisepsis was a more *conservative* approach to solving the problem at hand, and it was Lister who "resisted" substantial change. But even at the more technical level there were many alternatives to Lister's antisepsis. As Worboys states: "each surgeon had his own ideas and techniques,"[79] and each of these surgeons, "in their different ways, made wounds clean, halted sepsis, controlled inflammation and improved the healing power of the patient's constitution."[80] One the most influential alternatives to antisepsis was the so-called cleanliness and cold water school. Its protagonist, Thomas Spencer Wells, who was often portrayed as stubbornly resisting Lister's innovation, "emphasized the role of general sanitary principles and scrupulous cleanliness and purity.[81] Wells performed and documented thousands of invasive interventions, in particular ovariotomies, with minimal complications, without using antisepsis.[82] Spencer Wells is only one example. Historians can find a whole landscape of creative and rational innovations at the time. However, historiography lost sight of the diversity once Lister had been declared the founding figure of all the different methods of avoiding wound infection in the late nineteenth century. Following this teleological narrative, historians until recently cast the majority of these surgeons in the role of stubborn and conservative detractors of Lister's innovation.

We can see how the underlying teleology in much of the historiography conceals the fluidity and contingency of technical change in surgery, how it sanitizes and streamlines the diversity of human technical creativity and the varieties of use of new and old surgical technologies. In this volume we want to take a broader perspective. We want to "study the real, messy, contested and complex debates by which, over time, some procedures were accepted in preference to others," as Pickstone demanded in 1992.[83] We want to look at how surgical technologies exist in the setting of multiple and heterogeneous agents and structures, including doctors, patients, manufacturers, objects, institutions, regulations, etc., and how specific technologies and their uses emerged in such settings, how they were shaped by the settings, and, in turn, reconfigured them.[84] Within such a scenario the context is as variable and fluid as are the technologies themselves. As we have seen, this fluidity includes the newness of technologies, which varies according to perspective, context, and rhetoric. Novelty as such should therefore not be the main rationale for historical interest: a narrow focus on innovation understood as the introduction of new technologies makes it difficult to do justice to the full dimensions of the uses of technology. Similarly does the adherence to the simple dichotomy of acceptance versus rejection obscure choices and consequence, as do the value-laden categories of success and failure. Resistance, inertia, blindness, etc., are not the most useful categories to describe and explain why historical actors did not use certain new technologies.

With this volume we thus want to go beyond innovation studies. The papers here widen the view to take in multiple, simultaneous variations on tools and procedures, old and new. They explore the manifold choices that were available to historical actors as they sought to solve their problems. As we have seen, at closer examination such alternatives emerge wherever one looks in the history of surgery. Whole worlds of alternative versions of modern surgery open up, for example, concerning the multiple ways of dealing with wound infection through the surgeon's hands described above. Alternative technologies could be old or new, surgical or nonsurgical. Taking these alternatives into account helps understand the choices and decisions made by historical actors. It helps to explore the "paths not taken," the multiple parallel roads, the narrow trails and dirt tracks, as well the main highways. This makes it possible to appreciate also the diversity of technologies in the present time. It puts us in a better position to take notice of alternative forms of understanding and solving problems today, and to beware of "overblown claims of a one best way"[85] of dealing with technical, surgical, and medical challenges. In the chapters that follow the authors make use of these insights concerning technological change in surgery to explore a productive range of case studies.

The Book

One of several authors in the book who adds a layer of complexity to the notion of innovation is Lisa Haushofer. Her study of the celebrated early nineteenth-century surgeon Johann Friedrich Dieffenbach raises questions about the nature of innovation. Dieffenbach's reputation for innovation belies the ability of subsequent observers to point to a distinct technical advancement that he established. This insight leads Haushofer to explore Dieffenbach's role in advancing a different form of surgical innovation, in which new procedures were—paradoxically, from a modern point of view—difficult to teach and replicate. As Haushofer shows, the German surgeon intentionally emphasized the personal, inimitable character of the surgical technologies he developed. This move can be understood against the background of Dieffenbach's economic and professional context as well as the ideological climate of academic surgery in his time. In this context,"success" in innovation had a very different meaning from later times. Successful innovation is thus not always synonymous with standardized reproduction and diffusion of a new procedure—an idea that has been part a specific way of defining innovation in more recent times. Haushofer identifies the influence of the broad scholarly and cultural movement of *Naturphilosophie* in Dieffenbach's ambitions to create a new physiological surgery founded on the power of surgery to build and promote bodily healing, as against its ability to disassemble and excise bodily pieces. Dieffenbach's vitalist and antireductionist way of innovation in surgery thus embodies the holistic and universalist claims of the contemporary German university scholars and scientists that went very well with an individualizing approach to the transfer of new techniques.

Looking at nineteenth-century ovariotomy, Sally Frampton finds that the definition of this revolutionary surgical procedure remained unstable for decades after its introduction. Although widely practiced and discussed, the meaning of ovariotomy remained in flux, with different forms and applications of the procedure referred to as ovariotomy, oophorectomy, and "Battey's operation." By going beyond the common focus on the operation as merely an expression of the gender relations of the time, Frampton adds a crucial factor to understanding the use of ovariotomy in that time period. The history of ovariotomy is a good example of how the very identity of a surgical procedure is not necessarily a given but often a matter of negotiation. This means that the judgment about whether a particular operation is new and distinct is also contingent on a variety of factors. Frampton also shows how the issue of the identity and novelty of a surgical operation carries over into the writing of its history.

How the character of a surgical procedure as a novelty depends on its historical context is also demonstrated by Delia Gavrus. The techniques that were used in her example of surgery for juvenile delinquency were often centuries old. What made them novel was their purpose, which Gavrus locates in the interests of the users within the cultural climate of the time. For Gavrus, it was a progressive enthusiasm for a treatment to fight juvenile delinquency that renewed interest in the technology of trepanation and similar procedures for the release of pressure from the skull cavity. Surgeons with the backing of reform-minded agencies were eager to promote this project to create new forms of protopsychosurgery in the 1920s. Here, surgery appears as an alternative to nonmedical ways of dealing with the problem of juvenile delinquency in the legal and pedagogical domain. Instead of punishment or reeducation, delinquents undergo surgery.

Several authors have drawn on David Edgerton's insight that the "newness" of a technology derives from its ability to win usage in certain preferred locations, among certain preferred users. Versions of both a "new" and an "old" technology may have been long in use and continue in use outside an area of special interest. The alternative use of existing procedures, techniques, and instruments for new purposes thus makes up a significant part of innovative practice.

Other chapters combine the focus on the material dimension of surgery with a thorough exploration of the setting of surgery's use within the multitiered configuration of user demand from surgeons, manufacturers, and patients. Looking at the creation of the surgically implanted Harrington Spinal Rod in the 1950s, Beth Linker finds that patients seeking treatment were especially influential in establishing the Harrington Spinal Rods as a successful innovation. In a postwar period filled with bold technological innovations, people suffering from spinal deformities expressed optimism about Harrington's ability to free them from a lengthy process of restrictive casting and rehabilitation. Linker also demonstrated how even the case of a single inventor with a single device reveals a set of branching choices and decisions. In her analysis, the novel Harrington Rods used to treat spinal deformities arose out of the gradual refinement of devices worked out between engineering and surgery, as Harrington relied initially on the skills of the engineer Thorkild Engen, followed by a partnership with the firm of Zimmer Manufacturing.

The collaboration of engineering and surgery in innovative treatments was also at the core of the creation of the left ventricular assist device (LVAD), a partial version of the artificial heart, whose development is examined in the chapter by Shelley McKellar. She examines the spread of the LVAD in the context of a variety of therapeutic options and demonstrates how developments of this context influenced the adoption of the device. One example is the way that the improved prognosis of cardiac transplantation redefined the LVAD as a bridging technology at one point and thus broadened its area of indication—an observation that points to the dynamics between different treatment rationales in surgery. McKellar's essay also demonstrates how the spread of surgical innovations depends on processes of clinical evaluation. The clinical adoption of the artificial heart was strongly influenced by testing in a single large experimental clinical trial. It featured the Randomized Clinical Trial (RCT) as a key tool that through its general adoption as a gold standard has become crucial even in the field of surgery, which for a long time did not accept RCTs as its main assessment tool. This look at the artificial heart also exposes a tension between the need to establish a fixed, standard version of treatment for valid experimental testing against the surgeon's desire to tinker and improve.

This theme figures prominently in Christopher Crenner's chapter examining competing means for the clinical evaluation of new surgical technologies. Although in surgery the standards of outcome assessment were traditionally based on case reports, beginning in the mid-twentieth century this long-standing method was challenged by the randomized clinical trial. This clash of methods appears with particular clarity in controversies about placebo surgery. Crenner makes use of this example to explore alternative ways of judging surgical innovation and to make visible how these technologies of assessment interacted with contextual factors, inside and outside of the field of surgery. The examination also shows how different evaluation techniques are related to different ways of understanding surgical innovation itself: The case series method is associated with an understanding of innovation as gradual and continuous; by contrast, clinical trials conceptualize the transformation of surgical techniques as a series of distinct discoveries that can each be assesssed in turn through rigorous testing. The case of placebo surgery demonstrates how the evaluation of new surgical developments also depended on their historical context and not just on their inherent characteristics.

Authors in this collection examine surgery over a wide span of eras, exposing some large-scale changes in the societal context of innovation. Whereas among nineteenth-century surgeons benefits from a successful new procedure came largely through gains in reputation and influence, as well as perhaps traffic in new patients, by the twentieth century the linking up of industrial production and surgical innovation meant that firms like Zimmer for spinal rods, as discussed by Linker, or Thoratec for artificial hearts, as discussed by McKellar, created large commercial stakes. Crenner's chapter reminds us that such alliances were not always successful. He tells the story of the firm NMT Medical, Inc., that closed its doors after it lost a gamble on an innovative surgical device being tested in clinical trials.

The contributions to this book focus on the nineteenth and twentieth centuries, with special attention given to the United States. Although this emphasis is in part due to the natural limitations of a brief edited volume, it also reflects the changing geography of surgical innovation, in which the major centers of innovation shifted to North America,[86] as well as, in terms of chronology, the accelerated pace of technological change in surgery in the late nineteenth and in the twentieth century, accompanied by an increasingly confidence in technological progress.

These shifts are especially notable in the developments in cardiac surgery. In analyzing the success of coronary artery bypass surgery (CABG) in the 1970s and 1980s, David Jones provides a model for understanding the relationship between technological change and change in disease concepts. He notes how coronary artery disease was not simply a preexisting problem awaiting solution. Instead, the definition of the disorder varied according to the strategies of treating it: disease understanding and therapy were mutually constitutive. Jones compares his view with the concept of the "ecological niche" in recent evolutionary biology. Such a niche is successfully populated by a novel species. However, an environment is not made up of preexistent niches; instead the ecologic niche is defined and shaped by its successful evolutionary occupant. Applied to technological change in surgery, this means that by demonstrating successful application in clinical practice, the procedure of CABG secured and reinforced a conception of coronary artery disease as a localized defect that could be "bypassed." Yet alternate treatments for coronary disease such as cholesterol-lowering medications were being deployed simultaneously. So in this case two contradictory disease concepts—one that sees the problem as local, and the other that considers it systemic—have been used in parallel, as have the respective treatments: one surgical, the other pharmaceutical. This demonstrates to what extent the understanding of disease in modern medicine is being shaped by therapeutic considerations, even in the face of patent inconsistencies.

The chapters thus use a range of case studies to explore the ways that technological change comes about in surgery. They investigate the eclectic nature of surgical innovation and follow the manifold influences in larger society as well as within medicine and technology that have shaped changes of surgical practices and thus broaden and often transcend the notion of "technological innovation."

Notes

1. Wiebe E. Bijker, Thomas P. Hughes, and Trevor Pinch, "General Introduction," in *The Social Construction of Technological Systems: New Directions in the Sociology and History of Technology*, ed. Wiebe E. Bijker, Thomas P. Hughes, and Trevor Pinch (Cambridge, MA: MIT Press, 1987), 4. For the use of this concept in surgery, see Thomas Schlich, *Surgery, Science, and Industry: A Revolution in Fracture Care, 1950s–1990s* (New York: Palgrave MacMillan, 2002).

2. John V. Pickstone, "Introduction," in *Medical Innovations in Historical Perspective*, ed. John V. Pickstone (Basingstoke, England: MacMillan Press, 1992), 1.

3. Trevor J. Pinch and Wiebe E. Bijker, "The Social Construction of Facts and Artifacts: Or How the Sociology of Science and the Sociology of Technology Might Benefit Each Other," in Bijker, Hughes, and Pinch, *Social Construction of Technological Systems*, 22–24; and Jennifer Stanton, "Making Sense of Technologies in Medicine," *Social History of Medicine* 12 (1999): 437–48; also Schlich, *Surgery, Science, and Industry*, 239.

4. Pickstone, "Introduction," 1, 9; Ilana Löwy, "Medicine and Change," in *Medicine and Change: Historical and Sociological Studies of Medical Innovation*, ed. Ilana Löwy et al. (Paris: INSERM), 1–4. For a survey, see Jennifer Stanton, "Introduction," in *Innovations in Health and Medicine: Diffusion and Resistance in the Twentieth Century*, ed. Jennifer Stanton (London: Routledge, 2002), 1.

5. Löwy, "Medicine and Change," 1; see also Stanton, "Making Sense of Technologies in Medicine."

6. Pickstone, "Introduction," 1.

7. Stanton, *Innovations in Health and Medicine*, 438.

8. Ibid., 448.

9. Löwy, "Medicine and Change," 3.

10. Thomas Schlich, "Risk and Medical Innovation: A Historical Perspective," in *The Risks of Medical Innovation: Risk Perception and Assessment in Historical Context*, ed. Thomas Schlich and Ulrich Tröhler (London: Routledge, 2006), 1–19.

11. Pickstone, "Introduction," 1. J. B. McKinlay, "From 'Promising Report' to 'Standard Procedure': Seven Stages in the Career of a Medical Innovation," *The Milbank Memorial Fund Quarterly* 59, no. 3 (1981): 374–411.

12. Sally Wilde, *History of Surgery: Trust, Patient Autonomy, Medical Dominance and Australian Surgery, 1890–1940* (Byron Bay, Australia: Finesse Press, 2010), 61. See discussion in Sally Frampton, "'The Most Startling Innovation': Ovarian Surgery in Britain, c. 1740–1939" (PhD diss., University College London, 2013), 223–24.

13. Frampton, "'Most Startling Innovation,'" tonsillectomy on 226–27; labels on 272.

14. Schlich, *Surgery, Science, and Industry*, 241.

15. Frampton, "'Most Startling Innovation,'" 70.

16. Michael Worboys, *Spreading Germs: Disease Theories and Medical Practice in Britain, 1865–1900* (Cambridge: Cambridge University Press, 2000), 73–107, 150–92. Thomas Schlich, "Asepsis and Bacteriology: A Realignment of Surgery and Laboratory Science," *Medical History* 56 (2012): 308–43.

17. Thomas Schlich, *The Origins of Organ Transplantation: Surgery and Laboratory Science, 1880s–1930s* (Rochester, NY: University of Rochester Press, 2010).

18. Schlich, *Surgery, Science, and Industry*.

19. Thomas Schlich, "Ein Netzwerk von Kontrolltechnologien: Eine neue Perspektive auf die Entstehung der modernen Chirurgie," *NTM Journal of the History of Science, Technology and Medicine* 16 (2008): 333–61.

20. John Law, "Technology and Heterogeneous Engineering: The Case of Portuguese Expansion," in Bijker, Hughes, and Pinch, *Social Construction of Technological Systems*, 112.

21. Schlich, *Surgery, Science, and Industry*, 241. See also Frampton, "'Most Startling Innovation,'" 269–70.

22. Stanton, "Introduction," 1.

23. Frampton, "'Most Startling Innovation,'" 14.

24. Clayton M. Christensen, *The Innovator's Dilemma: When New Technologies Cause Great Firms to Fail* (Boston, MA: Harvard Business School Press, 1997).

25. Jill Lepore, "The Disruption Machine: What the Gospel of Innovation Gets Wrong," *New Yorker*, June 16, 2014, http://www.newyorker.com/magazine/2014/06/23/the-disruption-machine (accessed February 8, 2016).

26. James R. Zetka, *Surgeons and the Scope* (Ithaca, NY: Cornell University Press, 2003). Interestingly, Zetka does not refer to Christensen but to a concept of the same name and very similar contents, which had its origins in occupational sociology.

27. Robert K. Merton, *The Sociology of Science* (Chicago: University of Chicago Press, 1973), 293, as discussed in Frampton, "'Most Startling Innovation,'" 138–39.

28. Löwy, "Medicine and Change," 3.

29. Frampton, "'Most Startling Innovation,'" 271.

30. Merton, *Sociology of Science*, 301–3.

31. David Edgerton, *The Shock of the Old: Technology and Global History since 1900* (London: Profile, 2006), 8.

32. Ibid.

33. Ibid., 9; similarly, Pickstone, "Introduction," 1; and Frampton, "'Most Startling Innovation,'" 134: "Writing an historical account on an ostensibly 'successful' innovation— . . . always runs the risk of characterising detractors along the way as conservative or even backwards looking."

34. Edgerton, *Shock of the Old*, 9.

35. Ibid., 6.

36. Ibid., 7.

37. David Edgerton, "From Innovation to Use: Ten Eclectic Theses on the Historiography of Technology," *History and Technology* 16 (1999): 123.

38. G. Basalla, *The Evolution of Technology* (Cambridge: Cambridge University Press, 1988), 204, as cited by Edgerton, "From Innovation to Use," 123.

39. Edgerton, "From Innovation to Use," 123.

40. Edgerton, "From Innovation to Use," 135n67.

41. Edgerton, *Shock of the Old*, 9.

42. Stanton, "Introduction," 13.

43. Ann Dally, *Women under the Knife: A History of Surgery* (London: Hutchinson Radius, 1991), 210, as quoted by Frampton, "'Most Startling Innovation,'" 223.

44. Frampton, "'Most Startling Innovation,'" 265.

45. Wilde, *History of Surgery*, 61, as discussed in Frampton, "'Most Startling Innovation,'" 223–24.

46. Frampton, "'Most Startling Innovation,'" 226–27, 269.

47. S. J. Srirangam et al., "Nephroptosis: Seriously Misunderstood?," *BJU International* 103, no. 3 (2009): 296–30.

48. Frampton, "'Most Startling Innovation,'" 224–25.

49. Even the first successful transplants in the 1960s circumvented the immunological obstacles by choosing identical twins as donor and recipient; Schlich, *Origins of Organ Transplantation.*

50. Frampton, "'Most Startling Innovation,'" 221, 269.

51. Thomas Schlich, "How Gods and Saints Became Transplant Surgeons: The Scientific Article as a Model for the Writing of History," *History of Science* 33 (1995): 311–31.

52. David Hamilton, *A History of Organ Transplantation: Ancient Legends to Modern Practice* (Pittsburgh, PA: Unversity of Pittsburgh Press, 2013).

53. Schlich, "How Gods and Saints."

54. For this and the following, see Schlich, *Surgery, Science, and Industry.*

55. David Edgerton, "Innovation, Technology, or History: What Is the Historiography of Technology About?," *Technology and Culture* 51 (2010): 682.

56. Edgerton, *Shock of the Old*, 8.

57. Edgerton, "From Innovation to Use," 123.

58. For a case example, see Frampton on ovariotomy, "'Most Startling Innovation,'" 127.

59. Edgerton, *Shock of the Old*, 8.

60. Justine Randers-Pehrson, *The Surgeon's Glove* (Springfield, IL: Charles C. Thomas, 1960), quotes on 3, 14, 30. See also Thomas Schlich, "Why Were Surgical Gloves Not Used Earlier? History of Medicine and Alternative Paths of Innovation," *Lancet* 386, no. 10,000 (2015): 1234–35.

61. Thomas Schlich, "Negotiating Technologies in Surgery: The Controversy about Surgical Gloves in 1890s," *Bulletin for the History of Medicine* 87 (2013): 170–97.

62. William Stewart Halsted, "Ligature and Suture Material," *Journal of the American Medical Association* 60 (1913): 1123.

63. J. M. T. Finney, *A Surgeon's Life: The Autobiography of J. M. T. Finney* (New York: G. P. Putnam's Sons, 1940), 90.

64. Halsted, "Ligature," 1124.

65. Randers-Pehrson, *Surgeon's Glove*, 58.

66. W. G. MacCallum, *William Stuart Halsted, Surgeon* (Baltimore, MD: Johns Hopkins University Press, 1930), 233, also 86–87.

67. W. S. Halsted, "The Treatment of Wounds," *Johns Hopkins Hospital Reports* 2, no. 5 (1891): 305.

68. MacCallum, *William Stuart Halsted*, as cited by Michael Bliss, *Harvey Cushing: A Life in Surgery* (New York: Oxford University Press, 2005), 101.

69. Carl Ludwig Schleich, *Neue Methoden der Wundheilung, ihre Bedingungen und Vereinfachung für die Praxis* (Berlin: Springer, 1899), 106–9. See, e.g., Theodor Kocher, "On Some Conditions of Healing by First Intention, with Special References to Disinfection of Hands," *Transactions of the American Surgical Association* 17 (1899): 116–42.

70. See, e.g., Albert J. Ochsner, "Aseptic Surgical Technique: Minimum Requirements for Aseptic Surgical Operating in a Hospital in Which the Personnel of the Operation Room Is Permanent," *Annals of Surgery* 40 (1904): 456.

71. William A. Lane, *The Operative Treatment of Fractures*, 2nd ed. (London: Medical Publishing Company, 1914), 126. Anon., "'Knife and Fork' Surgery," *The Star*, Lyttleton, New Zealand, May 4, 1903, 3.

72. Carl S. Haegler, *Händereinigung, Händedesinfektion und Händeschutz* (Basel: Schwabe, 1900), 167.

73. Ibid., 170–74.

74. Schleich, *Neue Methoden*, 108.

75. Miller, Benjamin F., Richard Abrams, Dorothy Ann Huber, and Morton Klein, "Formation of Invisible, Non-Perceptible Films on Hands by Cationic Soaps," *Proceedings of the Society for Experimental Biology and Medicine* 54 (1943): 175.

76. Erwin Payr, *Die physiologisch-biologische Richtung der modernen Chirurgie* (Leipzig: Hirzel, 1913), 29, more in n. 9, on 50–51. Johann von Mikulicz-Radecki, "Experiments on the Immunization against Infection of Operation Wounds, Especially of the Peritoneum," *Lancet* July 2, 1904, 1 1.

77. Worboys, *Spreading Germs,* 77.

78. Ibid., 84.

79. Ibid., 76.

80. Ibid., 102.

81. Ibid., 80.

82. Ibid., 186, see also, e.g., Peter J. Kernahan, "Causation and Cleanliness: George Callender, Wounds, and the Debates over Listerism," *Journal of the History of Medicine and Allied Sciences* 64 (2008): 1–36.

83. Pickstone, "Introduction," 16.

84. Schlich, *Surgery, Science, and Industry,* 241.

85. Edgerton, "From Innovation to Use," 129.

86. Thomas Schlich, "'One and the Same the World Over'—The International Culture of Surgical Exchange in an Age of Globalization, 1870–1914," *Journal of the History of Medicine and Allied Sciences* (online February 16, 2016), doi:10.1093/jhmas/jrw003.

Chapter Two

Inimitable Innovation

Johann Friedrich Dieffenbach and the Renewal of Surgery, 1822–1847

Lisa Haushofer

The surgeon Johann Friedrich Dieffenbach is often referred to as one of the most innovative characters in the development of German surgery during the early nineteenth century, particularly in the area of plastic surgery. But for a figure that has become almost emblematic of surgical innovation, Dieffenbach's case also challenges two common assumptions about innovation in surgery. One is that innovation in surgery during the nineteenth century was largely the product of technological change, particularly the introduction of anesthetic and aseptic techniques.[1] The other, that a vital factor in the success of surgical innovations is the degree to which they can be reproduced and diffused.[2] As for the first, Dieffenbach's work is located in the early part of the nineteenth century, rendering explanations of the growth of surgery based solely on technological determinism problematic, and opening up new questions about the driving forces behind innovation in surgery. With regard to the second, Dieffenbach's brand of innovation was formulated in a way that made it essentially inimitable. Dieffenbach's writings therefore provide an opportunity to reexamine these assumptions and offer alternative explanations.

The flourishing of plastic surgery in the early nineteenth century is a particular puzzle. Why would a technique dedicated to non-life-threatening conditions gain such momentum in the pre-anesthesia world? Many histories of plastic surgery avoid this question altogether and merely chart the diffusion of plastic surgical techniques, from the moment of the "rediscovery" of a technique for reconstructing the nose developed in India in the late eighteenth century, to the uptake of this and similar techniques by a number of surgeons in the German states and other countries in the early decades of the nineteenth century.[3] More analytically oriented works have vaguely relied on a certain spirit of the age for answers. "Innovation was in the air," writes Roy Porter about the introduction of a number of new plastic surgical techniques by the German surgeon Johann Friedrich Dieffenbach.[4] Other authors have expressed surprise that plastic surgery boomed *in spite of,* not because of, the Zeitgeist. "The German enthusiasm for plastic surgery was a puzzling development," observes David Hamilton, "because German-speaking thinkers were the origin of Naturphilosophie and the Romantic movement, whose antiscience stance rejected the scholarly achievements of Enlightenment thinking and substituted a free-floating theorizing and philosophical stance. Somehow," he concludes, "plastic surgery, a fundamentally mechanistic human endeavor without the slightest hint of the mystical, flourished."[5]

Dieffenbach is cited in Porter's chapter on the development of surgery as a particularly ridiculous example of the "craze" of surgical innovations, which seemed to grip surgery in this period.[6] Indeed, the seemingly eclectic spectrum of Dieffenbach's surgical ventures—ranging from plastic and orthopedic surgical techniques to operations for stuttering and strabismus—have earned him a place in the occasional collection of "strange medicine" or "weird cures."[7] In histories of the development of the discipline of plastic surgery, Dieffenbach appears instead as a "pioneer,"[8] "founder,"[9] or "father"[10] of the field. In these accounts, Dieffenbach's innovativeness is usually told as a series of pragmatic technical additions to surgical procedures and the introduction of new techniques, taking the motivation for these innovations as self-evident. For example, he is credited with "improving" the Indian method of rhinoplasty, a technique in which a skin flap was mobilized from the forehead and rotated downward to cover the nose.[11] Dieffenbach modified the technique by using a larger, slightly differently shaped skin flap. He is also acknowledged for "reducing blood congestion with leeches and reducing the compression of vessels in the pedicle (skin bridge) of the forehead flap by insetting the pedicle."[12] Given that these alterations are arguably minute, some of the foundational narratives of the discipline of plastic surgery struggle to determine in what Dieffenbach's "pioneering" role consisted exactly.[13]

A different approach is taken by Sander Gilman, whose cultural history of aesthetic surgery understands the development of techniques like rhinoplasty in this period as a response to particular social and cultural pressures. According to Gilman, the expansion of plastic surgical procedures must be understood in the context of changing cultural fears surrounding the stigmatized syphilitic nose, and later, the "Jewish" nose.[14] One of the pitfalls of writing the history of plastic surgery from a cultural perspective has been to assume the existence of a distinct category of "plastic surgery" with particular characteristics and concerns that align astoundingly well with those of contemporary plastic surgery. In this vein, historians have associated Dieffenbach most strongly with the distinction between aesthetic and reconstructive surgery. According to these interpretations, Dieffenbach sought to distinguish a useful reconstructive surgery from a frivolous unnecessary surgery for purely cosmetic purposes.[15] At the same time, Dieffenbach appears as practicing "aesthetic surgery."[16] Yet the distinction between aesthetic and reconstructive operations does not appear as a prominent concern in Dieffenbach's writings. Instead, the *plastic* of Dieffenbach's surgery, I suggest, reflected contemporary *Naturphilosophie*-inflected thinking about processes of growth and change in living beings. If there is a distinction Dieffenbach was concerned with, it is not one between cosmetic and reconstructive operations, but one that delineates a *physiological* surgery based on those principles of life formation from a *mechanistic* surgery that treats the body as lifeless material. Dieffenbach sought to create a new approach to surgery in its entirety, a *plastic* surgery.

While Hamilton's surprise at the development of plastic surgery in a period rife with Naturphilosophie-inspired thinking is understandable, I suggest it is exactly this intersection that should serve as the point of departure for understanding the particular brand of innovation Dieffenbach was championing. Dieffenbach sought innovation not through the development and naming of new surgical techniques or through the modification of existing ones. Instead, his goal was a renewal of the surgical approach in its entirety. Drawing on debates among his contemporaries about medical education and the role of the university, Dieffenbach envisioned surgery as based entirely on the principles of physiology, oriented toward the restoration of bodily forms and functions rather than their destruction or removal. Plastic surgery offered a particularly apt platform to formulate these larger goals, as it was governed by general physiological principles, while at the same time it demanded consideration of idiosyncracies and tested surgical ingenuity. However, this made Dieffenbach's surgical innovations essentially inimitable, a characteristic generally thought incompatible with "successful" innovations. Solving the paradox of Dieffenbach's "inimitable innovation" is only possible, I suggest, when considered within the professional and institutional context of early nineteenth-century Prussian university medicine.

Knowledge, Practice, and Medical Education

Of the numerous developments that brought profound transformations for the German-speaking territories at the turn from the eighteenth to the nineteenth century, the most significant was perhaps the indignity of the defeat of Prussia's undefeatable army. In the wake of this symbolic humiliation, Prussian state officials grew more attentive to calls from education reformers whose vision of a nonutilitarian university dedicated wholly to *Bildung* and *Wissenschaft* promised to reaffirm Prussia's leading role in a politically fragmented yet culturally consonant Germany united by a critical "public sphere."[17] However, when put into practice in the form of the University of Berlin in 1810, and later the university of Bonn in 1818, these ideals remained contested, and just how much a university should serve the purposes of the state by providing professional training, or form the individual into a truth-seeking, autonomous, free citizen by encouraging research, remained a point of contention. In medicine, the debate over useful versus pure knowledge materialized in the form of recurring tensions between theory and practice as the supreme goals of a university medical education.[18]

One of the most promising fields to bridge the gap between medical knowledge and its application was the science of physiology. At the end of the eighteenth and the early nineteenth century, physiology was understood as a theoretical and reflective science that served to uncover the fundamental principles and laws of life. This theoretical orientation distinguished it from its sister discipline, anatomy (or morphology), which was an investigative and often experimental discipline, and provided the empirical phenomena that physiology interpreted and synthesized. It was, in the words of Andrew Cunningham, a science performed with the pen, and not with the hand or scalpel (or sword, as Cunningham poetically suggests).[19] The physiology of the period was profoundly shaped by German Naturphilosophie-inspired thinkers such as Johann Friedrich Blumenbach and Johann Wolfgang von Goethe, who sought to explain the phenomena of human life as manifestations of universal natural principles and forces.[20] Physiology was a true philosophy of nature, a "Wissenschaft par excellence," and as such it had been able to claim a position for the study of life at the German universities.[21]

Efforts to emphasize the *Wissenschafts* character of the study of life had prompted a response by physicians who instead stressed the connection between physiology and pathology, and therefore the practical importance of a medical education steeped in the *Wissenschaft* of physiology.[22] One such physician was Dieffenbach's teacher Karl Friedrich Burdach, who saw in physiology the key to understanding clinical pathology. Only an acquaintance with the fundamental formational properties of life could provide insight into their dysfunction. According to Burdach, physiology was "the basis for the art of preserving the present normal state in its integrity, and bringing it closer to its ideal." It was also fundamental for therapeutics, or the "art of returning the abnormal state of life to normality."[23] Physiology had the potential of mediating between medicine's scientific aspirations and its imperative for use.

Whereas reconciling the goals of science and application produced a number of productive strategies in medical faculties, the situation looked bleaker for surgery. The military and civil needs of the state had long ensured that high-quality surgical education was available to medical practitioners, university educated or otherwise, at military and governmental training schools, and surgery had become firmly established as a university discipline at nearly all German medical faculties by the end of the eighteenth century.[24] Yet the delineation between surgery and medicine remained clearly defined professionally and socially. The Prussian state distinguished between several classes of practitioners on the basis of different kinds of professional training and varying areas of practice, ranking graduate physicians and graduates with both medical and surgical training, practical surgeons, military physicians, specialists such as midwives and dentists, and apothecaries.[25]

What was more, although surgery seemed to approach equality with university medicine institutionally, it was by no means considered on a par with it conceptually. The linguistic separation between "medicinal" and "operative" surgery was still in use, and occasionally calls were voiced for its translation into practice, even by practicing surgeons themselves. Reflecting on ways to optimize medical teaching, Ferdinand von Ritgen, professor of medicine and obstetrics at the university of Giessen, confessed that he saw benefits in a separate instruction of the nature of surgical diseases on the one hand, and of their surgical treatment on the other. Medical surgery, the doctrine of disturbances of organic tissues in processes of external formation, was to be distinguished from mechanical and chemical modes of their cure, as this would greatly facilitate the task of gaining a comprehensive overview of surgical pathology, he believed. Shrugging off the discussion of surgical diseases in a mere one and a half pages, Ritgen went on to elaborate on medical surgery for the remainder of his fifty-five-page article.[26] Across the Elbe, the physician and first director of the medical faculty at the University of Berlin, Christoph Wilhelm Hufeland, added a theoretical distinction to Ritgen's practical argument for a separation of two different kinds of surgeries. As much as the "business of healing" in its "foundational principles" was "one," Hufeland argued, it was true that the treatment of internal and external woes required a different "orientation of the mind" (*Richtung des Geistes*). "Inner curing," an activity that dealt with invisible ailments, required a propensity to envision the invisible, a capability for "abstraction, for profound research and reflection." Curing external afflictions, by contrast, challenged the practitioner to sensual perception (*sinnliche Wahrnehmung*) and to a culture of sensibility (*Kultur der Sinnlichkeit*); it required the comprehension of external objects (*Auffassen äußerer Gegenstände*) and manual dexterity. Even within surgery, a distinction was to be made between a kind of surgery that did not require any science of healing (*Wissenschaft der Heilkunde*), merely a mechanical craftsmanship, and a surgery that was informed by the principles of medicine as taught by the university faculties. These two different kinds of surgery, according to Hufeland, should find expression in different forms of surgical careers: surgeons, educated in surgical training schools and performing a broad range of duties mainly in the countryside, and barbers, performing only menial manual tasks.[27]

Johann Friedrich Dieffenbach: A New Method of Surgery against Surgical Methods

It is within this turbulent historical context, shaped by profound political and structural transformations, by debates about the organization of the medical profession and state healthcare, about the balance of theory and practice, *Wissenschaft* and utilitarianism, and about the place of surgery within medicine, that Dieffenbach's career and writings must be placed. Dieffenbach was born in 1792 in the Prussian town of Königsberg. Because of the early death of his father, Dieffenbach grew up in limited financial circumstances and was dependent on financial benefactors during his education and much of his life, especially after the death of his mother in 1814. Like many German physicians of the period, Dieffenbach joined the wars of liberation against Napoleon's troops. After his dismissal, Dieffenbach took up studying medicine, first at the University of Königsberg, then at the newly founded University of Bonn. During this time, Dieffenbach is said to have worked as a physician at duels, a common yet illegal practice at the time.[28] The majority of his years were spent in Berlin, where Dieffenbach worked as a practical physician from 1823 and 1829, and then as director of the surgical department of the Charité hospital. In 1832, Dieffenbach was promoted to Extraordinary Professor before he finally became a full professor and director of the university surgical clinic in 1840. Dieffenbach died unexpectedly in 1847 at the age of fifty-five.[29]

While he was in Berlin, Dieffenbach had worked under the auspices of Carl Ferdinand von Graefe, a surgeon who had himself gained considerable notoriety for introducing the recently rediscovered method of rhinoplasty to the German speaking world in 1817. Graefe had merged the so-called Indian method, in which the nose was reconstructed through rotation of a skin flap taken from the forehead, with the so-called Italian method, a technique that used a skin flap attached to the forearm to cover the nose defect. Graefe's technique used skin from the forearm, but in contrast to the Italian method, the flap was immediately attached to the nose after separation, so that the time during which the arm needed to stay attached to the nose was considerably shortened. He called this method the "German method." Graefe also placed great emphasis on the formation of the nose, and demanded that the surgeon study the exact features of the patient's face and calculate the size and form of the nose accordingly.[30]

If Graefe had sought to obtain notoriety by creating a new method of operation and giving it a name, Dieffenbach was not going to follow his example. He reserved only ridicule for such practices. If every surgeon was to "name a surgical method invented by him, or even merely slightly modified by him, after his country of origin," what were his successors to do? "Resort to names of provinces or towns?"[31] Dieffenbach's contempt for methods was not limited to their patriotic nomenclature, however. In the general section of his multivolume work on plastic surgery, *Surgical Experiences, in Particular about the Restitution of Destroyed Parts of the Body according to New Methods,* he dismissed the current use of "methods" in plastic surgery, despite the prominent position of the term, and his promise to produce new ones, in the title of his book. Methods alone were not sufficient, he cautioned, instead the aspiring plastic surgeon had to "study the peculiar self-formation (*eigenthümliche Selbstgestaltung*) of the new body part, and draw from it the doctrine of organic formation (*Lehre der organischen Formbildung*)."[32] The sentiment expressed in this passage is at the heart of Dieffenbach's ambitions for surgery and holds the key to understanding the seeming paradox of a surgeon advocating new methods in surgery while distancing himself from a method-based surgery.

Physiology: A New Surgical Epistemology

Dieffenbach's critique of Graefe's method of rhinoplasty may have been a petty professional sneer in part, but it was also rooted in a fundamental disagreement about how surgical knowledge ought to be obtained and how new surgical procedures ought to be devised. For Dieffenbach, the guiding principle for the innovative surgeon was the study of physiology, both as a deductive discipline concerned with the laws of nature and as an experimental enterprise investigating its idiosyncracies.

In his doctoral dissertation, composed in 1822, Dieffenbach had been examining the general principles of tissue formation and regeneration, while also investigating their individual manifestations in the body. The reason for all regeneration of tissue, Dieffenbach wrote, was what Johann Friedrich Blumenbach had described as the "formative drive" (*nisus formativus* or *Bildungstrieb*).[33] In Dieffenbach's words, this "drive of all organized bodies to retain their proper form, and to substitute and restitute lost lesions"[34] was a regular and predictable force, whose lawlike character could help anticipate and control the behavior of tissues. Among its characteristics was a gradient in potency from "less perfect" organisms to greater perfection, a scale that in turn corresponded to the degree of sophistication of the nervous system. This ordering principle of the animal kingdom could also be applied to different parts of the human body. Just as lower, less perfect animals regenerated more completely, so did less differentiated, less innervated parts of the body exhibit a tendency to more complete regeneration, such as the nails, hair, teeth, and skin.[35] Dieffenbach distinguished between two variants of the formative drive, the "ordinary regenerative force," which was at play in regular regeneration processes of the body, such as in the regular regeneration of the feathers of birds and the skin, nails, and hair of humans, and the "extraordinary, healing" regenerative force, which acted after injuries to the integument.[36] Quoting Goethe, Dieffenbach emphasized the role of the external layer or "envelope" of organic matter, the skin of humans, in effecting this healing force.[37] A surgeon relying on the properties of the skin to regenerate and form healing bonds thus had to know the general laws of this process in order to operate in accordance with the body's mechanism to heal itself.

While emphasizing the general laws underlying the regeneration of tissue, Dieffenbach also insisted on the individual conditions acting on the potency of the regenerative force. To a degree, individual variations were themselves the result of general principles. For instance, the regenerative force varied "according to different life stages," and so was regularly found more active in young people than in older generations.[38] Similarly, the principle of greater regenerative drive in less differentiated and externally located tissues dictated that particular body parts, such as the skin, and in particular, the nose, were more prone to perfect regeneration than other body parts.

But Dieffenbach also sought to explore the multiple variations of the regenerative force's manifestation in individuals. To this purpose, he complemented his analysis of Naturphilosophical physiological texts with a number of experiments in animals and even humans. Dieffenbach had performed experiments since his medical studies under Burdach and Karl Unger in Köngisberg, specifically on the question of the transplantability of feathers and hairs between animals.[39] For his dissertation, he used a variety of animals (doves, chickens, dogs) to transplant feathers, hairs, and pieces of skin into skin wounds of the same animal or an animal of a different species.[40] He also performed several transplantation experiments on himself.[41] During his time as practical physician in Berlin, Dieffenbach continued his transplantation experiments on animals, publishing some of his results in the *Journal der Chirugie und Augenheilkunde* in 1824.[42] Once he was established at the Charité, Dieffenbach had easy access to animals through the Royal Veterinary School of Berlin, which also provided him with experimental space.[43] He also performed skin transplantations on a forty-year-old woman who was suffering from anesthesia on one side of her body. Dieffenbach reasoned that since the therapy for anesthesia was to set "irritations" (*Reize*) for the spinal chord, transplantation experiments on the woman's skin would not only be interesting to himself but also benefit the patient. Seeking to investigate the potential for survival of a piece of skin in which the "life potential had been artificially heightened" by rubbing the skin into a less "vital" (*lebenskräftig*) skin area, and vice versa, Dieffenbach excised two pieces of skin in the patient's forearm and inserted them into the respective other wound. The result showed good healing in the rubbed skin and partial healing in the other skin area.[44] In the same article, Dieffenbach reported the successful reattachment of a piece of skin from the cheek of a young man that had been separated from his face in a duel.[45]

Dieffenbach combined his insights gained through the study of physiological texts and experiments into a summary of the general phenomena of skin transplantations, from which followed a series of principles for plastic surgery, rooted entirely in physiology. These were hinted at in Dieffenbach's dissertation and described in detail in his *Surgical Experiences*, as well as in his textbook on surgery, *Die Operative Chirurgie.* To begin with, physiology had made clear that transplanting skin was possible, not only when a connecting bridge of tissue existed between the separated part and the remaining skin, but also in those cases where the flap had been separated completely from the body's surface. The latter issue was by no means undisputed. It hinged on the question of whether the vitality of the skin depended on its connection with the organism or whether there was vitality within body parts irrespective of their ties to the body. In essence this was a question about the precise nature and localization of the vital force: was vitality a function of the organization of the body, a mechanical force that was conducted, or was it an inherent component of matter? Although Dieffenbach had observed that transplantation of not entirely separated skin flaps was by far more successful than that of completely separated parts, he attributed this success not merely to the connecting bridge and its function as a "conductor" of blood and innervation. Instead, the flap retained "in and of itself a high degree of vitality and autonomy."[46]

In his experiments, Dieffenbach had also observed a number of striking phenomena regarding the color of the flap and its blood flow, which ought to guide the precise moment the surgeon chose to reunite the separated skin. Immediately after separation, the skin flap revealed a striking pallor, which was occasioned, in Dieffenbach's opinion, by the "spastic" contraction of blood vessels, not because of the blood loss occasioned by the cut. A short time after, blood was flowing from the skin flap as a result of an active "contractive force" of the venous blood vessels in the flap.[47] Both of these phenomena hindered the insertion of the flap, however; contracted, spastic blood vessels were incapable of establishing new connections with surrounding tissue, and the venous blood expulsion formed a "membrane" that hindered the merging of tissue mechanically. Hence the surgeon had to let the flap rest for a few minutes before joining it to the surrounding tissue.[48] From these observations resulted another important principle for plastic operations. Whereas previous surgeons had attributed the pallor of the skin flap to a loss of vitality within the separated tissue, and had attempted to reawaken the vital power of the flap through "spirituous unctions, tapping, rubbing," or through "camphor," Dieffenbach recommended the use of leeches and the application of coldness in order to reduce blood flow and lower vessel spasticity.[49] Finally, Dieffenbach's observations on regenerative processes of the skin had revealed a number of characteristic changes in the flap's shape immediately after its removal. Typical was a contraction, reeling, and reduction of the flap's form, followed by the formation of a rounded elevation in its center.[50]

Yet although plastic operations could be based on these general physiological principles, surgeons also had to take into account the idiosyncracies of these lawful manifestations in the individual. With regard to the color of the flap, Dieffenbach did not specify a length of time that would indicate when the flap was ready to be transplanted. Instead, the surgeon had to observe the precise transformations of the color of the flap to allow him to determine the onset of a more "passive state" and hence the stop of blood expulsion and vessel contractility. This was the "right condition for union."[51] Similarly, although the changes in shape could be predicted by general laws, the precise manifestation of form phenomena depended "solely on the consistency of the skin of the individuum,"[52] with stronger contractility "in young strong individuals," and slighter form changes in persons with "loose, delicate, blond skin."[53] The general and individual characteristics of skin formation made the "incredibly careful preparation of a nose model,"[54] as recommended so insistently by Graefe, futile. The skin followed its own laws of formation and would defy efforts to press it into a desired form. Instead, the surgeon had to learn to form the skin in accordance with the peculiarities of living matter.

Dieffenbach's approach to physiology is peculiar and deserves a brief discussion. The period of Dieffenbach's activity saw a profound transformation not only with regard to the meaning of physiology itself, but also with regard to the relationship between physiology and experiment. Historians have argued that it was during the last decades of the eighteenth and the first decades of the nineteenth century that the "old physiology," with its experiments or *experiences* that demonstrated observable manifestations of general laws, was gradually replaced by "experimental physiology." This self-conscious new approach, proclaimed famously by François Magendie, and later Claude Bernard, centered on the experimental phenomena first, and inducted conclusions later. Experiments were performed in controlled conditions with repetitions and slight variations, leading to idiosyncratic conclusions about the nature of life phenomena.[55] Historians of surgery have argued that this new experimental physiology became the basis of a "physiological surgery" that looked to experimentation as an epistemic rationale as well as a form of applied surgery toward the late nineteenth century.[56] Dieffenbach's call for a surgery based on physiology could be interpreted as an anticipation of that later trend. On the other hand, the work of Mary Terrall has recently suggested that eighteenth-century naturalist experimental culture was much more interventionist than previously assumed.[57] In this sense Dieffenbach's conception of physiology and of physiological experimentation might be seen as continuing an already established eighteenth-century tradition of experimentation.

But rather than seeing Dieffenbach merely as continuing eighteenth-century experimental traditions or anticipating nineteenth-century experimental physiology, or being exemplary of a kind of "stage of transition," I suggest that his surgical epistemology reflects a variety of seemingly competing but often overlapping approaches to physiology as a *Wissenschaft* that reigned at the turn of the eighteenth and nineteenth centuries in the German medical context. Passages engaging with Blumenbach's *Bildungstrieb* and Goethe's *Morphologie* reveal a desire typical of *Naturphilosophie* to grasp and describe the fundamental laws underlying the formation of organic structures.[58] This version of physiology as *Wissenschaft* is accompanied by a number of observations of the manifestations of these laws in nature, and a number of experiments (partly undertaken by Dieffenbach himself, partly summarized from other authors' accounts) that demonstrated the validity of the principle of organic regeneration in different animals. In the description of his experiments forming the basis of his *Surgical Experiences*, Dieffenbach assured his readers that he had sought to act "merely in an observing capacity, describing nature."[59] This variation of physiology-as-science evokes Cunnigham's "old physiology" and a deductive experimental approach. But it is also reminiscent of Dieffenbach's teacher and lifelong friend Burdach's attempt to integrate experience and science, creating a conception of physiology as *Erfahrungswissenschaft*.[60] On the other hand, Dieffenbach's use of experimental variation, and the idiosyncratic conclusions that could be induced by them, is also characteristic of the principles of the new experimental physiology, which Dieffenbach had studied under Magendie during his stay in Paris in 1821.[61] For instance, resecting parts of the ear of dogs and rabbits, and then reattaching them, Dieffenbach varied the instrument he was using (scissors or knife), the form and size of the tissue piece, the location of removal on the ear, and the kinds of sutures and dressings he used to close the wound.[62] In the preface to his book on blood transfusion, Dieffenbach elaborated on his experimental technique, emphasizing that few physiologists paid sufficient attention to minimizing the pain of the experimental animal. The animal's muscular contractions during the experiment as well as his state of shock and dismay once the procedure had been performed were likely to influence the result of the experiment, and ought therefore to be minimized.[63] Dieffenbach was clearly concerned with the idiosyncratic variables determining the results of an experiment and took great care to vary the circumstances of the experiment to account for these. But Dieffenbach's experiments and his emphasis on the idiosyncracies of the properties of organic tissues also bring to mind a current in late eighteenth- and early nineteenth-century medical thought, which under the intellectual leadership of Christoph Hufeland and others reacted against the abstract tendencies of *Naturphilosophie* and sought to reestablish a science of medical practice centered around direct observation, empiricism, and the individuality of the patient.[64] By adopting an eclectic conception of physiology, Dieffenbach managed to mediate a tension between physiology as a pure science and an applied science, between the need to establish general rules of "natural" processes on the one hand, and to account for their idiosyncracies on the other. This conception also pervades his approach to the practice of plastic surgery, where it proved to be highly productive.

The seemingly minute changes Dieffenbach made to the technique of rhinoplasty appear in a new light when viewed through the physiological principles Dieffenbach advocated. The larger size of the forehead triangle ought to be made in recognition of the peculiar contractive properties of separated skin. The slight transposition of the incisions of the bridge followed Dieffenbach's observation of the importance of reducing vessel contractility in the flap and enabling maximum contact between the surfaces of the two wounds. Finally, his instructions on the timing of the flap insertion, and on the intraoperative and postoperative cooling of the flap, reflected his insight into the phasic phenomena of increase and decrease of contractive activity in the tissue. Yet while recognizing these isolated technical improvements as part of an integrative system of physiological thought is certainly illuminating, it only inadequately characterizes the kind of innovation Dieffenbach had in mind. The role of physiology was not merely to improve individual techniques, but to challenge notions of how surgery should be done and what it meant to be a surgeon. The task of demonstrating this new vision of surgery would fall to plastic surgery.

A New Kind of Surgery

If this chapter has so far used the term "plastic surgery" for pragmatic purposes, it is important to point out that this term did not hold the same meaning then as it does today, charged with the associations of the aesthetic-reconstructive binary. Neither was it the only term used to describe the same group of operations or even the most commonly used one.[65] The demarcation of the field was not based on the result or motivation of the procedures (improving or neutralizing appearance) but on the approach that characterized this branch of surgery. Graefe had first used the word "rhinoplasty"

(*Rhinoplastik*), drawing on the Greek word for *forming* in his 1818 description of a successful operation. The emphasis placed on the constructive element of the procedure compared a surgery that removed parts of the body in order to heal, often disfiguring the body, with a surgery that instead "substituted organic loss organically."[66] Like Graefe, Dieffenbach emphasized the "reconstructive" character (*Wiederherstellen*) of plastic surgery, and contrasted the compensative, replacing nature (*wiederersetzend*) of the "organic plastic" with the mutilating effect of regular surgery (*verstümmelnde Operationen*).[67] The title of his major 1829 work *Surgical Experiences, in Particular about the Restitution of Destroyed Parts of the Body according to New Methods,* which deals with plastic operations, reflects this emphasis. Whereas "*Chirurgia curtorum,*" the title Dieffenbach chose for a chapter on plastic operations in Rust's *Handbook of Surgery,* had emphasized the "mutilated parts" (lat. *Curta*) as the object of the procedures, the reprint of the same article, titled "On Organic Substitution" (Über den organischen Ersatz), foregrounded the reconstructive and physiologically informed approach Dieffenbach was advocating.[68] Organic substitution, organic plastic, and finally plastic surgery were Dieffenbach's preferred categories in later years.[69]

The range of operations discussed in Dieffenbach's *Surgical Experiences*—including, for example, injuries to the urethra and perineal tears—equally suggests that Dieffenbach sought to classify the procedures he was describing according to their common methodology—a reconstructive rather than a destructive approach—and not according to the ability of the operations to restore appearance or function.[70] The same distinction makes it possible to see the seemingly arbitrary range of Dieffenbach's career in a new light. Operations like the surgical cure for stuttering through incisions of the tongue, or the various separations of tendons for limb deformities, can be understood as variations of the same principle: to base surgical interventions on the physiological laws of nature, be they the regenerative forces of tissues or the contractive properties of muscles.[71]

In addition to being a constructive rather than a destructive form of surgery, plastic surgery also stood out as the branch of surgery that was most closely modeled on a *Naturphilosophie*-based physiology, and thus dealt with the properties of the living body. The term "plastic force" *(Plastische Kraft)* was sometimes used as a synonym for Blumenbach's formative drive (*Bildungstrieb*) to describe the processes by which living bodies acquired their characteristic *organized* form.[72] More specifically, Hufeland used the term "plastic force" to describe one of the subcomponents of the *formative drive,* that part which "regulates the binding, development, and formation of already organized parts according to certain purposes and forms." This included the "ongoing regeneration during life and finally the new reproduction in a pathological state."[73] A surgery that was truly *plastic* promised to act analogous to the plastic force of *living* nature by creating new forms, and by settling on the terms *Organische Plastik* and *Plastische Chirurgie,* Dieffenbach emphasized the centrality of physiological insight into the plastic formation of the living body in guiding his surgical approach.[74]

The term "plastic" therefore also evoked a stark contrast to a surgery that had based its insights on the study of the *dead* body, a surgery rooted in morbid anatomy. Surgical approaches derived from the handling of dead matter in cadavers were inferior, according to Dieffenbach, to those plastic operations that required that surgeons master the dynamic behavior of living matter. "Such a surgery," Dieffenbach told his students in one of his clinical lectures, "has physiology as its basis, it adjusts its steps according to the laws of the eternal, natural healing processes, which older surgery was unaware of, since it was based only on mechanics, and created its operational methods using cadavers."[75] The rhetorical contrast between the automated, mechanic nature of cadaver-based surgery, and the flexible, organic character of physiology-based plastic surgery not only satisfied the criticism voiced by Hufeland about the different intellectual abilities required to do different kinds of surgery, one a "science of healing," the other a mere "mechanical craftsmanship."[76] It also elevated the "raw, craft-like" character of regular surgery to the state of a "*Wissenschaft*"[77] that was capable of development. "A surgery based on mechanics," Dieffenbach warned, "is a rider on a wooden horse: it remains in one place and would be immutable if worms would not gnaw away at it. A surgery based on physiology, by contrast, flies through deserts like an Arabian horse."[78] Plastic surgery, as a truly physiological approach, was the key to true innovation in surgery.

A New Kind of Surgeon

The new kind of surgery Dieffenbach was advocating demanded a new kind of surgeon.[79] The special position plastic surgery occupied within the realm of surgery, and its close connection to physiology, meant that it was not sufficient to simply transfer principles and skills acquired from other areas of surgery to the domain of plastic operations. "From the observation of the physiological phenomena of transplanted skin parts," Dieffenbach claimed, "results the necessity for a very specific surgical method (*Verfahren*) for plastic operations in general. Very little is to be gathered from the other, more familiar areas of surgery. Here, the finding and assembling of completely different principles is needed, which are only to be found by way of physiology."[80] Neither was it sufficient to simply follow the recipe-like instructions so common in the description of new surgical techniques, such as rhinoplasty. "Surgery teaches how incisions are to be made in general, and rhinoplasty in particular specifies how one is to proceed when excising the flap of the arm or forehead, it even prescribes to measure the lines that the knife should draw on the skin, but will not the main part, that which is not drawable in lines, remain to be done?"[81]

It is important at this point to distinguish between two different uses of the word "method" in Dieffenbach's writings. On the one hand, method is used to describe the instructions for a single operative technique, such as the method of rhinoplasty. As pointed out earlier, Dieffenbach occasionally ridiculed the practice of inventing new methods and naming them. He used the second meaning of method in order to draw a contrast between this, an approach overly reliant on specific instructions, and a comprehensive, systematic approach to operations in general, based on the principles of the regenerative properties of matter. Innovating surgery based on *a multitude* of recipe-like methods was an inferior form of innovation, as it required future surgeons to merely follow instructions. Reforming surgery on the basis of an entirely new and systematic approach, *a* new method, would demand that the surgeon use those capacities of intellect previously reserved for nonsurgical physicians the likes of Hufeland: a capability for "abstraction, profound research, and reflection."[82]

Hence a surgeon could not merely learn the "method" for rhinoplasty and think that he could now perform rhinoplastic operations. The idosyncracies of skin physiology required him to first learn the physiological laws governing the behavior of organic matter, and then adjust his technique according to the specific circumstances of each individual case. Exactly what enabled the surgeon to go beyond his learned repertóire of techniques and rules, and apply them skillfully in individual cases, remained obscure in Dieffenbach's writings, but it was clear that there was ample room for interpretation. On several occasions Dieffenbach stressed the interplay of general rules based on physiology, and the need for situational interpretations of these principles. In a chapter titled "General Surgical Principles for Plastic Operations," Dieffenbach explained that the skin flap used in transplant operations could be "sometimes small, sometimes big, sometimes short, sometimes long, round, oval, triagonal, or lobed with a small appendix. It consists sometimes of thin skin, which is transplanted into thick skin, or vice versa. It is made to heal in a flat or arched way, either entirely or in part." In addition, the surgeon had to decide on the position of insertion ("into the skin, or above, or below"), the thickness of the layer ("single or double"), and even the method of removal ("through extraction, stretching, pulling, and auxiliary cuts").[83] Although Dieffenbach prefaced the large series of cases in his *Surgical Experiences* with the step-by-step description of a new rhinoplastic method, and a brief synopsis of alternative techniques introduced by other surgeons, the case descriptions themselves often illustrate the necessity to deviate from this established principle. Describing the case of an eighteen-year-old girl with "scrofular deformities of the nose," Dieffenbach recalls that, "at first glance, the idea that this case was ideally suited for a reconstruction of the missing nose fragment from the arm had to suggest itself to every physician. . . . Then she asked my advice, and after I had made myself aware precisely of everything that was still there, and everything that was missing from the nose, I recognized the possibility of reconstructing the nose wing from the depth, enlarge it through additions from neighboring parts, and re-create the face in such a way that one was hardly able to discern anything alien in it."[84] Sometimes Dieffenbach even chose to deviate from what he had acknowledged to have been the indicated procedure for the individual case based on the general principles of plastic surgery. Introducing the case histories of two young male patients who had experienced injuries of the nose in a duel, Dieffenbach declared that "the mutilation of both individuals presented itself in such a manner that according to the general established principles of rhinoplasty, the reconstruction of the missing nose fragments should have been performed using the skin of the arm." Instead, both cases were operated using a variation of the Indian method.[85] Students who, intending to learn and emulate rhinoplasty and other techniques in plastic surgery, looked to Dieffenbach's writings for instruction, were constantly reminded of the limitations of this way of learning.

Recurring insistence on the limitations of imitation, and on the inadequacy of a one-size-fits-all approach to plastic surgery, also appears in Dieffenbach's clinical teachings. Dieffenbach's student Karl Theodor Meier had recorded Dieffenbach's clinical surgical lessons in the Charité hospital from May to August 1840. Addressing his students on the first day of class, Dieffenbach dismissed the reliance of some surgeons on fancy instruments and empirical methods. "The instrument," he frowned, "is only the pen with which the surgeon charts down his thoughts; he forms and creates not according to an old, established method, but he improvises the method according to the individuality of the case."[86] He warned his students, therefore, not to expect to be given precise methods that they could simply follow. "I will not," he insisted, "dictate hundreds of recipe formulas into your wallets, with which you can cure for the rest of your life. In doing so I would cut off your own thoughts for the future. I have no recipe formulas, just as I have no formulas for letters."[87]

In order to navigate such precarious dichotomies as science versus empiricism, knowledge versus expertise, acquired skill versus talent, Dieffenbach drew on nuanced variations of familiar metaphors from the realm of arts and crafts.[88] Emphasizing the difference between the mechanical manipulation of dead matter and the challenging task of forming live body parts, he insisted: "The skin is very different from wax, it forms itself idiosyncratically during the healing process, shrinks here and dies off, proliferates there, and so . . . the artist needs the talent to repair the damage happily. The surgeon is so-to-speak a sculptor, who has to be able to calculate exactly form and relationship of the parts, on their own as well as in relation to their surrounding parts."[89] If a combination of knowledge and artistry was required for the calculated and creative formation of tissue, it was only the artist's individual ingenuity that would distinguish the true artist from the skilled craftsman. "The painter learns to draw thoroughly, and to mix and apply colors, to copy correctly—then he paints from within (*aus sich selber*), he paints his thoughts, his fantasies. One can learn how to build verses, but not how to write poetry, it is an innate ability of the poet. One can learn how to cut, but often one has to cut differently from what has been learnt. That is operative surgery."[90]

Resonating within these statements was a conception of the acquisition of surgical learning and skill as a path to self-expression and self-realization, an ideal that was also at the heart of the German notion of *Bildung*. Thomas Broman has pointed out that the ideal of *Bildung*, meaning the attainment of true freedom through the cultivation of the character of an individual, had replaced older notions of "learnedness" by the late eighteenth century, and had also mediated the debates around the nature of creative genius.[91] A surgical education according to Dieffenbach's vision was not a mere apprenticeship, nor was it a form of utilitarian, practical instruction in the vein of the surgical training schools. It promised to allow the talented and physiologically schooled surgeon to unfold his full potential. Once he had abandoned the methods and instruments of old surgery, he would be able to attain true "surgical freedom."[92] Studying plastic surgery was therefore no easy path, and the beginner was discouraged from venturing into the field too soon; indeed, he might even find it frustrating. Only once he had become acquainted "through many other operations with the plastic processes of nature, her strengths, her weaknesses, and her own will to take shape in particular forms" would he "find in the organic plastic a higher form of inner satisfaction."[93]

But he may also have been discouraged for another reason. Dieffenbach's use of artistic metaphors evoked those notions of the innate, creative genius so paramount to the literary movements of the period.[94] Central to this debate was the dualism between imitation (*Nachahmung*) and creation (*Schöpfung*). The literary movement of *Sturm und Drang* heralded a shift from representations of nature as expressions of rule and reason to a creative conception of the natural world.[95] Dieffenbach's surgical instructions express a similar preference for a creative rather than a rule-bound approach to the natural material he handled. Whereas *Bildung* had contributed to democratize the access to medical education to an extent,[96] plastic surgery would serve to exclude those without creative ability. Even if the surgeon had mastered the rules of plastic surgery, each individual case demanded that he combine his scientific knowledge of the laws of nature with a more intangible quality: ingenuity. "Though general rules for plastic operations can be given," Dieffenbach cautioned in his surgical textbook, "it will always be left to the talent and judgment of the surgeon which method he chooses in one or the other case."[97] A plastic surgeon thus needed both, a profound knowledge of physiology and the ability to judge how it should be applied, as well as a capacity for improvisation and creativity.[98] "Without a certain natural gift (*Anlage*) for the discipline," Dieffenbach warned, "whoever studies it will always remain a beginner. May he have studied all branches of the healing sciences thoroughly, may he know all surgical operations according to their acts and masters, and be able to perform them on the cadaver and on the living body, he will always remain inadequate in his actions." A true surgeon, by contrast, knew and mastered "even that which is not written," and was able to "again and again create something new"—a true "innovative (*erfindungsreicher*) Ulysses."[99]

Inimitability

Both the variability and unpredictability of Dieffenbach's physiological approach to operations and his insistence on the centrality of surgical ingenuity introduced an element of inimitability into Dieffenbach's writings and clinical teaching. This seems counterintuitive. Should not an easily reproducible method have been more conducive to the "diffusion" and therefore to the "success" of the technique? In order to solve this seeming paradox, it is necessary to understand the notion of "success" in relation to Dieffenbach's career and the broader context of university medicine in early nineteenth-century Germany.

In their struggle to regain cultural preeminence in the aftermath of the defeat and symbolic humiliation of Prussia through Napoleonic troupes, Prussian universities were crucially aware of the importance of attracting illustrious faculty. Thus cultivating a reputation was a central imperative for obtaining and retaining a university position in medicine.[100] Dieffenbach himself was very preoccupied with the hiring and firing landscape of German universities, in fact, it is one of the major recurring themes in a majority of his letters to friends and colleagues. With his correspondent and friend Karl Ernst von Baer, for instance, Dieffenbach speculated about the possible candidates for a position in Berlin, discussed the attempts of one of his colleagues to find a position, and updated von Baer about his own professional situation.[101] Similar concerns appear frequently in Dieffenbach's correspondence with Georg Stromeyer.[102] Attracting a large number of medical students was one way of increasing one's notoriety. But student numbers also directly impacted the livelihood of a university employee in the Prussian medical system. University professors, who depending on their rank were not always paid for the general public lectures they were expected to give, could significantly increase their income and reputation if they could offer so-called *Privatissima*—small-sized private clinical teaching sessions that were often highly valued by students as they tended to emphasize hands-on experience.[103] Dieffenbach had been Extraordinary Professor of Medicine for four years before he was able to teach his first *Privatissimum* on operative doctrine (*Operationslehre*) in the winter semester 1835/36.[104] A year later, he managed to offer a *Privatissimum* on organic plastic.[105]

Given the importance of creating a reputation and attracting students to private courses (two factors that were also mutually enforcing), a "successful" form of innovation, from Dieffenbach's point of view, would have been one that amplified the role of the surgeon and attracted many students to his private lessons. The new plastic operations he promoted, with their emphasis on the inadequacy of methods and book learning, and on the centrality of the operator, fit the bill.

Dieffenbach's biographers have at times been puzzled by what they perceived to be a lack of clarity in Dieffenbach's writings, especially in his descriptions of operations. Richard Lampe, a surgeon himself, confessed that, even with the "greatest attentiveness" and "vivid use of the imagination," he had often been unable to follow Dieffenbach's descriptions.[106] Dieffenbach's contemporary and friend Eduard Zeis commented that Dieffenbach's writings on plastic surgery "contained many attractive descriptions of individual cases, while his descriptions of operations often lacked the necessary clarity."[107] Lampe attributed this lack of clarity to a shortcoming of Dieffenbach's writing abilities, and suggested that Dieffenbach could have increased the intelligibility of his communications had he only divided his operative descriptions into acts and included illustrations.[108] Yet there is some evidence that the intelligibility of his descriptions is not a shortcoming, but the result of a deliberate effort, and must be understood in the context of the potential benefits of inimitability. Dieffenbach explicitly expressed his contempt for divisions of operations into acts, a sentiment that he articulated using the same metaphor he had used to voice his dislike of methods. "I have a peculiar aversion against all acts within surgery," he lamented. "They tear apart the subject (*Gegenstand*), and transform a living body into the bones of a skeleton."[109] Dieffenbach also claimed to use the potential incomprehensibility of his writings in order to sift out lesser able surgeons, whom he advised not to imitate his procedures. In fact the first exposition of his own "method" for rhinoplasty is followed by the caveat, "I did not find it necessary to be more elaborate in the descriptions of the particulars of the operation. Whoever finds the description of the procedure not to be cumbersome enough, and who cannot imagine the rest that automatically results from it, should best not attempt the operation."[110] The paucity of images in Dieffenbach's publications may in part have been due to editorial constraints, at least Dieffenbach expressed the wish that he had been able to provide "copper or wood cuts" instead of case histories.[111] But more striking than the lack of illustrations is the choice of images when images were added to his works. The twenty-six plates appended to the four volumes of Dieffenbach's *Surgical Experiences* contain almost exclusively images of patients before and after the operation. Details about the operative procedures themselves are rare, and if they are featured, they tend to emphasize a stage within the operation, without specifying how the result was obtained. The illustrations are therefore not a visual tool meant to facilitate emulation of procedures, but serve to document the favorable results of Dieffenbach's operations. In other words, images, like the texts to which they were attached, confirmed and performed the talent of the operator.

Compared with other surgical texts at the time, the peculiarity of Dieffenbach's inimitable style is even more striking. Herrmann Fritze's and O. Reich's 1845 work on plastic surgery, for instance, contains a large number of images, including detailed colored visualizations of operative steps, which are referred to at the relevant stages in the description of the operative method.[112] Fritze and Reich also regularly used exact measurements in their operative instructions.[113] Dieffenbach's contempt for measurements and acts may have been most explicitly directed at Graefe, whose text on rhinoplasty made copious use of acts and contained several pages of instructions on measurements,[114] but many surgical textbooks at the time used the division of surgical techniques into acts, and specified measurements.[115]

If Dieffenbach's rhetoric and choices emphasized and showcased instances of inimitability, this does not mean that his writings were useless compilations of incomprehensible, obfuscated prose. There are many moments where the attempt to be clear and intelligible is visible, where Dieffenbach formulates distinct "methods" of operations and structures them, if not in explicit acts, then at least in discernible stages. But the distribution of these moments of clarity is significant and underscores the importance of the professional context in which he wrote. First, there is a development throughout his career: Dieffenbach's writings are more explicitly clear and easier to emulate toward the later stages of his professional life when he was already an Ordinary Professor at Berlin University and less dependent on private teaching. Where earlier writings emphasize the individual variations and idiosyncracies of rhinoplastic operations, Dieffenbach's 1845 textbook on Operative Surgery contains a crystallized, singular rhinoplastic method, of which he claims ownership. Second, detailed explanations appear more frequently in Dieffenbach's clinical lessons than in his published writings. Although Dieffenbach still emphasized the need to adjust the physiological principles underlying plastic procedures in each individual case, he demonstrated variations in his clinical teachings more clearly, and most importantly, he specified the reasons for having chosen a particular variation. Demonstrating the rhinoplastic reconstruction of the nose of a sixteen-year-old girl in front of his students, for example, he described in detail the sequence of cuts he undertook and elaborated on the relationship between his choices ("I must separate the skin of the nose a few lines away from the bone") and the underlying considerations ("in order to obtain enough room for the reception of the nourishing bridge").[116] This discrepancy in pedagogical effort between his published writings and his clinical teachings is not surprising considering that plagiarism, both from published works and clinical lectures, was not an uncommon practice in the competitive culture of the medical university. In the preface to his work on nutrition, Friedrich Tiedemann lamented the widespread practice of copying a professor's lectures and then publishing them as a book without the professor's knowledge and profit. This "unexpected honor" had also been bestowed on his own lectures, he lamented sarcastically.[117] The surgeon Ernst Blasius even hastened the publication of his *Lehrbuch der Akiurgie* because a certain Dr. Eulenburg, who had already acquired notoriety for having published someone else's clinical lectures, had recently published a surgical manual that was almost entirely an "excerpt" of Blasius's earlier surgical works.[118] Dieffenbach himself complained that the "miserable Blandin" had "almost copied" his *Surgical Experiences,* and acknowledged Dieffenbach only insiginificantly.[119]

The discrepancy between Dieffenbach's written works and his clinical lectures might also have been a product of the pressure on university educators to make their courses attractive for students. If a textbook was too comprehensive, or a clinical lesson not different enough from the published writings of that faculty member, students might choose not to attend lessons at all. Nicolai Pirogow, who wrote a detailed account of his medical studies as a traveling student in a number of German universities, claimed that he had meant to visit a physiology lecture with Johannes Müller, but had decided not to, not only because it clashed with his clinical lectures but also because he would be able to read everything in Müller's textbook, with the exception of the demonstrations with animals and with the microscope.[120] Pirogow also experienced one of Dieffenbach's *Privatissima.* His report is illuminating. Although it was very expensive, Pirogow found the experience mostly not worth his expense, not least because Dieffenbach "spoke very muffled and uttered individual words with apparent unwillingness." But Pirogow was still content to have had the opportunity to watch Dieffenbach perform "a number of remarkable and, at the time, new plastic operations." "In fact," he wrote, "with regard to plastic operations, he was practically an original genius. Dieffenbach's inventive spirit in this surgical specialty was infinite. Each of his plastic operations stood out through something new and improvised."[121] If Dieffenbach had meant to perform his own ingenuity without revealing too many imitable surgical techniques, he had certainly succeeded with Pirogow.

Conclusion

"*Nomen, omen!*" (it's all in the name) announced Dieffenbach's first biographer Rohlfs in the opening sentences of his eulogy on Dieffenbach's life and career in 1883. Translating the word Dieffenbach (*tiefer Bach*) as "profound creek," Rohlfs sought to locate Dieffenbach's significant and transformative effect on the development of German surgery in his name. The discipline had needed Dieffenbach, the profound creek, in order to grow into "a majestic stream." His name, Rohlfs continued, was "so intimately connected to German surgery that he felt justified in declaring Dieffenbach "the first German surgeon."[122] Though Rohlfs may have been exceptional in his euphoria, his portrayal is nevertheless telling as to the extent to which Dieffenbach was successful in conjuring a vision of a new kind of surgeon, one that would provide a form of identification not only for future plastic surgeons but for surgeons of all disciplines.

The factors shaping the intense period of innovation in surgery prior to the advent of anesthesia are multiple and complex, and cannot possibly be adequately exhausted by this chapter. Developments such as urbanization, the transformation of the political landscape after the Napoleonic Wars, and the establishment of the research university certainly contributed to the growth and rapid development of surgical practice. Cultural and social influences like the framing of disfiguring diseases and the growing popularity of physiognomy may also have played a role in promoting the development of plastic surgery in particular. The case of Dieffenbach and plastic surgery invites historians to consider more seriously the impact of physiology, of professional pressures, and of theoretical debates about the function of medicine as major driving forces in the development of new surgical approaches in this period.

In a context in which surgery's place within medicine, as well as the relationship between medicine and *Wissenschaft* itself, were precarious, and where the meaning of physiology was unstable, Dieffenbach championed a new approach to surgery. By promoting truly *plastic* operations, that is, surgical approaches based on physiological laws of the living body and their idiosyncratic manifestations, he was able to emphasize surgery's basis in scientific, Naturphilosophical principles, and stressed its healing potential rather than its mutilating character. Yet the same context also gave Dieffenbach's innovation a peculiar form, one that seemingly contradicted one of the most fundamental conditions for an innovation's diffusion or success: its potential to be learned and emulated by others. This *inimitability* of Dieffenbach's brand of innovation was a crucial component of the form of success he sought to achieve, as it had the potential to accommodate the particular professional exigencies of the early nineteenth-century Prussian university context. Dieffenbach's case reminds historians of innovation to historicize not only the social and cultural conditions that produce the needs for certain new techniques, but also the expectations of what constitutes a successful innovation at a given point in time.

Notes

Translations from Latin and German below are my own. I am grateful to Christopher Crenner, Thomas Schlich, Allan Brandt, Sophia Roosth, David Jones, Janet Browne, Kate Womersley, Paolo Savoia, Roksana Filipowska, the history of surgery group at the Department of Social Studies of Medicine at McGill University, and the participants of the History of Medicine Working Group at Harvard University for reading drafts of this chapter and providing valuable comments and suggestions. My warmest thanks to Gotthard Haushofer, Ingrid Haushofer, and Runhild Laubmann for helping me to learn old German script and assisting me in the transcriptions of letters in Kurrent, and to Gotthard Haushofer for his valuable assistance with translations from Latin.

1. For examples of recent histories of surgery that combine a notion of "technological determinism" with a sense of advancement through self-evident progress (against resistance), see Harold Ellis, *A History of Surgery* (Cambridge: Cambridge University Press, 2001); Leo Zimmerman and Ilza Veith, *Great Ideas in the History of Surgery* (San Francisco: Norman Publishing, 1993). Histories of plastic surgery written in this manner include Paolo Santoni-Rugiu and Philip Sykes, *A History of Plastic Surgery* (New York: Springer, 2007); David Hamilton, *A History of Organ Transplantation* (Pittsburgh, PA: University of Pittsburgh Press, 2012). These narratives are reproduced in cultural studies approaches to plastic surgery, for example, Kathy Davis, *Dubious Equalities and Embodied Differences: Cultural Studies on Cosmetic Surgery* (Oxford: Rowman & Littlefield, 2003), 24.

2. For example, Royal College of Surgeons, *From Innovation to Adoption: Successfully Spreading Surgical Innovation* (London: Royal College of Surgeons, 2014).

3. For a detailed yet largely descriptive history of plastic surgery, see, for example, Santoni-Rugiu and Sykes, *History of Plastic Surgery*.

4. Roy Porter, *The Greatest Benefit to Mankind: A Medical History of Humanity* (New York: W. W. Norton, 1999), 362.

5. Hamilton, *History of Organ Transplantation*, 59.

6. Porter, *Greatest Benefit to Mankind*, 362–63.

7. Nathan Belofsky, *Strange Medicine: A Shocking History of Real Medical Practices through the Ages* (New York: Penguin, 2013), 113; Joel Fram and Sandra Salmans, *Weird Cures: The Most Hilarious, Disgusting and Downright Dangerous Medical Treatments Ever* (Philadelphia: Running Press, 2006), 53.

8. A. Mau and Edgar Biemer, "Johann-Friedrich Dieffenbach: The Pioneer of Plastic Surgery," *Annals of Plastic Surgery* 33, no. 1 (1994): 112–15; discussion 115–16; Wibke Knoener and Dirk Schultheiss, "Johann Friedrich Dieffenbach (1792–1847) Pioneer in Oral Maxillofacial Surgery," *Journal of the History of Dentistry* 50, no. 3 (2002): 117–21, quotation 302.

9. Dirk Schultheiss et al., "Johann Friedrich Dieffenbach (1792–1847) als Begründer der Plastischen Chirurgie," *Mund-, Kiefer- Und Gesichtschirurgie* 2, no. 6 (1998): 309–15.

10. U. Ulrich and C. Lauritzen, "Johann Friedrich Dieffenbach (1792–1847): 'Vater der Plastischen Chirurgie' in Deutschland," *Deutsche Medizinische Wochenschrift* 117, no. 30 (1992): 1165–67.

11. "Verbesserte": Schultheiss et al., "Johann Friedrich Dieffenbach," 312.

12. Deborah Sullivan, *Cosmetic Surgery: The Cutting Edge of Commercial Medicine in America* (New Brunswick, NJ: Rutgers University Press, 2001), 38.

13. In a dissertation discussing Dieffenbach's influence on modern medicine, Patricia Hellerström concluded that Dieffenbach had contributed new "insights, theories and methods" to the field, and was therefore rightly called a pioneer, even if many of his operative techniques were no longer in use in contemporary plastic surgery. Patricia Hellerström, "Johann Friedrich Dieffenbach: Leben und Wirken und sein Einfluß auf die moderne Medizin," Freie Universität Berlin, 1997, 75, 77, 85–86, 111–12. Wolfgang Genschorek acknowledges that "the surgery of [Dieffenbach's] main creative period consisted less in new epochal achievements than in the broadening of the experiental treasure trove, and in the perfection of operative technique." Wolfgang Genschorek, *Wegbereiter der Chirurgie: Johann Friedrich Dieffenbach, Theodor Billroth* (Leipzig: S. Hirzel, 1983), 10.

14. Sander Gilman, *Making the Body Beautiful: A Cultural History of Aesthetic Surgery* (Princeton, NJ: Princeton University Press, 2001).

15. Ibid., 12–13; Sander Gilman, *Creating Beauty to Cure the Soul: Race and Psychology in the Shaping of Aesthetic Surgery* (Durham, NC: Duke University Press, 1998), 42; Knoener and Schultheiss, "Johann Friedrich Dieffenbach (1792–1847)."

16. Gilman, *Making the Body Beautiful*, 91; Blair Rogers, "The Development of Aesthetic Plastic Surgery: A History," *Aesthetic Plastic Surgery* 1, no. 1 (1976): 3–24; according to Santoni-Rugiu and Sykes, Dieffenbach "recognized the beneficial cosmetic effects done primarily for pathological reasons" (*History of Plastic Surgery*, 308).

17. David Blackbourn, *History of Germany, 1780–1918: The Long Nineteenth Century* (Malden, MA: Blackwell, 2002), 37–68; Thomas Broman, *The Transformation of German Academic Medicine, 1750–1820* (New York: Cambridge University Press, 2002), 159–73.

18. Broman, *Transformation*, 180–85; Broman, "University Reform in Medical Thought at the End of the Eighteenth Century," *Osiris*, 2nd ser., 5 (January 1, 1989): 36–53.

19. Andrew Cunningham, "The Pen and the Sword: Recovering the Disciplinary Identity of Physiology and Anatomy before 1800—I: Old Physiology—the Pen," *Studies in History and Philosophy of Science* 33, no. 4 (2002): 631–65; Andrew Cunningham, "The Pen and the Sword: Recovering the Disciplinary Identity of Physiology and Anatomy before 1800—II: Old Anatomy—the Sword," *Studies in History and Philosophy of Science* 34, no. 1 (2003): 51–76.

20. Robert Richards, *The Romantic Conception of Life: Science and Philosophy in the Age of Goethe* (Chicago: University of Chicago Press, 2002), 207–37, 434–57.

21. Lynn Nyhart, *Biology Takes Form: Animal Morphology and the German Universities, 1800–1900* (Chicago: University of Chicago Press, 1995), 52–59, quotation 52; Broman, *Transformation*, 73–101.

22. Broman, *Transformation*, 102–27.

23. Karl Friedrich Burdach, *Die Physiologie* (Leipzig: Weidmann, 1810), 6; Nyhart, *Biology Takes Form*, 51–62; Broman, *Transformation*, 180–92.

24. Thomas Neville Bonner, *Becoming a Physician: Medical Education in Great Britain, France, Germany, and the United States, 1750–1945* (New York: Oxford University Press, 1995), 53–58; Broman, *Transformation*, 52–54, 67–68.

25. Bonner, *Becoming a Physician*, 67.

26. Ritgen's conception of "external" is not a designation describing disease location on the surface of the body, but refers to one of two different modes of organization of organic tissue: their interconnectedness through inner composition and their separatedness through external manifestation in "form" (Gestalt). Only the latter is the domain of the surgeon. Ferdinand Ritgen, "Ueber den Begriff und das Gebiet der Chirurgie, und über die Grenzen und die Eintheilung des chirurgischen Lehrvortrags," *Magazin für die gesammte Heilkunde* 4, no. 1 (1829): 3–58.

27. Christoph Wilhelm Hufeland, "Zusätze," *Journal der practischen Heilkunde* 60, no. 1 (1825): 112–26; Hufeland is recalling here an earlier debate with his colleague Johann Christian Reil over the best education of medical personnel in light of the needs and financial means of the Prussian state between 1804 and 1807. The degree to which medical practitioners in different positions should and could be confronted with research and *Wissenschaft*, or with practical skills and clinical teaching, also had implications for how surgery as a science or practice was envisioned and how surgical training could best be implemented. Speaking here in 1825, Hufeland confessed that his views had not changed much since the earlier debate with Reil. Johann Christian Reil, *Pepinieren zum Unterricht ärztlicher Routiniers als Bedürfnisse des Staats nach seiner Lage wie sie ist* (Halle, 1804); Christoph Wilhelm Hufeland, "Ueber Aerzte und Routiniers," *Journal der practischen Heilkunde* 21 (1805); Christoph Wilhelm Hufeland, "Bemerkungen über die Reilsche Schrift: Pepinieren zum Unterricht ärztlicher Routiniers," *Journal der practischen Arneykunde und Wundarzneykunde* 26, no. 1 (1807): 9–57; for a thoughtful summary and analysis of the debate, see Broman, *Transformation*, 119–25.

28. Nicolai Pirogow, *Lebensfragen: Tagebuch eines alten Arztes* (Stuttgart: Cotta, 1894), 396.

29. For biographical accounts of Dieffenbach, see Heinrich Rohlfs, "Johann Friedrich Dieffenbach," *Deutsches Archiv für Geschichte der Medicin und medicinische Geographie* 6 (1883): 452–89, Heinrich Rohlfs, "Johann Friedrich Dieffenbach," *Deutsches Archiv für Geschichte der Medicin und medicinische Geographie* 7 (1884): 44–143; Richard Lampe, *Dieffenbach* (Leipzig: Barth, 1934); Bodo Mros, "Der Arzt Johann Friedrich Dieffenbach (1792–1847) in seiner Zeit" (Humboldt Universität, 1965); Genschorek, *Wegbereiter der Chirurgie.*

30. Carl Ferdinand von Graefe, *Rhinoplastik, oder die Kunst, den Verlust der Nase organisch zu Ersetzen* (Berlin: Realschulbuchhandlung, 1818).

31. Johann Friedrich Dieffenbach, *Chirurgische Erfahrungen, besonders über die Wiederherstellung zerstörter Theile des menschlichen Körpers nach neuen Methoden*, vol. 2 (Berlin: T. C. F. Enslin, 1830), 151.

32. Ibid.

33. Johann Friedrich Dieffenbach, *Nonnulla de Regeneratione et Transplantatione* (Würzburg: Richter, 1822), 11.

34. Ibid.

35. Ibid., 12–14.

36. Ibid., 14–17.

37. Ibid., 16.

38. Ibid., 13.

39. Rochus Freiherr von Liliencron, Franz X. von Wegele, and Anton Bettelheim, eds., "Johann Friedrich Dieffenbach," in *Allgemeine deutsche Biographie*, vol. 5 (Leipzig: Duncker & Humblot, 1877), 120–26.

40. Dieffenbach, *Nonnulla de Regeneratione et Transplantatione*, 35–42, 48–50.

41. Ibid., 50–52.

42. Johann Friedrich Dieffenbach, "Transplantationsversuche bei Thieren," *Journal der Chirurgie und Augenheilkunde* 6 (1824): 122–35.

43. Lampe, *Dieffenbach*, 116, 196.

44. Johann Friedrich Dieffenbach, "Ueberpflanzung völlig getrennter Hautstücke bei einer Frau, und Wiederanheilung einer grösstentheils abgehauenen Wange," *Journal der Chirurgie und Augenheilkunde* 6 (1824): 482–86.

45. Ibid.

46. Johann-Friedrich Dieffenbach, *Die operative Chirurgie*, vol. 1 (F. A. Brockhaus, 1845), 317.

47. Dieffenbach, *Chirurgische Erfahrungen*, 2:173.

48. These considerations by Dieffenbach about blood and the contraction of blood vessels has been interpreted by his biographers as a prescient recognition of the damaging effect of venous stasis and the "antiphlogistic" principles of surgical wound care. However, these interpretations overlook the conceptual context of vital forces and the physiological laws of tissues amidst which Dieffenbach formulated his recommendations. See, for example, Genschorek, *Wegbereiter der Chirurgie*, 58; Schultheiss et al., "Johann Friedrich Dieffenbach," 309.

49. Dieffenbach, *Chirurgische Erfahrungen*, 2:165, 168.

50. Ibid., 2:175–85.

51. Ibid., 2:162–63, 172–75; Dieffenbach, *Die operative Chirurgie*, 1:317–21.

52. Dieffenbach, *Chirurgische Erfahrungen*, 2:175.

53. Ibid., 2:175–76.

54. Ibid., 2:177.

55. Andrew Cunningham, *The Anatomist Anatomis'd: An Experimental Discipline in Enlightenment Europe* (England: Ashgate Publishing, 2010), 371–79; Cunningham, "Pen and the Sword" (2002); Cunningham, "Pen and the Sword" (2003).

56. Peter C. English, *Shock, Physiological Surgery, and George Washington Crile: Medical Innovation in the Progressive Era* (Westport, CT: Greenwood Press, 1980); Ulrich Tröhler, *Auf dem Weg zur physiologischen Chirurgie: Der Nobelpreisträger Theodor Kocher 1841–1917* (Basel: Birkhäuser, 1984); Thomas Schlich, *The Origins of Organ Transplantation: Surgery and Laboratory Science, 1880–1930* (Rochester, NY: University of Rochester Press, 2010), especially 150–62; Thomas Schlich, "'Physiological Surgery': Laboratory Science as the Epistemic Basis of Modern Surgery (and Neurosurgery)," unpublished manuscript, 2014. Many thanks to the author for making the manuscript available.

57. Mary Terrall, *Catching Nature in the Act: Réaumur and the Practice of Natural History in the Eighteenth Century* (Chicago: University of Chicago Press, 2014).

58. Timothy Lenoir, "Teleology without Regrets: The Transformation of Physiology in Germany: 1790–1847," *Studies in History and Philosophy of Science*, Part A, 12, no. 4 (1981): 293–354; Nyhart, *Biology Takes Form*, 35–47. For the most part the

morphological elements of Dieffenbach's physiological reflections seem to be compatible with Timothy Lenoir's characterization of teleomechanism, an approach that accepted the need for teleology in the formation of organic tissue but found teleology in mechanical and organizational, not strictly vitalistic, properties of matter.

59. Dieffenbach, *Chirurgische Erfahrungen*, 2:174.

60. Nyhart, *Biology Takes Form*, 47–64; Olaf Breidbach, "Karl Friedrich Burdach," in *Naturphilosophie nach Schelling*, ed. Thomas Bach and Olaf Breidbach (Stuttgart: Frommann-Holzboog, 2005), 73–106.

61. Dieffenbach explicitly pondered the challenges of the new experimental approach, in particular the challenges posed by the suffering of the animal, and the need to control for this, in the context of his transfusion experiments. Johann Friedrich Dieffenbach, *Die Transfusion des Blutes* (Berlin, 1828), ix–xii.

62. However, the specific result of all these variations remains unclear in the text. Instead, Dieffenbach seems to have attempted to establish certain generalizable rules resulting from his experiments, for instance that the likelihood of perfect regeneration was greater in tissues with a cartilaginous component (such as the nose) and a high blood flow, or in those with a known large reproductive force (such as the scrotum). Dieffenbach, *Chirurgische Erfahrungen*, 2:164–65, 171.

63. Dieffenbach, *Die Transfusion des Blutes*, ix–x; in fact, Dieffenbach was one of the first enthusiastic users of ether anesthesia when it became available. See Johann Friedrich Dieffenbach, *Der Aether gegen den Schmerz* (Berlin: Hirschwald, 1847).

64. This current is discussed in detail by Thomas Broman. Broman, *Transformation*, 102–27. Though, as Broman himself points out, the boundaries between thought systems were never as clearly drawn, Broman's characterization of the debate is an extremely useful crystallization of the major themes and groups.

65. Regularly discussed were, among others, the terms "Morioplastik," "Organoplastik," "Chirurgia curtorum," and "Transplantation." For a discussion of these terms, see Eduard Zeis, *Handbuch der plastischen Chirurgie* (Berlin: G. Reimer, 1838), 5–7; Friedrich-August von Ammon and Moritz Baumgarten, *Die plastische Chirurgie nach ihren bisherigen Leistungen kritisch dargestellt* (Berlin: G. Reimer, 1842), 3–7.

66. Graefe, *Rhinoplastik*, vi–vii.

67. Johann Friedrich Dieffenbach, *Chirurgische Erfahrungen, besonders über die Wiederherstellung zerstörter Theile des menschlichen Körpers nach neuen Methoden*, vol. 3 (Berlin: T. C. F. Enslin, 1834), v.

68. Johann Friedrich Dieffenbach, "Chirurgia Curtorum," in *Theoretisch-praktisches Handbuch der Chirurgie*, ed. Johann Nepomuk Rust, vol. 4 (Berlin: Enslin, 1831), 496–599; Johann Friedrich Dieffenbach, *Ueber den Organischen Ersatz* (Berlin: Enslin, 1831).

69. The use of different terms at different periods in his career may indicate an increasing crystallization of the kind of surgery Dieffenbach sought to establish, especially his emphasis on the plastic, living properties of the skin. The advantages and disadvantages of different terms were also explicitly debated by other authors, making deliberate choices more plausible. Zeis, *Handbuch*, 5–7; Ammon and Baumgarten, *Plastische Chirurgie*, 3–7.

70. Johann Friedrich Dieffenbach, *Chirurgische Erfahrungen, besonders über die Wiederherstellung zerstörter Theile des menschlichen Körpers nach neuen Methoden*, vol. 1 (Berlin: T. C. F. Enslin, 1829).

71. Johann Friedrich Dieffenbach, *Die Heilung des Stotterns durch eine neue chirurgische Operation* (Berlin: Förstner, 1841); Johann Friedrich Dieffenbach, *Ueber die Durchschneidung der Sehnen und Muskeln* (Berlin: Förstner, 1841).

72. Johann Friedrich Pierer, ed., "Bildungstrieb," in *Medizinisches Realwörterbuch*, vol. 1 (Leipzig: Brockhaus, 1816).

73. Christoph Wilhelm Hufeland, *Ideen über Pathogenie und Einfluss der Lebenskraft auf Entstehung und Form der Krankheiten* (Jena: Academische Buchhandlung, 1795), 65.

74. This meaning of plastic as the potential for the manipulation of living tissue, and its limits due to the unpredictability of the behavior of living matter, is echoed in the notion of "plasticity" that scholars have developed for the twentieth century. See, for example, Hannah Landecker, *Culturing Life: How Cells Became Technologies* (Cambridge, MA: Harvard University Press, 2009), 1–10; Hannah Landecker, "Living Differnetly in Time: Plasticity, Temporality and Cellular Biotechnologies," in *Technologized Images, Technologized Bodies*, ed. Jeanette Edwards, Penelope Harvey, and Peter Wade (New York; Oxford: Berghahn Books, 2010), 211–36.

75. Karl Theodor Meier, *Vorträge in der chirurgischen Klinik der königlichen Charité zu Berlin gehalten von Dieffenbach* (Berlin: Duncker, 1840), 5.

76. Hufeland, "Zusätze," 115..

77. Dieffenbach, *Chirurgische Erfahrungen*, 2:3.

78. Ibid., 3:vi.

79. For a thoughtful discussion of the historic specificity of certain surgical "styles" and the role of performance and metaphors in fashioning surgical identities, see Thomas Schlich, "'The Days of Brilliancy are Past': Skill, Styles and the Changing Rules of Surgical Performance, ca. 1820–1920," unpublished manuscript, 2014. Many thanks to the author for making the manuscript available.

80. Dieffenbach, *Die operative Chirurgie*, 1:324.

81. Dieffenbach, *Chirurgische Erfahrungen*, 1:4–5 This is very likely a stab at Graefe, who insisted on the creation of detailed drawings and models for his rhinoplastic operations.

82. Hufeland, "Zusätze," 115.

83. Dieffenbach, *Die operative Chirurgie*, 1:324–25.

84. Dieffenbach, *Chirurgische Erfahrungen*, 1:18.

85. Ibid., 2:38.

86. Meier, *Vorträge in der chirurgischen Klinik*, 5.

87. Ibid.

88. Thomas Schlich has described similar rhetorical strategies for the case of operative fracture care, in which proponents of the practice drew on notions of surgery as a science, and opponents emphasized the status of surgery as an art. Dieffenbach's case is interesting as he uses nuanced variations of familiar metaphors from the realm of the arts in order to argue that surgery was both, a science and an art. Thomas Schlich, "The Art and Science of Surgery: Innovation and Concepts of Medical Practice in Operative Fracture Care, 1960s–1970s," *Science, Technology & Human Values* 32, no. 1 (2007): 65–87.

89. Dieffenbach, *Chirurgische Erfahrungen*, 1:4.

90. Dieffenbach, *Die operative Chirurgie*, 1:1–2.

91. Broman, *Transformation*, 71–72.

92. Dieffenbach, *Die operative Chirurgie,* 1:18.

93. Ibid., 1:390–91.

94. The so-called genius movement (Geniebewegung) of the second half of the eighteenth and early nineteenth centuries, in reaction to the rational tendencies of the Enlightenment, emphasized the notion of a creative, irrational, enthusiastic, godlike genius. Jochen Schmidt, *Die Geschichte des Genie-Gedankens in der deutschen Literatur, Philosophie und Politik, 1750–1945: Von der Aufklärung bis zum Idealismus,* 3rd ed., 2 vols. (Heidelberg: Winter, 2004), vol. 1; Jochen Schmidt, *Die Geschichte des Genie-Gedankens in der deutschen Literatur, Philosophie und Politik, 1750–1945: Von der Romantik bis zum Ende des Dritten Reichs,* 2 vols. (Heidelberg: Winter, 2004), vol. 2; Günter Peters, *Der zerrissene Engel: Genieästhetik und literarische Selbstdarstellung im achtzehnten Jahrhundert* (Stuttgart: Metzler, 1982).

95. Schmidt, *Geschichte des Genie-Gedankens [Von der Aufklärung bis zum Idealismus],* 1:10–13.

96. Broman, *Transformation,* 71.

97. Dieffenbach, *Die operative Chirurgie,* 1:390–91.

98. Dieffenbach's demand for the surgeon to learn the laws of living tissue and know in each case how they ought to be applied can thus be said to lie at the intersection of a form of "trained judgment" and a more intuitive form of evaluation, leaving it unclear how exactly the surgeon could acquire this kind of judgment. Lorraine Daston and Peter Galison, *Objectivity* (Cambridge: Zone Books, 2007), 309–62.

99. Dieffenbach, *Die operative Chirurgie,* 1:1.

100. Broman, *Transformation,* 168–73.

101. Four letters from Johann Friedrich Dieffenbach to Karl von Baer, Berlin, October 10, 1929–January 1, 1843, call number ADB, 5, 120–26; BLÄ, 2, 262–64, Karl von Baer Fonds, University Library Giessen.

102. Bruno Valentin, ed., *Dieffenbach an Stromeyer: Briefe aus den Jahren 1836–1846* (Leipzig: J. A. Barth, 1934).

103. On professional hierarchies and internal competition in university faculties, see Awraham Zloczower, *Career Opportunities and the Growth of Scientific Discovery in Nineteenth-Century Germany* (New York: Arno Press, 1981), 11–38; Nyhart, *Biology Takes Form,* 15; Stefan Brüdermann, *Göttinger Studenten und akademische Gerichtsbarkeit im 18. Jahrhundert* (Göttingen: Vandenhoeck & Ruprecht, 1990), 310–16; Walter Rüegg, *A History of the University in Europe,* vol. 3, *Universities in the Nineteenth and Early Twentieth Centuries (1800–1945)* (Cambridge: Cambridge University Press, 2004), 141; *Privatissima* were sought out explicitly by traveling students like Pirogow: Pirogow, *Lebensfragen,* 383, 388, 390, 396.

104. Friedrich-Wilhelms-Universität Berlin, *Verzeichnis der Vorlesungen WH 1835/36,* 1835. Universitätsbibliothek der Humboldt-Universität zu Berlin, http://www.digi-hub.de/viewer/resolver?urn=urn:nbn:de:kobv:11-D-1072088.

105. Friedrich-Wilhelms-Universität Berlin, *Verzeichnis der Vorlesungen WH 1836/37,* 1836. Universitätsbibliothek der Humboldt-Universität zu Berlin, http://www.digi-hub.de/viewer/image/DE-11-001717043/8/.

106. Lampe, *Dieffenbach,* 125.

107. Eduard Zeis, *Die Literatur und Geschichte der plastischen Chirurgie* (Leipzig: Engelmann, 1862), 222.

108. Lampe, *Dieffenbach,* 125–26.

109. Dieffenbach, *Chirurgische Erfahrungen,* 1:135.

110. Ibid., 1:14–15.

111. Dieffenbach, *Die operative Chirurgie,* 1:x.

112. Hermann Eduard Fritze and O. F. G. Reich, *Die plastische Chirurgie in ihrem weitesten Umfange dargestellt und durch Abbildungen erläutert* (Berlin: Hirschwald, 1845), for example, 21.

113. Ibid., for example, 23.

114. Graefe, *Rhinoplastik,* esp. 37–45.

115. For example, Ernst Großheim, *Lehrbuch der operativen Chirurgie* (Berlin: Enslin, 1830); Ernst Blasius, *Lehrbuch der Akiurgie* (Halle: Anton, 1835).

116. Meier, *Dieffenbach's Vorträge,* 48.

117. Friedrich Tiedemann, *Untersuchungen über das Nahrungs-Bedürfniss, den Nahrungs-Trieb und die Nahrungs-Mittel des Menschen,* vol. 3 (Darmstadt: Leske, 1836), v–vi.

118. Blasius, *Lehrbuch der Akiurgie,* Vorrede.

119. Philippe Frédéric Blandin had published a book titled *Autoplastie, ou restauration des parties du corps qui ont été détruites etc.* in 1836. Valentin, *Dieffenbach an Stromeyer,* 21. In the letters to Stromeyer, Dieffenbach also complained about having been betrayed by Eduard Zeis, Friedrich Baumgarten, and Friedrich von Ammon, all of whom published works on plastic surgery during Dieffenbach's lifetime.

120. Pirogow, *Lebensfragen,* 392.

121. Ibid., 396.

122. Rohlfs, "Johann Friedrich Dieffenbach" (1883): 455.

Chapter Three

Defining Difference

Competing Forms of Ovarian Surgery in the Nineteenth Century

Sally Frampton

Introduction

"The perfecting of ovariotomy has resulted in saving and prolonging the lives of multitudes," the British surgeon John Halliday Croom declared in 1896.[1] Croom was reflecting on an operation that had, over the preceding fifty years, irrevocably altered the landscape of surgery. In the second half of the nineteenth century virtually no other operation garnered as much attention in Britain as that for the removal of diseased ovaries, and during which the operation undulated between controversy and accolade. In the mid-decades those who performed it were frequently lambasted, ridiculed, and even condemned as criminals by opponents who considered its high mortality rate unjustifiable.[2] By the 1890s, with a drastic diminution in the operation's mortality, and a rich archive of printed material now circulating among the medical community that showed hundreds of cases of the operation where the patient had been cured, ovariotomy had ascertained not just respectability but was viewed as emblematic of Victorian progress in medicine. The fruit of ovariotomists' labor was manifest in the many numbers of patients who had survived the operation and could now return to a life free of ovarian disease. In 1877 Thomas Spencer Wells (1818–97), Britain's most eminent and well-known ovariotomist, gave the address in surgery at the annual meeting of the British Medical Association in Manchester. In his speech Wells proclaimed that his ovariotomy operations alone had added eighteen thousand years to the lives of European women.[3] Such sentiments fitted in with broader understandings Victorian surgeons had of themselves as a civilizing force, both an intellectual and a moral one, their life-saving work a melding of sagacity and selflessness, augmented by the fact that it was women—the wives, mothers, and daughters of Britain—who were being drawn away from the clutches of disease.

Looking back, the history of ovariotomy might initially be viewed as simply one more example of a typically successful medical innovation: the resistance its advocates encountered before improvements in the procedure, and subsequent acceptance among the majority of the profession, marked its introduction into mainstream medicine. Certainty as the first major abdominal procedure to come into practice, ovariotomy raised difficult questions about the propriety and management of innovation as surgeons began to venture into the peritoneal cavity. For these reasons, and as I will show in this essay, ovarian surgery is a singularly good example of how the politics of surgical innovation was negotiated in the nineteenth century.

However, a close reading of the operation also suggests the limits of ascribing any kind of "career" model of innovation to ovarian surgery. I show that because the meaning and definition of "ovariotomy" was continually changing, the narrative of its innovation was (and is) unstable; while "ovariotomy" might ostensibly have been one operation, it was also many, and how exactly it was defined was constantly in flux, as the meaning of the operation was renegotiated. Of particular focus in this essay are the later decades of the nineteenth century, when different techniques and objectives for ovarian surgery proliferated. What happens when a surgical innovation develops a further innovation, and to what extent were these understood as distinct? What role does nomenclature play in this? Although the British experience of the operation is this essay's focus, international—and particularly transatlantic—connections between surgeons play a pivotal role. Difficulties in defining ovariotomy were heightened by the fact that new forms of ovarian surgery were arising from different countries, and concerns regarding priority and propriety motivated some to forge national distinctions between the various types.

Ovariotomy provides a useful way of unpacking not just the process of surgical innovation but also the usefulness of innovation as an analytical category in the history of medicine. How might we pin down the meaning of "innovation"—let alone "alternative innovation"—in surgery when these innovations themselves are unstable, changing entities that are difficult to define? Through the example of ovariotomy I show that alternative innovation need not necessarily imply competition between diverse innovations, but that such a framework might also be used to consider how different versions of the "same" operation arise.

"The Most Startling Innovation": The Invention of Ovariotomy

The powerful gender dynamics at play in ovariotomy have been the primary concern of most twentieth-century and contemporary historians who have examined the operation. In the 1980s and 1990s social and gender historians began to extricate the operation from the confines of triumphalist narratives (the formation of which was itself a critical aspect of ovariotomy's identity as an innovation), and the issue of women's submission to the operation became integral to a new historicization of it. Work by Ornella Moscucci stressed the role of gynecology—of which ovariotomy was the surgical showpiece—in forging constructions of Victorian femininity in Britain.[4] Through this reading, ovariotomy's status as a radical and innovative procedure was not merely a testament to surgical heroism, but instead revealed an operation implicitly tied to societal expectations regarding the role of women, which in turn helped legitimize a culture of novel and experimental surgery focused on the female body. The historiographical shift divulged not only historians' questions about the gendered nature of this surgical innovation but also that of the historical actors under scrutiny: the gendering of ovariotomy was of as much consequence to opponents of the operation—who could emotively use the loss of female life in their campaigns against the operation—as it was to advocates arguing that they were saving women's lives.[5]

The impact of this work has been significant. But it has led to a tendency for gender to obfuscate other significant aspects of the operation;[6] ovariotomy was by no means controversial solely for that reason. The claim of its novelty relied not just on removing the ovaries, but that the operation also called for the abdomen to be opened by a large incision. During the mid-eighteenth century, the possibility of surgically removing diseased ovaries became a subject of increased debate among British and French practitioners as attention turned to that organ's pathology. In the burgeoning field of morbid anatomy, the frequency and array of tumors found in the ovaries postmortem warranted attention.[7] But the possibilities for treating the condition in the living patient were limited. Ovarian tumors, usually assumed to be a form of dropsy, were considered extremely difficult to diagnose—they were often mistaken for pregnancy—and almost invariably fatal. Although one might live with the disease for many years it was usually in great discomfort and with no hope of a cure.[8] This grim state of affairs had been underlined by the work of the Birmingham physician William Withering, who in 1785 had published on the curative effects of digitalis on dropsical swellings. Withering admitted that the remedy was ineffective on afflictions of the ovary because of the peculiarity of their pathological makeup; "the ovarian dropsy defies the power of medicine," concluded Withering in 1785.[9]

By then speculation had already begun in medical circles as to the possibility of using radical surgical means to cure the condition. In Britain, William Hunter cautioned against making large wounds in the belly, believing them too dangerous, although he conceded smaller incisions into the abdomen might be permissible in desperate cases.[10] In France practitioners were rather more optimistic about the prospects of the operation, some suspecting ovarian extirpation would soon be a reality, although those who predicted its introduction declined to perform it themselves.[11] That ovarian surgery lingered as an idea during these decades complicates our understanding of innovation. Today we often associate the word "innovate" with rapid, radical change, and yet surgical innovation of the ovary was a drawn-out process, a theoretical possibility for many decades before it became a material reality.

A turning point came in 1809, when the American surgeon Ephraim McDowell successfully extirpated a diseased ovary.[12] The operation was the result not just of the patient's bravery and the surgeon's fortitude, but also bore the imprint of a surgical culture that was turning its attention toward the internal organs.[13] After news of McDowell's landmark procedure, decades of sporadic experimentation with the operation ensued in Britain.[14] By the mid-1840s ovarian extirpation was still comparatively rare, but in Britain at least the operation was beginning to be performed with a degree of consistency. Nonetheless it remained a hazardous procedure and the operation continued to be highly controversial.[15] Performers of the operation were alleged to have been decried as "belly rippers" by opponents. The term embodied the repugnance that was felt toward opening the abdomen, with its echoes of human vivisection.

The vanguard of practice in the midcentury was led by the Manchester obstetrician Charles Clay. Clay's views of abdominal surgery were likely shaped by his mentor, Thomas Radford, who had been unusual in his advocacy of caesarean section at a time when the operation was considered unjustifiable by most.[16] Radford had been present when Clay performed his first ovarian operation in 1842 on forty-six-year-old Mrs. Wheeler, who over the past three years had noticed a gradual enlargement of her abdomen. Clay noted that upon her consultation with him, she was "as large as a female in the ninth month of gestation." A huge tumor within the pelvic cavity was suspected to have begun in the ovary. In consultation with Radford, Clay ruled that only extirpation of the tumor offered the chance of cure, and he proceeded to successfully removed it three months later, after Mrs. Wheeler had been given time to weigh the risks of the operation against the burden of her disease. In Clay's notes recorded after the operation, he appeared conscious of its significance for surgery at large: "At this moment, none, but those who have witnessed such a scene, could have any idea of the extent and formidable appearance of the operation—the incision from sternum to pubis over the bulky tumour could not be less than twenty-four inches (being eighteen when the parts were flaccid subsequently), perhaps as large an incision as ever was made in the living subject."[17]

Clay's first seven cases, of which there were five successes and two fatalities, were published that year as the pamphlet *Cases of Peritoneal Section for the Extirpation of Diseased Ovaria.* His concluding commentary attested to an already forming distinction between types of practice in ovarian extirpation. For Clay, incision size was what marked his practice apart. The striking length of the cuts he made into the abdomen put his work at the very edge of impropriety, the "belly ripping" that opponents feared, but it was also what made his work new, different, and daring. Clay was quick to draw distinction between his work and that of surgeons who erred on the side of caution when it came to incision size. Those like William Jeaffreson (1790–1865), a Suffolk practitioner, who had performed a number of ovarian extirpations in the 1830s and who made incisions of about an inch and a half, extending the cut only if necessary. Clay was adamant that this form of practice was an alternative to his own, and a poorer one at that, because the surgeon's view was obscured; "the mode pursued by Mr. Jeffreson (sic) is not only impracticable, but really absurd," Clay wrote, claiming a lower mortality in his operations with large incisions.[18] However, Jeaffreson appeared satisfied with a distinction being made between his and Clay's operations because it enabled him to claim priority on a separate procedure. In a letter to the *Lancet* in 1843, Jeaffreson described himself as "the originator of the minor operation."[19] Matters of priority such as this were often at the heart of deliberations over surgical taxonomy, and as we shall see, it would not be long before further debates about priority occurred.

In modern surgery, general understandings of how an operation should be performed, for instance, as might be defined through a surgical manual or through instructions from senior surgeons, are frequently at variance with the idiosyncrasies of individual practice and the specifics of a patient's pathology.[20] In the nineteenth century, idiosyncrasy in surgical technique was an accepted tenet of practice. However, it could also be a source of frustration to those wishing to subject an operation to statistical investigation, which relied on a certain degree of standardization so that comparisons could be made. In 1843 incidences of ovarian extirpation began to be assimilated under a neologism that was coined to describe the procedure—"ovariotomy"—a term created by the obstetrician James Young Simpson in response to Charles Clay's operations and first used by Clay in an article for *The Medical Times and Gazette.*[21] The word stuck, assured perhaps by the considerable professional influence of Clay and particularly of Simpson.

The coining of the term had implications for practice. The operation of ovarian extirpation had been performed by a rather disparate group of practitioners, only loosely connected. "Ovariotomy" suggested a shift from a collection of individual operations to a collective identity, in which all occurrences of ovarian operations were expected to be made public. Nonreporting of ovariotomy cases was increasingly taken as evidence of occlusion of failed cases, and publication became the fundamental marker of authenticity. For the next two decades, during which the place of ovarian surgery would remain deeply contested, statistical collations of all known ovariotomies would be used by both advocates and opponents of the operation to defend their position. This endeavor marked the permeation of statistical data into the culture of medicine; "statistics will settle the question," proclaimed one obstetrician confidently in 1844, in regard to the ovariotomy question.[22] And yet, although both a fixed nomenclature and statistics brought a degree of clarity to proceedings, the statistics themselves were replete with caveats, with practitioners proffering diverse notions as to which of their operations should be included. For example, some ovariotomists did not report operations where they had opened the abdomen only as an exploratory procedure, and had not proceeded to remove the organ.[23] This only added fuel to the fire of those opponents who were steadfastly convinced that failed ovariotomies were not being reported because of fears of reprobation from the profession.[24]

In the 1860s ovariotomy was still an uncommon operation, its practice mainly limited to private patients or those admitted to specialist hospitals for women. But it was beginning to receive wide-scale acceptance from the profession. A number of factors played into this turnabout in opinion. Time had proven that many women could survive the operation and remain cured in the long term. And some operators were beginning to achieve remarkable results, most notably the Edinburgh surgeon Thomas Keith, who in 1867 announced that four-fifths of his ovariotomy patients had survived the operation.[25] However, on general aggregate, the mortality for the operation remained high, at around one-third, which was similar to that of other capital operations.[26] More significant than any real decline in the operation's mortality was the publication of a lengthy series of meticulously detailed cases by Thomas Spencer Wells in 1865.[27] Wells's openness about his experiences did much to improve the reputation of the operation, alleviating fears that cases were being deliberately concealed. It suggests that the determination of a new operation's success was dependent not only on a diminished mortality rate but also on the manner in which the operation was conveyed through published material.

The degree of change that ovariotomy signaled was now beginning to impress itself on the surgical psyche. As the surgeon William P. Swain wrote in 1866, ovariotomy was "perhaps the most startling innovation in surgery of late years . . . our old notion, that it was death to the patient to interfere with the peritoneum, has been somewhat rudely swept away by the wholesale manner in which it is now cut through, and burnt through, and mopped out with sponges."[28]

Such meditations spoke to the still precarious position that innovation held within surgical culture. The rich history of "innovation"—both as a word and concept—is not reflected on as frequently as it should be by historians, and yet given its constant presence in today's world, it warrants attention. Benoît Godin has observed that "for most of its history the concept innovation, a word of Greek origin, carried pejorative connotations. As 'introducing change to the established order,' innovation was seen as deviant behaviour, forbidden and punished."[29] Often synonymic with notions of "revolution"—another word that would come to have important connotations for nineteenth-century surgeons—"innovation" had long been associated with political and social uncertainty. In the nineteenth century, as the inventor was recast from eccentric outsider to heroic Briton of the Smilesean mould, innovation began to be understood more positively, or at least less as a signal of radicalism or instability.[30] Surgeons were by no means immune to this cultural shift. And yet as Swain's words suggest, although ovariotomy was increasingly construed as a force of good, there were ripples of unease as to the extent to which surgery was being changed by the operation. Even if it was no longer considered an outright mischief, it remained shocking and somewhat brutal.

Wells's success at bringing ovariotomy into the mainstream meant the operation soon became entrenched in a narrative that imagined it as an invention of Victorian progress. As a consequence, it also catapulted him into the surgical elite. Wells had been quick to claim credit as the surgeon responsible for "reviving" ovariotomy, much to the chagrin of Charles Clay, whose own cases having been performed entirely in private practice outside of London, and published separately rather than in book form, Wells deemed to have had rather less impact. Clay was accorded priority as the first surgeon to perform a series of ovariotomies in Britain, but the value of that contribution was now under attack as Wells began to publicly denigrate his role in the operation's innovation.

The fluidity of definition was significant in their dispute. Initially Clay presented Wells as a poor-quality imitator, speaking almost nostalgically about the days gone by when "I had the operation to myself, when I had rather to originate than imitate plans of operation and after treatment," inferring that was what Wells was in fact doing.[31] Imitation, as the saying goes, is the highest form of flattery, and if acknowledged correctly, was considered acceptable behavior for surgeons. Tacit knowledge was a vital part of surgical education and new techniques were in part learned through witnessing the operations of others and subsequently imitating them.[32] But this also had to be carefully negotiated. Unacknowledged imitation still had the potential to look like mere copying.

In later letters, Clay changed tactic and emphasized the polarity in his and Wells's methods, arguing that their operations were "two distinctly different modes of proceeding, if faithfully carried out." Wells, for example, championed an abdominal incision of about 4 inches; Clay, as we have seen, favored making a much larger one. Wells completed the operation by securing a clamp to the remaining pedicle; Clay used ligatures. Wells treated the pedicle external to the peritoneum; Clay kept it within, and so forth.[33] Deconstructing their operating methods helped Clay differentiate between his work and Wells's and strengthened his claim that he had created his own operation, which he argued was an entirely different procedure from Wells's. Such priority disputes brought to the fore differences in practice, but Clay and Wells were not alone in having these differences. Surgeons' methods for separating the pedicle from the tumor, for example, varied considerably and played a prominent role in discussions about the techniques of ovariotomy throughout the second half of the century.

The dispute between Clay and Wells showed that "ovariotomy" could only ever be an umbrella term for the numerous methods of practice that were being employed. To some degree every performance of ovariotomy was unique, each was dependent on the way the surgeon performed it and the patient who underwent it. Diagnosis before an operation remained limited, and many cases saw unexpected adhesions and complications being discovered once the abdomen was opened and its mysteries revealed. These variations did not necessarily negate the usefulness of "ovariotomy" as an indicator of the procedure being performed, although they did draw attention to its limitations. However, the stability of ovariotomy as a clearly defined form of surgery was soon to be much more seriously challenged as new ovarian procedures began to emerge.

An American Import: The Introduction of Battey's Operation

In the late 1870s ovariotomists had never been held in higher regard. "Even now the most favourable ovariotomy is a marvellous liberty with the human body, and it is difficult to do justice to the courage and the faith of the men who first undertook it under every kind of discouragement from the heads of surgery," opined the *Lancet* in 1877, reimagining the history of resistance to the operation as a test of courage for surgical prophets like Wells.[34] That obstetricians and surgeons were beginning to develop new ways of performing the operation would have been of little surprise. Modifications were constantly occurring and, as we have seen, practitioners often had their preferences when dealing with various aspects of the operation. Reduced mortality rates meant more opportunities to operate and a safer testing ground for new techniques. But in the late 1870s a new development was to emerge from America that would radically alter ovariotomy because it involved not just a change in technique but also objective.

The practice of Robert Battey has already been well-explored by a number of historians.[35] Indeed his name has become rather notorious in the history of medicine, synonymous with the seeming excesses of nineteenth-century gynecologists. Born in 1828 in Georgia and trained in Philadelphia, Battey returned from his duties as a Confederate Army surgeon in 1865, settling into practice in Rome, Georgia. He began to perform ovariotomies in 1869, his interest in the operation having been piqued in the late 1850s when a tour of Europe had led him to meet many practitioners of the operation, including Wells.[36] Battey had begun to hypothesize the use of ovarian surgery for conditions other than tumors soon after his return to practice. Perturbed by the numerous physical and psychological problems suffered by his patients with menstrual irregularities, Battey had developed the theory that if both ovaries were removed, menopause would ensue, thus effecting a cure. He put theory into practice in 1872 when he removed both ovaries from his twenty-three-year-old patient Julia Olmberg, who was suffering from a range of gastric, rectal, and epileptic symptoms.[37] Battey and his advocates would go on to perform the operation for a wide range of conditions, including, most controversially, on women whose menstrual disorders were believed to be causing hysteria, nymphomania, or insanity. As Lawrence Longo has shown elsewhere, the indications for the operation were strikingly vague.[38]

The appellation Battey gave his operation was "normal ovariotomy," chosen to reflect a belief that his method was a "truer" ovariotomy than that usually performed—which he described as "irregular ovariotomy"—because the ovaries he removed were not diseased. As he rather arrogantly described it, "it was I who had really and truly done an ovariotomy rather than Dr. Ephraim McDowell."[39] Battey's peers were critical of his appropriation of the word "ovariotomy." Its inference that perfectly normal ovaries were being removed was liable to be misunderstood. This was far from ideal given that the propriety of ovariotomy had so often been questioned already. "Battey's term, *Normal Ovariotomy* is inapplicable," reasoned the St. Louis physician George Engelmann in an article analyzing forty-three cases of the operation published in 1878, Engelmann claiming that in the majority of cases the ovaries were in fact diseased, thus rendering the phrase even more misleading. As he further probed the nomenclature, conceptual and taxonomic confusion became apparent, for Engelmann then went on to argue that Battey's procedure was "ovariotomy proper, and *Ovariotomy* it should be called, were not that term now, by long continued usage, given to the operation for ovarian tumours."[40]

By this time Battey had already acquiesced to the concerns of his contemporaries regarding the name of the operation and had sought to change it. This had been done in collaboration with the gynecological surgeon James Marion Sims, who was to become an influential supporter of the operation, advocating its use under certain circumstances. At the end of 1877 Sims introduced the new procedure to Britain, by which time it had been performed by a variety of operators. His involvement with the operation warranted attention. Like Battey, Sims was from the South; his early medical practice had been in Montgomery, Alabama, where he had dedicated himself to improving the surgery for vesico-vaginal fistula. This brought him professional acclaim, but also left him with a dubious legacy, Sims having "perfected" his technique on enslaved black women, a number of whom were operated on multiple times.[41] By the 1850s Sims had left the South for New York, where he built a reputation sufficient enough to propel him on to the international stage. After the outbreak of the Civil War Sims moved to Europe and spent the rest of his life dividing his time between London, Paris, and New York.[42] Having succeeded in crafting an eminent reputation on both sides of the Atlantic—no mean feat—Sims was an integral figure in connecting American and European surgery and ideally placed to ease a new operation into the consciousness of British surgeons. In the final weeks of 1877, a series of articles by Sims was published in the *British Medical Journal* detailing twenty-eight cases where the procedure had been performed. Practices deviated considerably within these cases; some operators had used abdominal sections, others had extracted the ovaries vaginally, although this had a higher mortality. Battey's theory was that termination of ovarian function was required to enable cure. And yet on a on a number of occasions he had himself extirpated only one ovary, either deeming the removal of one sufficient or because of the impossibility of removing the second.[43] The result was an operation that was distinct more through objective—preventing ovarian function—than its technique. It differentiated from the operations of Wells and Clay because it was the ovary as a whole rather than ovarian tumor that was considered the seat of trouble.

Sims emphasized a genealogical connection between the two procedures, framing Battey's operation as the progeny of ovariotomy and citing the history of the first operation to forestall the profession rejecting the second too quickly. He wrote: "Without operative procedures, these cases are all hopelessly incurable. We must improve our methods or leave them where we found them. I see no reason why the operation should not be made safe and successful. Ovariotomy was once opposed because it was unsuccessful; but now it is accepted because it is successful . . . let us look back at our work, and see if it has always been well done."[44]

The connection between the two was thus leaned on to quell concerns about the new development, Sims reminding surgeons of the difficulties ovariotomy went through before it was accepted. Nonetheless the introduction of the operation to a British audience was also a convenient opportunity to rebrand the operation in a way that emphasized distinction. In his final paper in the series, Sims announced that Battey had asked his advice in renaming the operation and that he had conferred on it the name "Battey's operation," urging European surgeons to "unite with us in America in giving it the name of the man who originated the operation."[45] This renaming served a number of functions. First, it formed a connection between Battey and the procedure. In what was a calculated risk, Battey's professional reputation was now intertwined with the fate of the operation. Second, it was used to more firmly differentiate the procedure from ovariotomy, expunging the confusion that "normal" ovariotomy had brought. In both respects, Battey and Sims were only moderately successful; the term "normal ovariotomy" would still continue to be used sporadically in Britain and America. Other terms soon came into use that diminished Battey's proprietary hold on the procedure. In 1872 the American surgeon Edmund Peaslee had drawn attention to the failure of "ovariotomy" as an explanatory term and had suggested "oöphorectomy" as a more accurate one (the suffix "-ectomy" denoting removal, whereas "otomy" implied only incision).[46] Athough this suggestion was not taken up in relation to ovariotomy for tumors, the phrase reemerged at the tail-end of the 1870s to refer to the removal of both ovaries to cease ovarian function. Initially British practitioners used the phrase interchangeably with "Battey's operation," although by the late 1880s it was "oöphorectomy" that was more commonly used. It seems clear that many practitioners did not wish their work to be associated with Battey's. The Birmingham surgeon Robert Lawson Tait, for example, had begun removing the ovaries and fallopian tubes as a way of curing inflammatory disease (pyosalpinx) of the latter around the same time that Battey had begun performing his operation. His procedure was similar enough to Battey's that the two were frequently compared, but Tait repeatedly felt the need to emphasize their difference, denying that he would ever remove the ovaries for anything other than inflammatory disease; "what Dr. Battey has advocated and practised, I, for one, practically have never performed," he wrote to the *British Medical Journal*.[47] Tait eschewed both "Battey's operation" and "oophorectomy," instead describing the operation as "removal of the uterine appendages."

The change to "Battey's operation" was no doubt conceived to have another important role: it asserted the American identity of the operation. Though never overt, there had long been a degree of tension between American and British surgeons as to who should be credited for introducing ovarian surgery. There was a feeling on the American side that not enough had been done to build on McDowell's legacy in his home country.[48] The long series of operations performed by Clay, Keith, and Wells had shifted the central arena of ovarian surgery to Britain, and surgeons there claimed it was owing to British endeavors that the operation had flourished. Battey's operation, on the other hand, was undeniably an American invention and accepted as such by British practitioners. The British response to the procedure had been mixed. As we have seen, there was an expansion in home-grown gynecological surgery led by Robert Lawson Tait, who sought to distance himself from Battey. But other surgeons and obstetricians began to replicate Battey's model of operating, praising the American surgeon's enterprise in bringing the operation to the profession's attention. A glimpse into British patients' perceptions of Battey's operation—albeit one mediated through the narrative of the medical professional—was provided by the obstetrician Alexander Russell Simpson in 1879. Writing in the *British Medical Journal,* Russell recounted a patient with chronic menstrual pain who had implored Russell to perform Battey's operation on her after he had mentioned the developments occurring in American surgery. According to Russell, the patient claimed to have been "reading all about" the new operation, asking Russell, "Can't you do here what the doctors in America can do?"[49] It suggests that some patients were also schooled to recognize the distinct and distinctly American nature of the operation.

As Sims seemed to anticipate, resistance soon occurred in Britain. Anxieties were heighted by the mortality rate for the new operation, which, in the 1880s, was higher than that for ovariotomy. In 1883 Tait recorded mortality rates of 12.8 percent and 5 percent, respectively, although both had dropped to under 3.5 percent in his practice by 1888.[50] Critics both inside and outside the profession began to express concern about overoperating, much of which centered around fears that women were being "unsexed." A pejorative and highly loaded term was soon being used to describe the apparent craze for ovarian surgery: that it had become a "fashion." Such language not only pointed to the continued characterization of ovarian surgery as a novelty, but also the possibility of unthinking consumption of surgical trends on the part of both practitioners and patients. Ornella Moscucci has speculated that oöphorectomies may have even been sought by patients as a means of preventing unwanted pregnancies.[51]

The revelation that the operation was being used experimentally to treat insanity also startled many, even those who were themselves ovariotomists. Thomas Spencer Wells spoke out forcibly against the new operation. In an essay published in the *American Journal of the Medical Sciences* in 1886, and later reprinted as a pamphlet, he described the procedure as an "unnecessary mutilation of young women."[52] For Wells, this unwelcome development could only be understood through the framework of nationality, its roots in the "fanaticism" of American surgeons.[53] But, he warned, its implications were global. "The danger is now increasing as the operation is becoming world-wide," Wells wrote, "the oöphorectomists of civilization touch hands with the aboriginal spayers of New Zealand."[54] Wells picked his words carefully, crafting an image of oöphorectomy that suggested savagery, in stark contrast to ovariotomy, which he depicted as a model of colonial advance, likening it to "the discovery of the Californian diggings or the African diamond mines."[55] Wells titled the essay "On the Castration of Women," provocatively ignoring any of the more respectable terms to use instead a word that carried stigma and that suggested a violent, animalistic procedure rather than a progressive one. Regardless of the efforts of Battey and others, both "castration" and "spaying" would frequently be employed to describe operations to remove both ovaries. By doing so Wells showed the power such descriptive words had in conveying the precarious propriety of the operation.

"What Is Ovariotomy?" The Unravelling Nomenclature of Ovarian Surgery

"Conceptual history must start with lexical history," it has been observed.[56] Surgeons of the nineteenth century may not have been averse to such an opinion. Medical nomenclature was of increasing concern in the second half of the century. In 1869 the Royal College of Physicians published the first of what would be many editions of their *Nomenclature of Diseases.* The pamphlet had originally been conceived in the midst of concerns about classification during the midcentury as public-health reform became a central focus on the medical profession. Fixed categories allowed for easier statistical analysis, and it was hoped the handbook would help form a standardized nomenclature that could be used both nationally and internationally. Its orientation toward public health meant that the bulk of the text was given over to the classification of disease. Nonetheless an appended list of surgical operations appeared in the first edition and was then considerably expanded in a later version published in 1885. In the latter edition, "ovariotomy" and "oophorectomy" appeared with the following definitions:

> Ovariotomy. Removal of enlarged or diseased ovaries.
> Oöphorectomy. Removal of healthy ovaries. *Syn.*, Spaying.[57]

These definitions gave the impression that there was now a clear demarcation between the two types of operation. But in the everyday of surgery, no such clarity existed. By the end of the 1880s there was still considerable confusion surrounding the correct nomenclature for ovarian surgery. Generally "ovariotomy" indicated the treatment of tumors and cysts, and oöphorectomy, the treatment of inflammatory conditions, diseases of the fallopian tubes and the removal of the ovaries as a means of bringing on menopause. But the two terms were also sometimes used to indicate whether one or two ovaries had been removed, respectively. Thus, depending on the practitioner, the removal of *both* ovaries for ovarian cysts, for example, might be called "ovariotomy" or it might be called an "oöphorectomy" or even a "double ovariotomy," to indicate both had been removed. This could make gathering and comparing statistics for the operation complex, and Robert Lawson Tait often complained about the difficulty of making a distinction, particularly as in his experience ovaries were frequently afflicted with both tumors and inflammation.[58]

This state of affairs was displeasing; as one surgeon wrote to the *British Medical Journal* in 1886, "the nomenclature is so various, and some of its terms so ambiguous, that all will concur in the advisability for the adoption of certain words which will indicate clearly particular operations." At the end of his letter the correspondent simply asked, "What is 'ovariotomy'?"[59] A response came one week later from an anonymous Fellow of the Royal College of Surgeons, who replied, "With every succeeding advance, fresh difficulties in division and in nomenclature have arisen . . . the question, 'what is ovariotomy?' is one which, at the present moment, it is perfectly impossible to give a definite and scientific answer to."[60] The author's implication that the term "ovariotomy" failed to provide an adequately *scientific* definition suggested that the proliferation of procedures was not the only problem. By the end of the 1880s the term also appeared increasingly outdated and unhelpful, doing little to indicate the histology of the tumor being removed. Many terms in surgery failed to reflect precise pathology, but with the "infinite and endless gradations" of ovarian tumor that were thought to exist, the "ovariotomy" seemed especially to convey an old-fashioned type of surgery that was scientifically imprecise.[61]

On a lexical level, a decline in the use of the word "ovariotomy" ensued from the late 1880s, with a particularly sharp drop from the first to the second decade of the 1900s. During this time "oöphorectomy" was increasingly favored to describe all operations where an ovary had been removed (as it continues to do so today), while advances in conservative surgery meant that ovarian cysts and tumors could now be dissected out so that the rest of the ovary could be retained. And yet while its use declined, that decline was markedly slow considering the acknowledged imperfections of the term. "Ovariotomy" did not shift easily from medical language even as its meaning became uncertain and where "oöphorectomy" was a more accurate term. Medical nomenclature is not easily changed once it has become common parlance, and clarity is not the only factor that occasions its use; as one commentator reflected in 1940, medical terminology is a "mixture in which historical and sentimental factors play a large part."[62] Ovariotomy, which had come to represent a poignant and triumphant episode in surgery, and which was steeped in history and emotion, retained a powerful symbolic resonance that was not easily lost. Because of this, by the end of the century, even when ovariotomy no longer seemed to have any clear definition, its presence remained. Throughout this time "ovariotomy" had lain on far safer moral ground than "oöphorectomy," a word that continued to be associated with the overoperating controversies of the mid-1880s. The sensitivity surrounding oöphorectomy may explain why the term "ovariotomy" continued to be used.

Indeed, despite its decline, the term "ovariotomy" has never quite disappeared from scientific use. Today, medical publications stemming from China and India still use the term, demonstrating the subtle linguistic shifts that can occur transnationally in medicine.[63] The long and complex lexical history of ovariotomy shows how the ascription of surgical nomenclature is far from a self-evident process, where words inherently connect to procedures; rather, nomenclature has significant ethical and professional ramifications.

Conclusion

Can the problems of defining difference in surgical innovation, described above, be viewed as exceptional to ovarian surgery? Or are these complexities representative more generally of surgical practice? In many respects ovariotomy is a singular example. It was an operation performed wholly on women, which imbued it with cultural politics more marked than that of less-obviously gendered operations. As the first form of major abdominal surgery to be introduced into practice, it also had a peculiarly emotive power among the surgical community, symbolic of hopes and fears about the future of surgery. It was during the nineteenth century that innovation came to be closely connected to concepts of "progress," and yet concerns remained about the degree of change this might entail. That major abdominal surgery was being performed frequently, without clearly defined objectives or nomenclature, contributed to these anxieties.

This provides an interesting counterpoint to histories of twentieth-century innovation, revealing as it does the transitioning status of innovation in nineteenth-century surgery. But it also highlights strands of continuity. There has been a tendency to pinpoint the late twentieth century as the period when significant doubts arose as to whether innovation in medicine was beneficial.[64] Ovariotomy shows this is far from the case, the operation frequently giving rise to major concerns about the place of innovation in surgery. Its history also compels us to consider how managing surgical innovation today remains peculiarly complex. The aspect of performance that is central to surgery—which can make achieving uniformity in practice difficult—continues, and the difficulty in standardizing surgery makes it rather less compatible than other medical disciplines with prevalent frameworks of modern practice such as the randomized controlled trial.[65]

What then did "Battey's operation" represent? An alternative to ovariotomy or a version of it? In the late nineteenth century the boundaries were blurred. "Ovariotomy" was the term that had for many decades described the extirpation of diseased ovaries, and it was clear that the shift toward removing ovaries to treat other forms of disease was, in part, the product of this innovation. For that reason the terms were often used interchangeably. And yet there were important reasons for both advocates and opponents of the new operation to distinguish it from the old. For Battey and his supporters, framing it as a distinct form of surgery meant the possibility of attaining priority for its invention, with all the attendant social cachet that might come from that should the innovation prove a triumph. For those wary of the new developments, the distinction offered a certain amount of security against accusations of impropriety. In Battey's case his claim to ownership on the new operation would not entirely pay off. His name and operation would go down in history, but not for the reasons he would have hoped. As ovarian surgery became subject to greater criticism, Battey was the man irrevocably associated with the "fashion" for removing ovaries, even if he was not the only surgeon to do so. Battey had gambled his name in the hope that personal association with the innovation would bring enduring fame, but it would also bring enduring notoriety. Battey's fate in this regard is as much a historiographical issue as it is a historical one. It is striking that in most secondary literature on nineteenth-century ovarian surgery, the two forms of operation have been collapsed together and "Battey's operation" has frequently been constructed as the climactic endpoint of the ovariotomy narrative rather than an alternative to the original operation.[66] It is these excesses of ovarian surgery that have come to be seen as unveiling the true meaning of ovariotomy, that is, the use of experimental surgery as a means of controlling the behavior of women. In truth, the difference between these two practices remains just as debatable today, and their meaning just as unstable.

Such deviations in practice raise significant methodological questions; if surgical innovation often occurs in the manner suggested above, then one might question the usefulness altogether of constructing the history of a surgical innovation. To do so, after all, one tends to rely on a certain amount of stability to the innovation at hand in order to produce a narrative. And yet the history of ovariotomy draws our attention to the chronic instability of that procedure, linguistically and conceptually, and it is unlikely to be the only operation to reveal such a history. I would argue, however, that this does not negate the usefulness of "innovation" as an analytical category, as long as one does not premise it on a simplistic understanding of innovations as discrete entities that can be neatly categorized as successes or failures. Indeed it is through using the framework of innovation that a much richer history of nineteenth-century ovarian surgery is revealed, bringing into view the wide deviation in theory and practice that lingered under that one powerful term—"ovariotomy."

Notes

This essay was generously supported by the Wellcome Trust (grant number 063019).

1. John Halliday Croom, "Obstetrics," *Lancet* 148 (1896): 343.

2. Robert Liston, *Elements of Surgery* (London: Longman, 1835), 54.

3. Thomas Spencer Wells, "The Address in Surgery," *Lancet* 110 (1877): 193.

4. Ornella Moscucci, *The Science of Woman: Gynaecology and Gender in England, 1800–1929* (Cambridge: Cambridge University Press, 1990). For an account of ovariotomy in America, see Regina Morantz-Sanchez, *Conduct Unbecoming a Woman: Medicine on Trial in Turn-of-the-Century Brooklyn* (Oxford: Oxford University Press, 1999).

5. One of the most outspoken opponents of ovarian surgery in midcentury London was the surgeon Robert Liston. Liston evocatively described those women who had died undergoing the procedure as "sacrificed to a desire for false reputation." This idea of sacrifice, particularly of women, was powerful, conjuring up images of slavishness to unthinking ritual and of unnecessary death, quite contrary to any notion of progress. Liston, *Elements of Surgery*, 54.

6. This is not to detract from the value of Moscucci's and Morantz-Sanchez's nuanced accounts. Both authors deny that the operation can be viewed merely as an exercise in misogyny. Nonetheless their work is firmly situated within gender history.

7. Many eighteenth-century anatomists and practitioners noted the frequency with which ovaries were found to be diseased. In fact so often were pathological changes discovered upon dissection that it was sometimes difficult to establish what exactly should be considered a normal ovary. Jean Astruc, *A Treatise on the Diseases of Women*, vol. 3 (London: J. Nourse, 1767), 14. See also Sally Frampton, "The Debris of Life: Diseased Ovaries in Eighteenth-Century Medicine," in *The Secrets of Generation: Reproduction in the Long Eighteenth Century*, ed. Raymond Stephanson and Darren N. Wagner (Toronto: University of Toronto Press, 2015), 344–63.

8. The difficulty in treating dropsies of the ovary was often attributed to the tumors being "encysted," meaning they were made up of small sacs in which fluid was trapped. This rendered the diuretic effect of digitalis ineffective.

9. William Withering, *An Account of the Foxglove and Some of Its Medical Uses* (Birmingham: Swinney, 1785), 203.

10. William Hunter, "The History of Emphysema," *Medical Observations and Inquiries* 2 (1758): 41–45.

11. Jean Delaporte was probably the first surgeon to publicly express his desire to see the establishment of a more radical operation that involved removing the whole ovary. Jean Delaporte, "Hydropsie enkistée de l'ovaire attaquée par incision," *Mémoires de l'Académie Royale de Chirurgie* 2 (1753): 452–55.

12. McDowell published on the operation only in 1817. By then he had removed diseased ovaries from three women, all of whom had survived. Ephraim McDowell, "Three Cases of Extirpation of Diseased Ovaria," *Eclectic Repertory and Analytical Review* 7 (1817): 242–45.

13. In the eighteenth century the womb and the spleen were also mooted as possible targets for extirpation. In Britain in the 1820s these organs, along with the kidney and the bladder, would be subject to animal experimentation by the physician James Blundell, who concluded that the ovaries, spleen, and parts of the bladder might all

be feasibly removed, and that "moderate openings into the human peritoneum will not necessarily, or even generally, prove fatal from inflammation." James Blundell, "On the Surgery of the Abdomen," *Lancet* 12 (1829): 355.

14. In 1825 the Scottish surgeon John Lizars had published four cases where he had attempted the radical procedure. Lizars's results were not good: of his four cases, one died from peritoneal inflammation, another was discovered to have been misdiagnosed, with no tumor to be found upon opening the abdomen, and in a third the operation had to be abandoned because of extensive adhesions. A fourth woman was operated on successfully. John Lizars, *Observations on Extraction of Diseased Ovaria* (Edinburgh: Daniel Lizars, 1825). In the late 1830s a number of provincial surgeons performed the operation with rather more success, and shortly after a small number of London surgeons also took up its practice.

15. Sally Frampton, "Patents, Priority Disputes and the Value of Credit: Towards a History (and Pre-History) of Intellectual Property in Medicine," *Medical History* 55 (2011): 322.

16. Thomas Radford, "Two Cases of Impracticable Labour Arising from Malacosteon of the Pelvis, in Which the Caesarean Operation Was Performed," *Edinburgh Medical and Surgical Journal* 55 (1841): 71.

17. Charles Clay, *Cases of Peritoneal Section for the Extirpation of Diseased Ovaria* (London: Munro & Congreve, 1842), 4.

18. Clay, *Cases of Peritoneal Section*, 18.

19. William Jeaffreson, "Mr Jeaffreson's Operation for Ovarian Dropsy," *Lancet* 41 (1843): 217.

20. Thomas Schlich, *Surgery, Science and Industry: A Revolution in Fracture Care, 1950s–1980s* (Basingstoke, England: Palgrave Macmillan, 2002), 133.

21. Charles Clay, "Ovariotomy," *Medical Times* 9 (1843): 4–5.

22. Fleetwood Churchill, "Ovariotomy," *Medico-Chirurgical Review* 82 (1844): 528. For more on the "avalanche of printed numbers" in nineteenth-century culture, see Ian Hacking, *The Taming of Chance* (Cambridge: Cambridge University Press, 1990).

23. "Royal Medical and Chirurgical Society, November 13th, 1850," *Lancet* 56 (1850): 585–86.

24. This was the contention of William Lawrence, one of London's most eminent surgeons, who was vehemently opposed to ovariotomy. "Royal Medical and Chirurgical Society," 586.

25. Thomas Keith, "Fifty-One Cases of Ovariotomy," *Lancet* 90 (1867): 291.

26. The phrase "capital operation" was frequently used in the nineteenth century to describe those major procedures that carried a substantial risk to the life of the patient. Aside from ovariotomy, in the mid-decades this generally included lithotomy, ligation of aneurysms, amputation at the thigh, and hernia operations. For more on British surgery in the early to mid-nineteenth century, see Peter Stanley, *For Fear of Pain: British Surgery, 1790–1850* (New York: Penguin, 2003).

27. Thomas Spencer Wells, *Diseases of the Ovaries: Their Diagnosis and Treatment*, vol. 1 (London: John Churchill & Sons, 1865).

28. William P. Swain, "Transactions of Branches: On Recent Improvements in Surgery," *British Medical Journal* 2 (1866): 304.

29. Benoît Godin, "Social Innovation: Utopias of Innovation from c. 1830 to the Present," Project on the Intellectual History of Innovation, Working Paper no.

11, INRS, Montreal, 2012, 8, http://www.csiic.ca/PDF/SocialInnovation_2012.pdf (accessed October 15, 2014).

30. Christine MacLeod, *Heroes of Invention: Technology, Liberalism and British Identity: 1750–1914* (Cambridge: Cambridge University Press, 2007).

31. Charles Clay, "The Ovariotomy Controversy," *Lancet* 85 (1865): 380.

32. Schlich, *Surgery, Science and Industry*, 67–8.

33. Charles Clay, "On Ovariotomy and Ovariotomists," *Lancet* 85 (1865): 227.

34. "Mr. Wells's Address in Surgery," *Lancet* 110, no. 2816 (1877): 249.

35. Lawrence D. Longo, "The Rise and Fall of Battey's Operation: A Fashion in Surgery," *Bulletin of the History of Medicine* 53 (1979): 244–67; Morantz-Sanchez, *Conduct Unbecoming a Woman*, 94–100.

36. Longo, "Rise and Fall of Battey's Operation," 245.

37. Ibid., 247–48.

38. Ibid., 249–50.

39. As quoted in ibid., 249.

40. George J. Engelmann, "Battey's Operation: A Brief Summary of Results Achieved in the Forty-Seven Cases So Far Reported," *The Saint Louis Medical and Surgical Journal* 35 (1878): 101–2.

41. Durrenda Ojanuga, "The Medical Ethics of the 'Father of Gynaecology,' Dr. J. Marion Sims," *Journal of Medical Ethics* 19 (1993): 28–31; L. Lewis Wall, "The Medical Ethics of Dr. J. Marion Sims: A Fresh Look at the Historical Record," *Journal of Medical Ethics* 32 (2006): 346.

42. "Obituary: J. Marion Sims, M.D.," *British Medical Journal* 2 (1883): 1001.

43. Sims even highlighted this contradiction in Battey's practice. James Marion Sims, "Remarks on Battey's Operation," *British Medical Journal* 2 (1877): 916.

44. Ibid.

45. Ibid., 918.

46. Edmund Randolph Peaslee, *Ovarian Tumors: Their Pathology, Diagnosis and Treatment* (New York: D. Appleton, 1872), 225.

47. Lawson Tait, "Removal of the Uterine Appendages," *British Medical Journal* 2 (1882): 153. For more on Tait's operation, see Morantz-Sanchez, *Conduct Unbecoming a Woman*, 100.

48. Peaslee, *Ovarian Tumors*, 249–50.

49. Alexander Russell Simpson, "A History of Double Oophorectomy, or Battey's Operation: With Remarks," *British Medical Journal* 1 (1879): 763.

50. Lawson Tait, "An Account of Two Hundred and Eight Consecutive Cases of Abdominal Section Performed between Nov. 1st, 1881 and December 31st, 1882," *British Medical Journal* 1 (1883): 300–303, see 300; Lawson Tait, "General Summary of Conclusions from Second Series of One Thousand Consecutive Cases of Abdominal Section," *British Medical Journal* 2 (1888): 1096–97.

51. Moscucci, *Science of Woman*, 148–49.

52. Thomas Spencer Wells, *Modern Abdominal Surgery: The Bradshaw Lecture Delivered at the Royal College of Surgeons of England; With an Appendix on the Castration of Women* (London: J. A. Churchill, 1891), 35.

53. Ibid., 42.

54. Ibid., 43.

55. Ibid., 36.

56. Stuart Jones, "Review of *The Invention of Altruism*, by Thomas Dixon," *Reviews in History*, April 2009, http://www.history.ac.uk/reviews/review/757.

57. The Royal College of Physicians of London, *Nomenclature of Diseases* (London: Printed for H.M.S.O. by Harrison and Sons, 1885), 273.

58. Tait, "Account of Two Hundred and Eight Consecutive Cases," 301.

59. Charles Jennings, "Nomenclature for Operations upon the Ovaries," *British Medical Journal* 2 (1886): 49.

60. "F.R.C.S.," "Nomenclature for Operations upon the Ovary," *British Medical Journal* 2 (1886): 187.

61. Ibid., 187.

62. "H.E.M.," "Medical Nomenclature," *Canadian Medical Association Journal* 43 (1940): 597.

63. One such recent example is B. Chakrabarti and N. Mondal, "Adolescent Ovarian Malignancy," *International Journal of Gynecology and Obstetrics* 107, supplement 2 (2009): S138.

64. In regard to medical innovation, John Pickstone wrote: "We no longer have the high Victorian confidence that change is for the best." John V. Pickstone, "Introduction," in *Medical Innovations in Historical Perspective*, ed. John V. Pickstone (Basingstoke, England: Macmillan, 1992), 1.

65. Peter Angelos, "The Art of Medicine: The Ethical Challenges of Surgical Innovation for Patient Care," *Lancet* 376 (2010): 1046. See also Schlich, *Surgery, Science and Industry*, 133.

66. A key example would be Thomas Laqueur's *Making Sex*. In it, Laqueur argues that ovariotomy was "the clearest case in which cultural assumptions fuelled a research tradition whose results in turn confirmed those views." Like many other historians, it is the sporadic use of ovarian surgery to treat mental conditions in the latter part of the century that seems to guide his analysis of ovariotomy as a whole. Thomas Laqueur, *Making Sex: Body and Gender from the Greeks to Freud* (Cambridge, MA: Harvard University Press, 1990), 175.

Chapter Four

"Making Bad Boys Good"

Brain Surgery and the Juvenile Court in Progressive Era America

Delia Gavrus

At the turn of the twentieth century, an operation purporting to relieve "pressure on the brain" flourished at the unlikely intersection between a newly interventionist branch of surgery and a Progressive Era jurisprudence that was undergoing its own radical transformation. From the 1890s to the 1920s, hundreds of men, women, and children all over the United States were subjected to brain surgery as a means of "curing" "criminal tendencies" that were ascribed to injury-induced temporary changes in the brain.[1] The surgeons were appropriating a new surgical procedure called "decompression," itself based on older craniotomy techniques, which had recently been developed to alleviate acute intracranial pressure from brain tumors or life-threatening trauma, but was rapidly being applied to an array of other conditions. In a radically different context, the same procedure was reinvented as a "cure" for the misbehavior of children who appeared before juvenile court.[2] To relieve the alleged pressure and remake the social identity of the "delinquent" child, the surgeons permanently removed buttons of bone, or cut long furrows into their patients' skulls, or resected parts of the membranes that cover the brain. Thus they claimed they could instantly alter, with their scalpels and trephines, the complicated socially contingent human behaviors that society deemed problematic. Both the surgical practice itself and the rhetoric that sustained it draw attention to an unexplored continuity in the history of psychosurgery and demonstrate that lobotomy developed in the 1930s in a context in which the American public had already been exposed for decades to the idea of altering human behavior, thought, and emotion by surgical intervention.

For the surgeons of the Progressive Era, asserting expertise and claiming social relevance in questions of "delinquency" became a means of acquiring cultural and economic capital at a moment when science was conceived as a privileged tool for social and judicial renewal. These were often civically minded surgeons who were interested in Progressive reform, were part of the local elite, and had the eager attention of the Progressive judges they advised. Although Juvenile judges made their recommendation under the guise of parental consent, in making surgery a part of jurisprudence they created a coercive legal environment that mandated the medicalization of children's behavior and its aggressive and dangerous "treatment." This was happening in a larger context in which eugenic ideology unleashed a moral panic about the supposed heritability of crime and the ubiquity of "mental defects," a panic that led to other egregious surgical practices and social policies (involuntary sterilization, immigration restriction). At first glance, the supposedly curative surgeries on the skull and brain appeared to offer a challenge to the eugenicists and their theories of inheritance and "degeneracy." But by once again reducing socially unsanctioned behavior to the brain and by rooting a concept of "criminal tendency" in a physical state, the proponents essentialized and reified "delinquency," implicitly articulating a vision of "criminality" as a personal condition of the individual and not a structural one of the polity. While some of the surgeons claimed not to generalize, alleging that the surgical procedure was appropriate only in *some* cases, they also called for state intervention to screen and implement this procedure on a larger scale. And at the same time, many commentators in the newspapers, and potentially their readers, embraced a much more sweeping notion of the transformative promise of "moral surgery."

This essay aims to shed light on the technical and conceptual roots of this surgical procedure and show how it was closely tied to the rise of a new branch of surgery—the surgery of the brain and nervous system—whose early radical and interventionist ethos has not been adequately captured by historians. Buoyed by the hope that a decrease in mortality rates might be accomplished by observing strict asepsis, late-nineteenth-century surgeons attempted to trephine for a number of conditions that to them appeared to involve the brain under pressure or irritation (from a blood clot, a bone splinter, a prematurely "ossified" skull, etc.)—such as "traumatic insanity," "microcephaly," "feeblemindedness," or "epilepsy." None of these categories, whether the terms themselves have changed or stayed the same, map unproblematically onto current concepts and understandings. As historians have shown time and again, notwithstanding the possibility of a "biological event"[3] or underlying distress, all medical diagnoses reflect a powerful engagement with the unique environment in which they are made, with the social values of the day, with prevailing scientific theories that in turn depend on culturally laden institutional practices and technologies for measuring and quantifying, and with broader attitudes toward factors such as disability, race, gender, class, and the social value of the individual.[4]

Another aim of the essay is to illuminate this process of labeling human behavior and creating classifications, a process the philosopher Ian Hacking has called "making up people."[5] Among the children who engaged in behaviors the Progressive state found threatening to its order ("truancy," refusing to go to school, theft, "viciousness") or whose parents found difficult to manage, Progressive judges and surgeons thought they could identify some who had "criminal tendencies" due to a "pressure on the brain" that was curable by means of surgery. This was a new kind of child "delinquent" "made up" by means of a host of new moral, scientific, and legal concepts.

Juvenile Courts and the Medicalization of Children's Behavior

In 1903, through the work of the police magistrate George Stubbs and several women's clubs, Indianapolis became the second American city, after Chicago, to establish a juvenile court for children under the age of seventeen.[6] As historians have shown, the preoccupation with the welfare and well-being of children, which had deep roots in the nineteenth century, acquired a new urgency at the turn of the twentieth. Progressive reformers argued that desirable social change could be attained by government intervention with the help of science, and "juvenile justice" was one of their most ambitious projects.[7] Juvenile judges had a great deal of discretion in deciding each case brought before them either by the police or by parents, and relying on various officials and experts, the court investigated each child's circumstances and environment.[8] The sentences were tailored to each child, and, in principle, the primary focus was on rehabilitation without institutionalization. In some cases, and especially for first offences, the children were scolded and dismissed, sometimes under the supervision of probation officers.[9] But juvenile court judges could do much more. In Indiana, as elsewhere, state law empowered them to institutionalize children deemed "incorrigible" or who had committed offenses considered serious.[10] By 1905, Judge Stubbs had sent at least eighty-three boys to one such institution.[11]

"Juvenile justice" was part of larger legal changes that proponents called the "socialization of law" and that gave the state unprecedented and increasing ability to police and intervene in what they deemed to be social problems. Eugenic discourses and practices were part of this jurisprudence, reflecting and fanning the widespread moral panic over the supposed heritability of

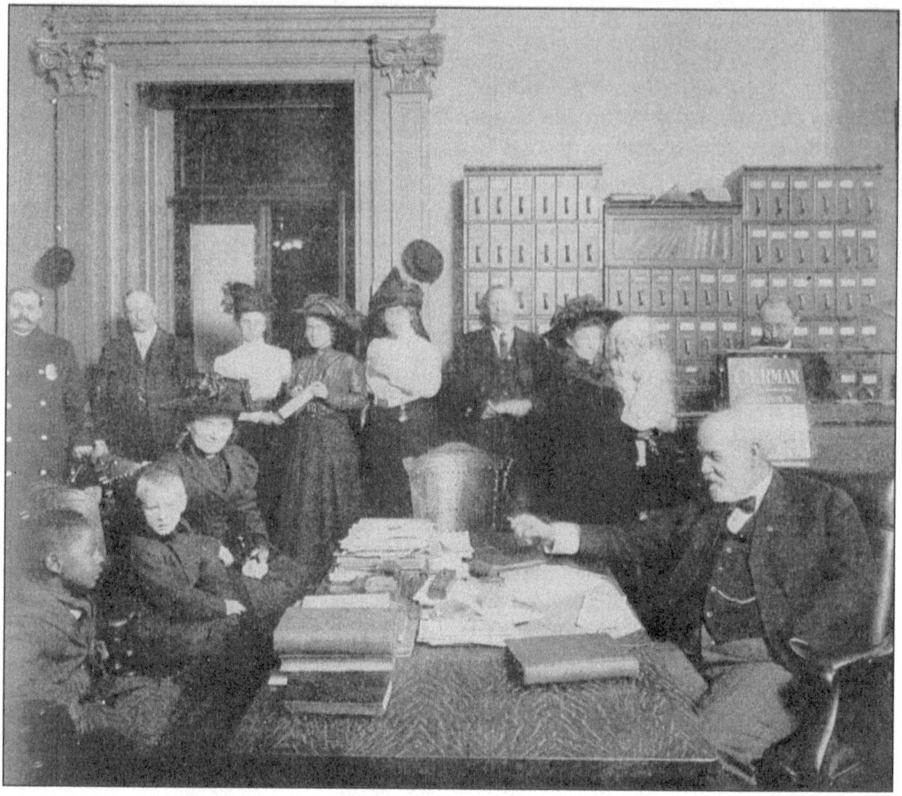

Figure 4.1. Judge Stubbs at the Indianapolis Juvenile Court in 1910. Childe Rheta Dorr, "The Child's Day in Court, *Hampton's Magazine*, November 1, 1910, 635.

crime and the imagined menace of the "defective delinquent," which led most egregiously to the enactment of compulsory sterilization laws in thirty American states, starting with Indiana in 1907.[12] Even before forced sterilization became a reality in Indiana, there existed a judicial culture that enabled coercive medical procedures, though under the guise of parental consent, as an alternative to institutionalization.[13] Medical inspection was an integral part of Judge Stubbs's court, and physicians could recommend invasive interventions such as the surgical removal of tonsils and adenoids, which, if "diseased," were thought to have "a very detrimental effect on [the] nervous system" and lead to "vice."[14] Even more invasive and dangerous, a surgical procedure on the skull, which was supposed to affect the brain and therefore the mind, was recommended and performed by a doctor who advised Judge Stubbs.

A graduate of the prestigious Jefferson Medical College, John Kolmer had probably been exposed to such surgical procedures in Philadelphia. In

1904, he operated on a fifteen-year-old boy who was deemed to have a "violent temper and criminal propensities."[15] The boy's mother, who brought him before the court, complained that he had run away from home, refused to go to school, and, when scolded, had threatened to kill her and the boy's sister. The chief probation officer referred the boy to Kolmer, and the surgeon uncovered the fact that the boy had fallen into a trench as a toddler. The mother initially hesitated to consent to surgery, and in the meantime the boy ran away again.[16] He was eventually taken to the hospital where Kolmer trephined his skull over the old injury and claimed to discover a "chronic inflammation of the brain covering" and "pressure on the brain." One newspaper reported that, with the supposed removal of the pressure, the boy "become kind and obedient and anxious to make up for the opportunities he had previously thrown away." "Science," the writer enthused in near-religious language, "opens up a way of salvation."[17]

By the following year, Kolmer had performed such operations on at least three additional children sent to him by juvenile court, receiving positive and widespread coverage in the local and national media.[18] By the time of his death in 1917, he was best remembered for being "the first surgeon of Indianapolis to introduce trephining surgery as a means of relieving bone pressure in cases of children where criminal tendencies were marked."[19] He may have been the first in Indianapolis, but, as I will show, he was certainly not the only one in the Midwest or the rest of the country. How could such a seemingly crude operation be associated with innovation, with modernity, with such exalted visions of personal salvation and social progress? And how did such a drastic and potentially dangerous surgical intervention come to be seen as an appropriate therapeutic technique in the first place? Part of the answer can be found in the changes—technical and conceptual—associated with the rise of a new branch of surgery.

An Interventionist Surgical Ethos and the New Brain Surgery

Prior to the last quarter of the nineteenth century, surgeons generally considered drilling or cutting into the skull a dangerous procedure to be employed only in desperate situations, if at all.[20] By the early 1880s, however, there had been such a radical shift in some circles that the Philadelphia surgeon John Bingham Roberts could declare that a surgeon's objection or refusal to open the skull in cases of trauma constituted "delusions of a most disastrous tendency."[21] After Listerian methods were seen to improve surgical outcomes, a number of American and European surgeons began to consistently open the skull when they thought symptoms indicated the presence of tumors, abscesses, or blood clots.[22] Localization of function, a subject much investigated and debated in the second half of the nineteenth century, in some cases provided these surgeons with an indication of where they might trephine.[23] Very soon, the new interest in opening the skull turned into a veritable enthusiasm for intervention that went beyond cases of blood clots and abscesses. Pleas for more "heroic surgical interference" were made, especially in the United States, in conditions such as "epileptic attacks, if . . . pointing to a localized lesion," "atrocious and incurable headaches," and "aphasia"—if these symptoms developed even "months or years" after a head injury.[24] The prominent Philadelphia physician D. Hayes Agnew declared that "all fractures of the skull attended with depression, however slight, and entirely irrespective of symptoms, should in the view of the late after effects be subjected to the trephine."[25] Roberts recommended intervention in cases of trauma that led to simple and complex fractures, as well as mere scalp wounds, because he argued that all these situations could potentially lead to "inflammation of the brain" caused by intracranial bleeding or by a splinter of bone driven into the brain.[26] He concluded that "the risk to subsequent mental health or to life," which manifested in "epilepsy or insanity . . . [or] mental impairment," was too great to not consider explorative trephining.[27]

At the turn of the century, doctors were employing a diagnostic category called "traumatic insanity," which they described as a condition caused by head injury that led to "striking changes in character," and which some doctors argued could lead certain sufferers to commit "crimes of violence."[28] For "traumatic insanity" too, an interventionist stance prevailed in some quarters. Prominent doctors, including the Philadelphia surgeon J. Chalmers Da Costa, advised operations.[29] The influential psychiatrist Adolf Meyer concluded on the basis of a literature review and his own clinical cases that "a chance should always be taken where there is sufficient evidence directing to a place of trephining; and in case of doubt, multiple trephining should be rather recommended than condemned."[30]

One of the most celebrated early surgeons who turned his attention to brain surgery, the Scottish surgeon William Macewen, suggested an explicit link between "pressure" exerted by a detached portion of the internal table of the skull, "homicidal tendencies," and potential therapy in a 1888 report in which he described a patient who, after an injury, began to suffer from a "deep melancholy" and "strong homicidal impulses" that manifested in an "almost irresistible impulse to kill his wife and children or other people."[31] Guided by the patient's neurological symptoms (rather than by what he saw as an irrelevant slight depression in the frontal region),[32] the surgeon opened the skull over the angular gyrus (in the parietal lobe) and found that "a portion of the internal table of the skull had exercised pressure on the posterior portion of the supramarginal convolution, while a corner of it had penetrated and lay imbedded in the anterior portion of the angular gyrus." Macewen removed the bone and reported that the patient improved, making no "further allusion to his homicidal tendencies."[33]

It was widely accepted within the medical community that significant injury to the brain could lead to changes in behavior,[34] but some doctors speculated that less severe trauma, even normal development under certain conditions, could produce dramatic effects. Writing just before the middle of the nineteenth century, one English physician claimed that a blow to the head could lead to inflammation that could in turn cause various character changes. He claimed that young people often engaged in meaningless crimes because during adolescence the growth of the brain outpaced that of the skull, which produced a kind of "cerebral congestion."[35] Increasingly in the nineteenth century causative explanations of behaviors, thoughts, or emotions deemed "pathological" in one way or another were rooted in conjectured lesions of the nervous system.[36] Though some doctors resisted generalizing such organicist interpretations, for others this physicalist view was given further impetus when a particular illness called "general paralysis of the insane," which was characterized by a cluster of psychological and neurological symptoms, was recognized to be caused by syphilis.[37]

Physicalist theories sanctioned somatic therapies. A few surgeons and alienists in Britain tested the utility of decompressive skull surgery in the case of general paralysis, on the assumption that it relieved a mechanical pressure that compressed the brain.[38] At first, the doctors claimed the operation to be curative, and promptly set off an acrimonious debate in the pages of the *British Medical Journal*. Unlike in Britain, however, the American medical profession appeared more open to this procedure: the editors of the *Journal of the American Medical Association* defended it by arguing that "the reckless use of powerful remedies experimentally and theoretically is common in nearly all cases, and the surgeon is equally justified in attempting means that give promise of relief."[39]

The interventionist ethos and the heady enthusiasm for the new brain surgery was articulated by surgeons like Emory Lanphear, who praised "the radical changes which have occurred in this department of operative surgery within the past few years" and noted unapologetically that "there are some who will contend that we are too aggressive—that we invade the cranium with too much impunity."[40] Like others, Lanphear aggressively opened the cranium for diagnoses of "epilepsy," "insanity," "cephalalgia" (i.e., headache "which proves refractory to other measures"), and "microcephalus."[41] For the latter especially, surgical intervention was tragically widespread.[42] On the theory that "premature ossification of the [skull's] sutures" impeded the brain's growth and affected "intelligence,"[43] prominent surgeons in Europe and North America made long linear incisions or removed circular parts of the patient's skull. One Philadelphia surgeon claimed that, after surgery, a patient with "a peculiar conformation of [the] skull" who suffered from seizures that "clouded" his "intellect" underwent "the greatest change that I

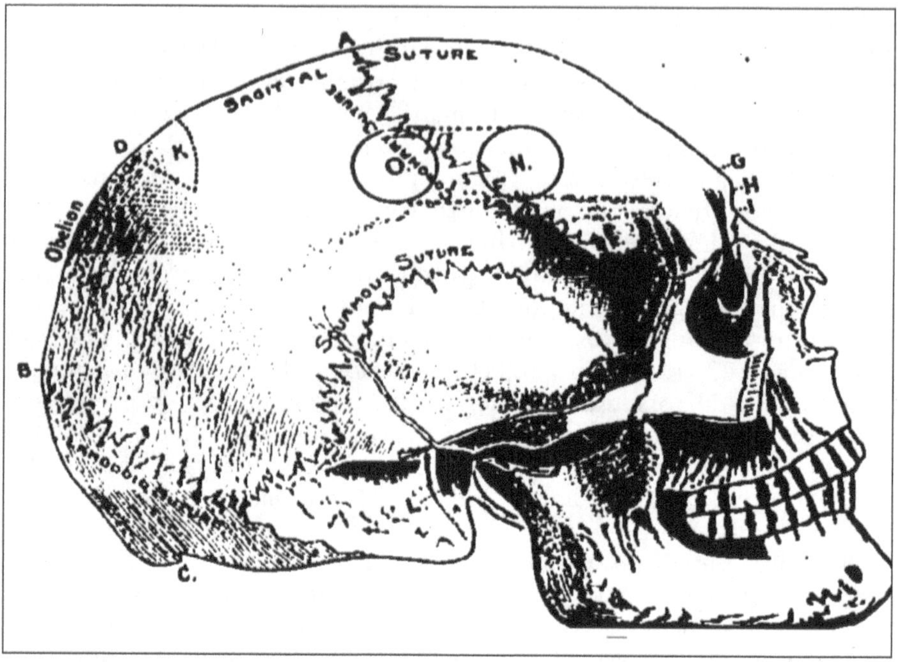

Figure 4.2. The points *O* and *N* denote the areas in which the bone was resected. Hugo Engel, "Mental Improvement following Operation of the Skull," *Medical News* 60, no. 17 (1892): 451.

have ever known to occur in the mental state of any individual, and not only the most marked but also the most sudden."[44]

Such claims were met with fierce resistance from a few doctors who considered the operation unethical and scientifically unjustified. In 1894 the New York physician Abraham Jacobi delivered a scathing attack on this procedure at an international congress, likening the surgeons' enthusiasm for intervention with a warlike frenzy: "When the brain of operative surgeons were taken with the *furor operandi* on the brains of luckless children, the war-cry was: microcephalus and idiocy."[45] Jacobi deconstructed what he considered to be an enormous complexity in those two diagnostic categories, complexity that could not justify the blanket application of "linear craniotomies" or "circular craniotomies." He denounced the horrific mortality rate of the procedure—42 percent in one sample of 33 cases. He decried the "undue tendency to, and rashness in, handling the knife," and he warned the surgeons in the audience that "such rash feats of indiscriminate surgery . . . are stains on your hands and sins on your souls. No ocean of soap and water will clean those hands, no power of corrosive sublimate will disinfect the souls."[46]

Twelve of the cases Jacobi cited in his talk belonged to the very prominent Philadelphia surgeon William W. Keen. Keen recognized the procedure's extremely high mortality, but as late as 1894 he continued to believe that "the gain is moderate, but possibly worth the risk."[47] He had been one of the first American surgeons to remove a brain tumor and was committed to the innovative techniques that allowed intervention into the brain. But perhaps he was having second thoughts about performing craniotomy for microcephaly when, two years later, he discretely checked up on a Philadelphia colleague, Ernest Laplace, who appeared oblivious to the unsparing and well-reasoned objections raised by Jacobi. Laplace was performing these surgeries on patients of the Pennsylvania Training School for Feeble Minded Children, and Keen wrote a letter of inquiry to Martin Barr, the chief physician of the institution, asking for details about Laplace's patients. Barr responded scathingly that "as the [two] children did not die under the operation I presume it was called a success." He thought Laplace's operations were "not rational" and he decried the misleading of "the unsuspecting parents." In his estimation "there was not the slightest improvement in any way in either case. In fact, the second state is worse than the first as they are much more nervous." Barr found it particularly vexing that Laplace did not follow up after the surgery: "I do not know Dr. Laplace, and he never has even taken the trouble to make any inquiries from me in regard to those children mutilated by him."[48]

Despite the condemnations from physicians like Barr and Jacobi, despite objections that "operative interference in [skull fracture] cases has been carried to extremes,"[49] and despite the occasional plea for "conservative surgery" to temper the radical interventionist ethos that, in the words of one critic, was not "justified by the literature or experience of those most competent to judge," and amounted to "pyrotechnics near a powder magazine,"[50] skull and brain surgeries continued to be performed. In a striking connection, a number of surgeons like Laplace who were, in Barr's words, mutilating children who had been diagnosed with "microcephaly" and "feeblemindedness,"[51] some of whom died as a result of the operation, began to use the same surgical technique on children who appeared before juvenile courts.

Surgery and Juvenile Courts

In 1906, an eleven-year-old was sent before a judge for holding up his teacher and classmates with a 38-caliber revolver "in true Wild West fashion,"[52] and the judge placed him in the care of Mrs. Griffith of the Easton Charity Society, who consulted Laplace. The surgeon found a lump on the boy's head from a fall sustained the previous year, and he concluded that the

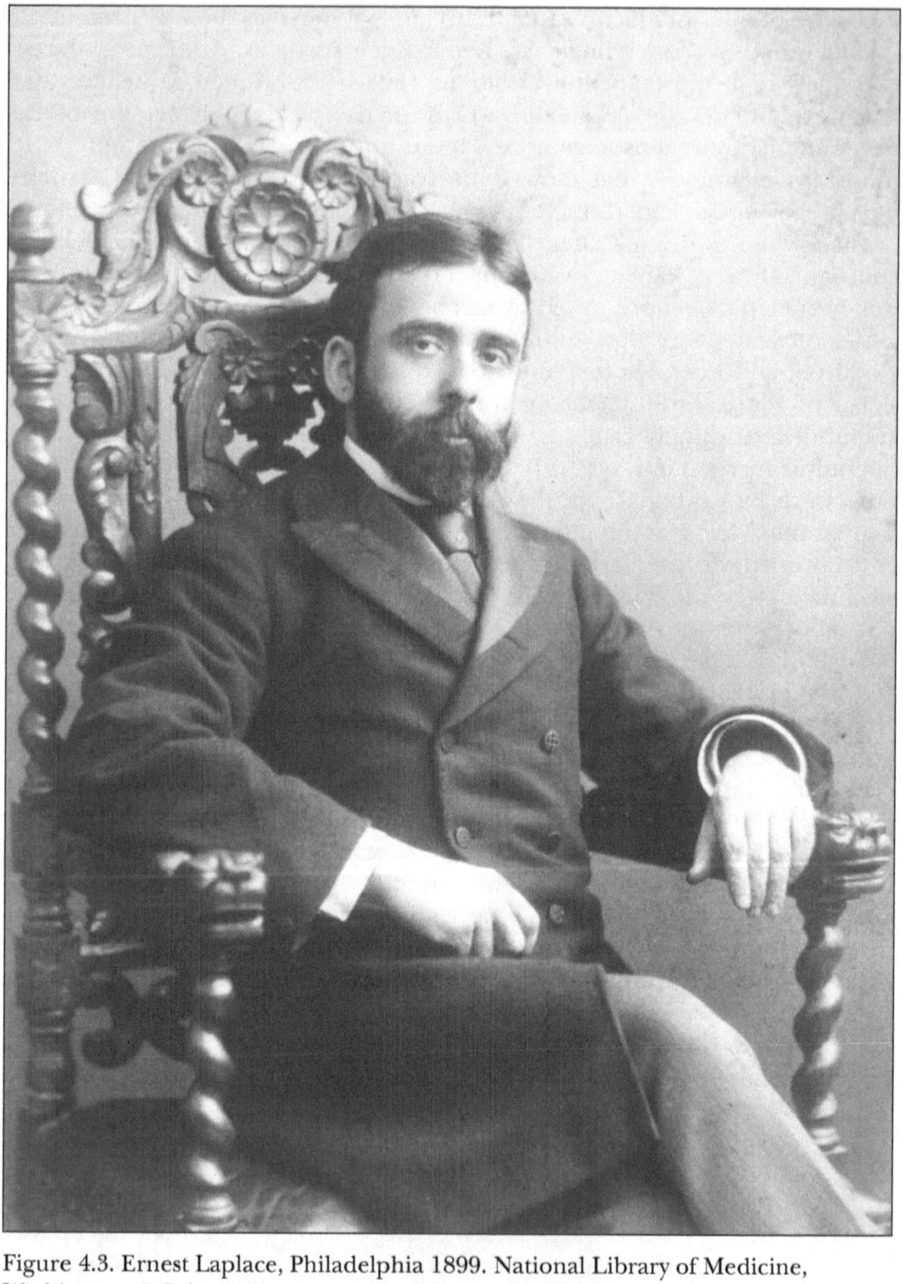

Figure 4.3. Ernest Laplace, Philadelphia 1899. National Library of Medicine, Washington, DC, http://resource.nlm.nih.gov/101421223.

damaged bone was pressing on the boy's brain and that surgery was needed to relieve the pressure that was supposedly affecting his behavior. Taking him to the hospital proved an ordeal; an ambulance had to be called for Mrs. Griffith, who fainted from the strain. The newspapers reported that, at the hospital, the boy chopped off the hair of other children on the ward, taught them to swear, almost asphyxiated nine of them by turning on the gas, and "grabbed a typhoid fever patient, threw him upon his back and raced wildly about the room."[53] The medical staff shackled him to his bed. Like other boys in his situation, he resisted being subjected to surgery; he was taken to the operating table by force.[54] Laplace performed the operation in front of a theater full of medical students at the Medico-Chirurgical College in Philadelphia, where he was professor of surgery and where he taught techniques for brain and skull surgery.[55] He removed a circular piece of the boy's skull, and later exhibited him at many clinics as a proof of what surgery could accomplish.[56] He declared him "positively cured," guaranteeing that since the boy had been good for seven weeks there was "not the slightest possibility of his badness returning."[57]

Ernest Laplace was well known in Philadelphia. He had attended the medical school at the University of Paris,[58] had studied with Louis Pasteur, and had returned from Europe with a keen appreciation for the importance of asepsis, a skill for performing "practically bloodless" operations,[59] and a preference for radical interventions.[60] In an 1897 address to the American Medical Association, Laplace described how "only a few years ago the surgeon scarcely dared to invade the sacred domain of the brain [but became] [e]mboldened by the triumph of aseptic methods in dealing with the surgery of the peritoneal cavity."[61] The brain, he claimed, could be irritated by four vectors—chemical, physical, biological, or mechanical. Subscribing to the principle of counterirritation, Laplace argued that "the mere traumatism incident to incising the scalp, trephining and irritating the dura over the region of impaired function, may at times suffice to alter by counterirritation the original pathologic process and be followed by an improvement in the case."[62] In the discussion that followed this paper, Laplace's colleagues were supportive and complimentary, with the exception of the surgeon J. William White, a member of the University of Pennsylvania medical school, who expressed incredulity vis-à-vis Laplace's extremely low mortality rate (2 percent) and advised a much more conservative stance toward brain surgery. Unperturbed by the criticism, Laplace appealed to the ethos of radical and progressive surgery and retorted that while one had to be careful, "we should not be backward."[63]

When Laplace performed skull surgery on the eleven-year-old in the care of the Easton Charity Society, he had been aware that similar procedures were being tried on children in other cities in the United States, and he specifically cited the case of a twelve-year-old from Toledo, Ohio.[64] The boy had been taken to juvenile court by his mother, who told the judge that the boy would run away from home and often sleep in downtown alleyways. He was just about to be sent to Lancaster Reform School when his probation officer noticed a scar on the boy's forehead. The boy had fractured his skull when he was five years old. A local surgeon, James Donnelly,[65] diagnosed "pressure on the brain," and the boy was sent to the operating room instead. His mother saw a transformation, and celebrated "the restoring of his affection" as the "most wonderful change" of all.[66] Only a few weeks later, the same probation officer recommended surgery for another boy—a ten-year-old.[67] The doctors claimed that they uncovered "a diseased condition of the membranes of the head, which was affecting the brain," and they removed a portion of the meninges, claiming a "complete cure." The probation officer vowed that in the future "all cases in which the mind seems to be demoralized in children will be submitted to the surgeons for careful examination into physical conditions before a sentence to reformatories is made."[68] Soon thereafter, another boy, a thirteen-year-old from Maumee, Ohio, was subjected to surgery.[69]

The same arguments were playing out in California.[70] As a juvenile court judge, Curtis D. Wilbur, whose career later included the position of Chief Justice on the California Supreme Court as well as an appointment as Secretary of the Navy, sent numerous children and adults to the operating room for various procedures such as the removal of adenoids, but also for trephining operations.[71] At the Congress of Mothers held in Los Angeles in 1907, where Wilbur told the audience that "in most cases there is some physical defect, largely in the throat, which causes truancy, delinquency, and so forth," and that "when the defect is relieved the child soon returns into bright normal boyhood again," his optimism was found by his audience to be inspiring and reassuring. "If he is correct in his conclusions," noted one commentator, "—and he may properly be termed an expert in these matters—science and common sense treatment may very often avail to transform a bad boy into a good one."[72]

Wilbur praised the physical examinations for California's child "delinquents," and he estimated that about 30 percent of them had been subjected to some kind of surgical intervention. Demonstrating the enormous trust he placed in the judgment of doctors, as well as an astonishingly cavalier attitude toward the children's bodily integrity and the law itself, Wilbur recounted:

> I was talking with the Governor of this State on the subject, and he asked me what authority we had to operate on these children. I hadn't thought of that before. Why worry over the law when a little common sense exercised in the right place will solve the problem. I do not want to detract from the law, but where a judge and a doctor advise that an operation will help the boy to be

> better, ninety-nine out of one hundred parents will want to have it done, and the only question is the question of expense. We must solve the problem in this common sense way.[73]

This judicial culture that did not "worry" about its authority to subject children to surgical procedures—a coercive process despite the veneer of parental consent—belonged to the very state that was on the brink of legalizing involuntary surgical procedures. Indeed, California would soon enact a forced sterilization law for persons the state deemed "unfit"—a law that was framed in distinctly public-health terms.[74] The surgeries on children were also framed in public-health terms.

"Crime Is a Disease"

As the historian David J. Rothman has noted "for all Progressives the most popular metaphors in criminal justice were medical."[75] The Progressives' philosophy of "respond[ing] to the criminal and not the crime,"[76] a confidence and pride in what they saw as their good intentions for both offender and society, as well as the medical metaphors of rehabilitation and cure, provided justification for the flexibility the reformers demanded in the judicial process. This flexibility—in sentencing, for instance—resulted in an expanding social control and in the state's ability to impose a particular vision of what constituted delinquency, criminality, and normative behavior. It was often the case that the medical language was not metaphoric at all: crime was, literally, imagined to be caused by disease. Behaviors deemed socially objectionable were criminalized *and* medicalized.[77] Armed with modern techniques (statistics and various standardized tests such as the newly invented Binet-Simon intelligence scale) psychologists, psychiatrists, and mental hygienists tested imprisoned populations and decreed that "mental disease," "mental defectiveness," "psychopathy," and "criminality" were related social problems that were increasing in prevalence. Clinics and laboratories such as Chicago's Juvenile Psychopathic Institute, which tested and classified children, were developed in conjunction with the juvenile court.[78]

General medicine was equally part of this trend. Temporary detention homes had mandatory medical examinations, and several even broader screening programs were instituted in some cities. In Minneapolis, a juvenile court judge reported that out of 204 "juvenile delinquents" who were "subjected to a thorough physical examination," 178 (87 percent) had "physical defects," such as phimosis, enlarged tonsils, bad teeth, adenoids, and "defective vision." He concluded that "here we have causes leading toward bad conduct as naturally as the tipping of the first of the line of dominoes."[79] Medical students were taught in their surgical training that enlarged tonsils would make the sufferer "dull mentally."[80] A probation officer in California explained that the "growth of adenoids . . . draws to the useless tissue blood that should go to the organs of sight and hearing, with the result that the boy is called dull."[81] The Pennsylvania Society to Protect Children from Cruelty (PSPC) noted that "it would be difficult to estimate the importance of this [medical examination] work,"[82] and noted in 1906 that out of 680 children who were examined ("physically" and "mentally") 585 were thought to need medical treatment, for which parents refused consent in 40 cases.[83] On the theory that "physical defects . . . are the direct cause of the criminal instincts that lead [children] into sin," the PSPC, working with the Children's Aid Society, the Board of Health, the juvenile court and other officials, attempted to screen ten thousand children living in "slums," and, with parental consent, offered various medical and surgical procedures.[84] A similar program was developed in New York.[85] Judges believed in the restorative power of medicine, or at least in its ability to determine if medical treatment was going to work: "I can see evidence of both crime and disease in habitual liars, persistent thieves, and in all those guilty of unnatural offenses. Such offenders should be kept under restraint in properly equipped hospitals until the attending surgeons and neurologists can advise the court as to whether or not operative surgery or continual medical treatment will serve any good purpose."[86] Most of these measures were directed toward the removal of adenoids, tonsils, and teeth, but brain surgeries for those who were deemed to have sustained injuries to the head received the lion's share of publicity, given the dramatic nature of the intervention.[87]

The surgeons who were performing the skull surgeries on boys sent to them by juvenile courts echoed these views. Kolmer declared: "Crime is a disease. It is not solely the choice of the individual," and "the management of criminals seems to me to be largely a question between physician and surgeon."[88] Peter Donnelly, who performed these surgeries with his brother James, urged the state to appoint a commission to investigate the possibility of making the procedure available on a large scale in penal institutions, for both fiscal and humanitarian reasons. "If by operation it can be established that incorrigibles can be cured, it will be a great blessing to humanity," Donnelly proclaimed publicly. "Brain surgery is in its infancy and experiments along the line of curing incorrigibles from pressure may lead to the discovery of a sure cure for cases from abnormality."[89] Another doctor in California (who diagnosed a twenty-two-year-old woman with "pressure on the brain" from a childhood fall), advised the Berkeley police department and was a close friend of Police Chief August Vollmer, one of the most prominent figures in early twentieth-century police reform.[90] The doctor convinced the court that "the prison cell is no place for [his patient]. She is sick; she needs medical attention to cure her passion for stealing."[91]

These surgeons can thus be accurately described as Progressive reformers. Kolmer was a Republican who was described by his contemporaries as having "a lively interest in the questions and issues of the hour and being well fortified in his convictions as to matter of public polity."[92] In 1897 he founded a hospital that offered free medical care to those who suffered from "nervous diseases" and could not afford to pay, a hospital designed for "suffering humanity without regard to religious or political creed, color or social condition."[93] Part of his motivation was to fight against what he perceived to be "the stigma of insanity which would have attached to [the patients] had they fallen into the hands of the insanity 'trust.'"[94]

For Kolmer that stigma may have been related to the widespread belief in the heritability of deeply complex and contingent human characteristics and behaviors—from intelligence to mental distress to aptitudes to "criminal behavior." Nineteenth-century theories of "degeneration" were adopted by psychiatrists and criminologists alike. Apparently contra the increasingly vocal eugenicists, Kolmer professed that "I never did believe much in hereditary criminality, which, heretofore, has been the only explanation of evil tendencies in young children."[95] Was this insistence on environment (in the form of accident or acquired disease by way of pressure, irritation, or infection) an explicit rejection of eugenicist ideas?

In the absence of rich historical and archival material, it is difficult to answer the question definitively and specifically for each individual doctor. Certainly they did not constitute a homogenous group, from this point of view and many others—for instance, some were allopaths, others were homeopaths and eclectics.[96] It is clear that an environmentalist position was not necessarily at odds with a commitment to eugenics. One surgeon who performed at least one skull procedure on an adult accused of breaking the law was the notorious and deeply committed eugenicist Harry J. Haiselden.[97] Historians have shown just how idiosyncratic were the beliefs, actions, and causes the eugenicists embraced (especially the doctors among them); many of them subscribed to Lamarkian ideas and thought that "degeneration" could be induced by the environment.[98]

This tension is displayed clearly in the stories that were told about the boys who underwent skull and brain surgery. At times Kolmer claimed to reject "hereditary criminality," but in other talks he allowed for the occasional role of "inheritance and social environment," and he emphasized the importance of a "careful tracing of the family history" in making a clinical decision about surgery.[99] His patients were repeatedly described as belonging to "an excellent family," a "family of high social standing,"[100] or to "respected residents"[101] of the city—families that were deemed to preclude hereditary degeneration by means of both inheritance and environment. Reporting on a case from London, the *New York Times* spoke of "a boy of good family who had developed brutal instincts."[102] In another case of supposed pressure on the brain, where "criminal" behavior was imagined by the doctor rather than pronounced as such by the court, the surgeon noted that the "family history showed no taint."[103] Other surgeons like Laplace appeared to subscribe to quasi-phrenological beliefs, such as the existence of a "center for selfishness" that he considered exaggerated in "criminality."[104]

But while some of these doctors appeared to echo such ideas about heredity that were common in the eugenics movement, they appear not to have voiced support for eugenicist policies (sterilization, marriage restrictions, etc.) and didn't display an interest in Mendelian genetics. Instead, they placed a relatively strong emphasis on accident resulting in disease at the expense of heredity and social environment: "I believe that more criminals are made so at birth than become so by environment," Kolmer pronounced, meaning specifically "that the skull is deformed when the child is brought into the world. . . . I have made extensive investigations at penal institutions and I find that, in a great majority of cases, the most brutal and violent criminals have skull deformations of varying degrees. Had this been corrected at birth, the result would have been altogether different."[105] This commitment to the role of the skull in exerting pressure meant that Kolmer faced situations in which the parents could not immediately remember a fall or injury, but after repeated prompting they might recall some incident, however insignificant it had appeared at the time.[106]

The parents themselves responded to the suggestion of surgery in different ways—many assented, some hesitated, several refused. More rarely, an appeal for surgery came from the parents themselves, and it was the judge who needed convincing.[107] Although the voice and agency of the parents should not be minimized—in many cases the parents were the ones reaching out to juvenile courts for help—it is nevertheless clear that given the expert recommendation of prominent local doctors and in the presence of judges who offered an alternative between institutionalization and the operating room, the parents were not making a simple choice; they were facing a calculus complicated enormously by issues of power and authority. The important role played by the local network of individuals of high social capital is evident from the fact that judges, doctors, and parole officers acted as negotiators and often convinced parents who were hesitating. One mother took her boy to the surgeon at the suggestion of the local priest.[108]

The children, meanwhile, resisted in their own ways. Some struggled in the hospital and refused to go willingly to the operating room.[109] A boy ran away, and after he was caught the judge "sentence[d] him to imprisonment instead of the scalpel."[110] During a consultation at Kolmer's office, "it required the services of three men to keep [one boy] from jumping out the window."[111] One of Donnelly's patients did manage to jump out a window. Eventually he returned, but his father, suffering from second thoughts himself, withdrew his permission at the very last possible moment, such that, as a newspaper reported, he ended up with "a very poor hair cut—and that was all."[112]

The newspapers, quick to announce that "science cures crime,"[113] also widely reported its failure to do so.[114] "Teaching morality with a surgeon's scalpel has failed," a reporter wrote, wondering: Had the boy "defied the scalpel" or had the "skull grown down into his brain cells again?" Perhaps, the writer concluded, "he is ripe for another operation."[115] When a boy from Toledo reoffended after his surgery, questions were asked about the same practices in nearby Cleveland, where Rev. Harris R. Cooley, a pastor and prominent reformer, had been instrumental in establishing a farm colony that functioned as a workhouse for boys.[116] Cooley believed that "the normal environment of the country life" was the best first step for the youths,[117] but he also looked to the curative power of medicine. To a reporter who was asking about the rationale of continuing such surgeries in light of their failure elsewhere, Cooley confidently reaffirmed his faith in the knife, "where the skull has been injured and a pressure against the brain is discovered."[118]

Such enduring faith was echoed widely in the American press, despite the numerous reports that belied it and that were printed in the same publications. Newspapers throughout the country editorialized about the transformative promise of these surgeries and imagined them applied on a broad scale. "As things are progressing," one newspaper prophesized, "the possibilities are that after a few years more, the jails and prisons of the country will be abolished, and when a man commits a crime, instead of being sent to jail, he will be sent to the hospital and put under the charge of 'character' surgeons."[119] Another took an even steeper flight of fancy into the imagined science of the future: "Does not this suggest infinite possibilities in the matter of mental improvement? . . . Suppose that a man is deficient in any particular mental quality. Call the phrenologist and the surgeon, hold a consultation, have a deft incision here, remove a trip of cranium there and the lack is no longer existent."[120] The *San Francisco Chronicle* expressed support for the procedure, noticing its ideological alignment with the Progressive ethos: "reformation, rather than punishment, should be the aim of our courts of justice."[121] In one letter to the editor published in the periodical *Health*, a female reader from Austin decried the many gynecological operations women suffered, while at the same time praising "one kind of surgery . . . that is seldom accompanied with danger or bad results, that is, "brain surgery," where pressure is removed from the brain by lifting the skull." She had "read quite a good deal about this, and have hoped that it would be a blessing to the world by being able to change the natures of criminals, or those whose brains are not well balanced."[122] Even a trade publication for lawyers applauded these developments, cautioning only that it would be too optimistic to hope that *all* criminal tendencies could be cured by brain surgery, and not just those due to head injury.[123]

The general enthusiasm for a potentially deadly operation deeply entangled with the justice system is surprising in a period in which some segments of the American public raised the issue of civil liberties in relation to forced treatment and medical experimentation.[124] Evidently Americans articulated complicated ideas and emotions toward surgery. As the historian Susan Lederer has argued about transplantation, "early twentieth-century Americans . . . were willing to try radical methods if they promised relief from suffering and the prospect of bodily improvement."[125] Dread, fear, hope, a belief in the miraculous remaking of the body by means of surgery,[126] and an equally potent anxiety about surgery's dystopian potential all coexisted more or less uneasily in the public imagination. Perhaps the reason why operations for "criminal tendencies" received such a positive reception in the public sphere was because in practice they never did become widespread enough to attract serious scrutiny from those concerned about civil liberties. And in the rare situations when parents resisted the ruling or when judges were publicly criticized for it, the court was quick to point out that the procedures were not "made compulsory"[127] and that the decision had been a matter between surgeon and parents.[128]

One group of professionals conspicuous by its silence was the small cadre of surgeons who were restricting their practice to the nervous system and who were setting the stage for the establishment of neurosurgery as a medical specialty. In comparison to their late-nineteenth-century colleagues, who had displayed, as I have shown, an interventionist and radical ethos, they took a more conservative approach.[129] As late as 1920, the premier brain surgeon Harvey Cushing declared that the most useful procedure that a brain surgeon had at his disposal was the decompression, which provided a means of alleviating the symptoms that accompanied inoperable brain tumors.[130] Meanwhile, in some of the decompressions on adults convicted of breaking the law, the doctors showed not only that they were aware of Cushing's technique, but also asserted that their own procedure "was conducted under methods followed by Dr. Horsley of St. Bartholomew's hospital, London, and of Dr. Cushing of Johns Hopkins."[131]

Although it is virtually certain that elite brain surgeons like Cushing, Ernest Sachs, and Charles Frazier would have strongly disapproved of these surgeries, it appears that they did not condemn them in the published literature or in a public forum. Some elite surgeons at the time did complain generally about the epidemic of unnecessary surgeries—such as the removal of the appendix—and when the American College of Surgeons was organized in 1913, one of its goals was to address this issue.[132] In 1908, in a chapter that, ironically, he wrote for Keen's surgery book, Cushing did echo Jacobi's strong opposition to linear craniotomy for microcephalus.[133] Nevertheless, there was no outcry from the first generation of neurosurgeons about the operations performed for "criminal tendencies,"[134] just as there had been no outcry from elite psychiatrists like Adolf Meyer about Henry Cotton's surgeries on asylum patients on the theory that focal infection caused insanity.[135] This lack of criticism may have constituted one reason why the procedure continued to be performed.

Conclusion

Scholars have shown how the notion of "criminal behavior" and the "criminal" as a type of person to be studied and classified emerged with the consolidation of the nineteenth-century nation-state and its reliance on statistics and the social and human sciences.[136] Medical testing in a legal context became an important part of the state's program of social control, and juvenile justice itself was tied to the professionalization of several medical fields: psychologists, social workers, sociologists, and psychiatrists were involved in the often-coercive activities of classifying, treating, and managing children who appeared before the court. In some instances, surgeons were part of this process as well. The idea of "criminal propensities," itself indebted to this transformation and to nineteenth-century notions of "criminal degeneracy," was also applied, as this essay shows, to a group of children who were seen not to have inherited but to have acquired a tendency toward crime through an accidental injury. On the theory that a blow to the head—whether mild enough to barely register in one's memory or severe enough to have caused at one time a fracture of the skull—led to pressure on the brain or to mechanical irritation, surgeons all over the United States advised juvenile judges on the therapeutic potential of trephining. The judges, in framing surgery as a choice, often in juxtaposition to institutionalization, were using the exceptional power of the state to pressure parents into considering the possibility of a dangerous procedure.

The concepts of "criminality" and "juvenile delinquency" were built on assumptions deeply influenced by theories of gender, race, and class.[137] Girls were more likely to be brought before the court for their sexuality and boys for theft, vagrancy, and "incorrigibility."[138] Perhaps the belief that boys were more likely to have suffered a head injury accorded with assumptions about masculinity and the ways in which boys engaged in risky physical activity, and for this reason it was overwhelmingly boys whom the judges sent to the operating room. Thus the collective tools of surgery, the law, and Progressive morality had "made up" a new kind of "delinquent" boy, one whose "bad" behavior was rooted in a brain temporarily under pressure.

Most prevalent in the first decade of the century, the procedure disappeared by the late 1920s, when the notions of "pressure on the brain" and "mechanical irritation" morphed into other scientific concepts and vocabulary, and when neurosurgery increasingly became the purview of a select and specialized community of surgeons.[139] What did not disappear, however, was the fantasy that an operation on the brain could redress intricately complex human emotions, behaviors, and illnesses, as well as social issues. A reductionist research program and a return to a radical surgical ethos enabled the proliferation of lobotomy—a surgical procedure that mutilated the brain, not just the skull, and which was applied in diagnoses of mental illness, but also in cases of "violent behavior" and "criminality."[140] The language of "cure" and "criminal tendencies" remained virtually unchanged,[141] and the rhetoric of the transformative scalpel and trephine would have been instantly recognizable to an earlier generation of Americans.

Acknowledgments

This research was supported by the University of Winnipeg and benefited from a Wood Institute travel grant from the College of Physicians of Philadelphia. For research assistance, I am grateful to Holly McElrea and Danna Slessor-Cobb. For comments on earlier drafts of this paper, I thank Michael Bliss, Thomas Schlich, Christopher Crenner, and the participants of the Asher Symposium on the History of Surgical Innovation held at University of Kansas Medical Center in September 2013, as well as James Hanley, Stephen Casper, and the volume's anonymous reviewers.

Notes

1. In the absence of statistics, this number is by necessity a (conservative) estimate based on the numerous newspaper reports and published medical case studies.

2. This paper focuses on American children, but there is a parallel story to be told about adults. At the time, newspapers also claimed that this practice occurred in other countries: "Unique Operation in Interests of Criminology," *Northern Advocate*, May 17, 1917, 2; "Prisoner Reformed by Cutting His Skull," *Boston Daily Globe*, October 17, 1920.

3. Charles E. Rosenberg, "Introduction, Framing Disease: Illness, Society, and History," in *Framing Disease: Studies in Cultural History*, ed. Charles E. Rosenberg and Janet Lynne Golden (New Brunswick, NJ: Rutgers University Press, 1992), xiii.

4. The literature is vast; for a conceptual overview, see ibid. While continuities are possible alongside discontinuities, I do not use contemporary terminology in order not to essentialize illness or social categories and to emphasize the inescapable historical contingency inherent in all such labeling. Like medical diagnoses, terms such as "criminality," "juvenile delinquency," etc., are likewise categories that were made in conjunction with and reflect the full complement of social and moral values, prejudices, scientific and legal theories, and expert knowledge in the Progressive Era.

5. Ian Hacking, "Making Up People," in *Reconstructing Individualism: Autonomy, Individuality, and the Self in Western Thought*, ed. Thomas C. Heller, David E. Wellbery, and Morton Sosna (Stanford, CA: Stanford University Press, 1986).

6. Childe Rheta Dorr, "The Child's Day in Court," *Hampton's Magazine*, November 1, 1910. The Chicago Juvenile Court was established in 1899, and within ten years, juvenile court laws had been passed in twenty-two states. See Joseph M. Hawes, *Children in Urban Society: Juvenile Delinquency in Nineteenth-Century America* (New York: Oxford University Press, 1971), 246.

7. Victoria Getis, *The Juvenile Court and the Progressives* (Urbana: University of Illinois Press, 2000). There is a large historical literature on juvenile courts: Robert M. Mennel, *Thorns & Thistles: Juvenile Delinquents in the United States, 1825–1940* (Hanover, NH: The University Press of New England, 1973); Anne Meis Knupfer, *Reform and Resistance: Gender, Delinquency, and America's First Juvenile Court* (New York: Routledge, 2001); Jennifer Trost, *Gateway to Justice: The Juvenile Court and Progressive Child Welfare in a Southern City* (Athens: University of Georgia Press, 2005); Elizabeth J. Clapp, *Mothers of All Children: Women Reformers and the Rise of Juvenile Courts in Progressive Era America* (University Park: Pennsylvania State University Press, 1998); Mary E. Odem, *Delinquent Daughters: Protecting and Policing Adolescent Female Sexuality in the United States, 1885–1920* (Chapel Hill: University of North Carolina Press, 1995).

8. Knupfer, *Reform and Resistance*, 80.

9. Odem, *Delinquent Daughters*, 76.

10. David J. Bodenhamer, Robert G. Barrows, and David Gordon Vanderstel, *The Encyclopedia of Indianapolis* (Bloomington: Indiana University Press, 1994), 858.

11. *Thirty-Ninth Annual Report of the Board of Control and Superintendent Indiana Boys' School to the Governor, Plainfield, Indiana, 1905* (Indianapolis: Wm. B. Burford, 1905), 17; https://babel.hathitrust.org/cgi/pt?id=mdp.39015074703649;view=1up;seq=3.

12. Michael Willrich, "The Two Percent Solution: Eugenic Jurisprudence and the Socialization of American Law, 1900–1930," *Law and History Review* 16, no. 1 (1998); Michael Willrich, *City of Courts: Socializing Justice in Progressive Era Chicago* (Cambridge: Cambridge University Press, 2003); Morton J. Horwitz, *The Transformation of American Law, 1870–1960: The Crisis of Legal Orthodoxy* (New York: Oxford University Press, 1992); Mark A. Largent, *Breeding Contempt: The History of Coerced Sterilization in the United States* (New Brunswick, NJ: Rutgers University Press, 2008); Nicole Hahn Rafter, *Creating Born Criminals* (Urbana: University of Illinois Press, 1997).

13. This culture of legal and medical coercion was much broader than the surgeries I discuss in this case study. Prior to 1900, before the introduction of eugenics policy that legally enforced involuntary sterilizations, castration and other coercive sexual surgeries were employed by doctors and prison officials as therapy or punishment for "sexual perversion." Largent, *Breeding Contempt*, 6.

14. "Tonsils Cause Vice," *Indianapolis Morning Star*, October 5, 1906.

15. "Moral Surgery," *Atlanta Constitution*, November 25, 1904; W.E., [no Title], *The Friend: A Religious and Literary Journal* 78, no. 13 (1904). Extensive searches of census forms and other government records were conducted and verified the claims made by the newspapers about the patients' identities, social status, and other details. Although all the names of the patients are in the public domain, after deliberation I have decided not to include them here.

16. "Surgeon's Knife Makes an Incorrigible Boy Obedient," *St. Louis Post-Dispatch*, October 9, 1904; "Bad Boy Is Made Good by a Surgical Operation," *Toledo News-Bee*, September 15, 1904.

17. "Moral Surgery"; Joe S. Miller, "Cut Out 'Bad Spots' in Boy's Brain," *Indianapolis Morning Star*, July 30, 1905.

18. "Cutting Crime Out," *Wenatchee Daily World*, August 1, 1905. He also attempted to operate on adults who had been arrested: "Flees from Operation," *Indianapolis Star*, October 15, 1910.

19. "Dr. John Kolmer, Pioneer in Trephining Surgery, Is Dead," *Indianapolis Star*, October 22, 1917.

20. For a brief history of the management of head trauma prior to 1867, see Eugene S. Flamm, "From Signs to Symptoms: The Neurosurgical Management of Head Trauma from 1517 to 1867," in *A History of Neurosurgery in Its Scientific and Professional Contexts*, ed. Samuel H. Greenblatt, T. Forcht Dagi, and Mel H. Epstein (Park Ridge, IL: American Association of Neurological Surgeons, 1997).

21. John Bingham Roberts, *Surgical Delusions and Follies: A Revision of the Address in Surgery for 1884 of the Medical Society of the State of Pennsylvania* (Philadelphia: P. Blakiston, Son & Co., 1884), 17.

22. In Europe, the prominent surgeons who opened the skull were William Macewen in Glasgow, Victor Horsley in London, Ernst von Bergmann in Berlin, and Antoine Chipault in Paris. For an overview of various aspects of the history of neurosurgery, see Greenblatt, Dagi, and Epstein, *History of Neurosurgery in Its Scientific and Professional Contexts.*

23. By "localization of function" I mean the nineteenth-century understanding that particular areas of the brain correlated with distinct functions such as speech production or vision. A reductive approach that located all mental function to discrete areas of the brain (at the expense of emphasizing the importance of connectivity within the brain) was already being challenged in the late nineteenth century: see Katja Guenther, *Localization and Its Discontents: A Genealogy of Psychoanalysis and the Neuro Disciplines* (Chicago: University of Chicago Press, 2015); Samuel H. Greenblatt, "Cerebral Localization: From Theory to Practice," in Greenblatt, Dagi, and Epstein, *History of Neurosurgery in Its Scientific and Professional Contexts*; Robert Maxwell Young, *Mind, Brain and Adaptation in the Nineteenth Century: Cerebral Localization and Its Biological Context from Gall to Ferrier* (Oxford: Carendon Press, 1970).

24. R. W. Amidon, "A Plea for More Heroic Surgical Interference in Affections of the Brain," *Medical News* 44, no. 25 (1884).

25. Society Proceedings," *Journal of the American Medical Association* (1891).

26. Roberts, *Surgical Delusions and Follies*, 20–21.

27. "The Field and Limitation of the Operative Surgery of the Human Brain," *Annals of Surgery* 2, no. 7 (1885): 12, 14.

28. Herbert A. Powell, "The Surgical Aspect of Traumatic Insanity (Presented for the Degree of Doctor of Medicine)," Oxford University, 1893, 10–11; A. B. Richardson, "The Symptomatology and Treatment of Traumatic Insanity," *American Journal of Psychiatry* 60 (1903).

29. J. Chalmers Da Costa, *Modern Surgery, General and Operative*, 7th ed. (Philadelphia: Saunders, 1914), 824–25.

30. Adolf Meyer, "The Anatomical Facts and Clinical Varieties of Traumatic Insanity," *American Journal of Insanity* 60, no. 3 (1904): 440. Meyer's education was deeply rooted in the German tradition of brain pathology, but he eventually adopted a more complex view of mental illness that emphasized environmental and psychosocial aspects. See Elliot S. Valenstein, *Great and Desperate Cures: The Rise and Decline of Psychosurgery and Other Radical Treatments for Mental Illness* (New York: Basic Books, 1986), 32–34; S. D. Lamb, *Pathologist of the Mind: Adolf Meyer and the Origins of American Psychiatry* (Baltimore: Johns Hopkins University Press, 2014).

31. William Macewen, "An Address on the Surgery of the Brain and Spinal Cord," *The British Medical Journal* 2, no. 1441 (1888): 306.

32. The neurological symptoms consisted in what Macewen called "psychical blindness"—the patient's inability to recognize objects by sight alone in the two weeks following his accident. Localizing this function to the angular gyrus, Macewen trephined in this particular region rather than in the area of the angular process of the frontal bone, where he noted a slight depression that he thought irrelevant given the lack of any neurological symptoms associated with that area. This is a very different approach from that of surgeons who embraced the surgery for "criminality," who did not seem to be bothered by the lack of neurological symptoms, and who usually trephined the area of the depressed bone.

33. Macewen, "An Address," 306.

34. See, for instance, the much-publicized case of Phineas Gage, an American railway construction worker who sustained a severe brain injury in 1948. Malcolm Macmillan, *An Odd Kind of Fame: Stories of Phineas Gage* (Cambridge, MA: MIT Press, 2000).

35. Anne Harrington, *Medicine, Mind, and the Double Brain: A Study in Nineteenth-Century Thought* (Princeton, NJ: Princeton University Press, 1987), 26.

36. There is a vast literature on this topic. Charcot, for instance, considered hysteria to be rooted in a lesion of the nervous system. For a recent overview of the increasingly physicalist tendencies of nineteenth-century psychiatry see Andrew Scull, *Madness in Civilization: A Cultural History of Insanity, from the Bible to Freud, from the Madhouse to Modern Medicine* (Princeton: Princeton University Press, 2015).

37. Ibid.

38. See, for example, J. B. Tuke, "The Surgical Treatment of Intracranial Fluid Pressure," *British Medical Journal* 1, no. 1514 (1890); German E. Berrios, "The Origins of Psychosurgery: Shaw, Burckhardt and Moniz," *History of Psychiatry* 8, no. 29, pt. 1 (1997).

39. "Surgical Treatment of General Paralysis," *Journal of the American Medical Association* 26, no. 19 (1891): 672.

40. Emory Lanphear, "What Can Be Done in Cerebral Surgery? Remarks Based Chiefly upon Personal Experience in Twenty-Three Cases," *Journal of the American Medical Association* 17, no. 25 (1891): 951–60.

41. Ibid. The prominent London-based surgeon Victor Horsley should be counted among the interventionist surgeons. See Victor Horsley, "Trephining," in Daniel Hack Tuke, *A Dictionary of Psychological Medicine* (Philadelphia: Blakiston, 1892), 1324–27.

42. Moshe Feinsod and Neil L. Davis, "Unlocking the Brain: Attempts to Improve Mental Function of Microcephalic Retarded Children by "Craniotomy," *Neurosurgery* 53, no. 3 (2003).

43. "Domestic Correspondence: Philadelphia Letter," *Journal of the American Medical Association* 18, no. 25 (1892): 788.

44. Hugo Engel, "Mental Improvement following Operation of the Skull," *Medical News* 60, no. 17 (1892): 452.

45. Abraham Jacobi, "Non Nocere," *Medical Record* 45, no. 20 (1894).

46. Ibid.

47. Ibid.

48. Letter from Martin W. Barr to W. W. Keen, September 29, 1896, Correspondence 1860–1931, box 1, ser. 1–2, MSS 2/076-01-06, William W. Keen Papers, Philadelphia College of Physicians and Surgeons.

49. N. Senn, "On Some of the Limits of the Art of Surgery," *Journal of the American Medical Association* (1896): 910.

50. S. V. Clevenger, "Conservative Brain Surgery," *Journal of the American Medical Association* 24, no. 26 (1895): 1004.

51. For example, Kolmer performed thirty-one such surgeries before 1906, with at least one death: "Submits to Surgery for Mind and Dies," *Indianapolis Morning Star,* August 26, 1906. Peter Donnelly did as well: "Surgeon Remedied the Depression in the Stupid Boy's Brain," *Cincinnati Enquirer,* September 13, 1906. And at least one of Laplace's patients died: "Domestic Correspondence."

52. "Operations to Prevent Crime? Urged by Surgeon Who Made Good Boy Out of a Bad One," *St. Louis-Dispatch,* April 19, 1906.

53. Ibid.

54. "Knife Lets Virtue Loose," *Chicago Daily Tribune,* September 30, 1906.

55. See the medical school notes of Milton Fraser Percival, *Notes on Medical Subjects: From His Student Days at Medico-Chirurgical College, Philadelphia, 1891–1905,* vol. 1., College of Physicians of Philadelphia.

56. "Surgery 'Cures' Bad Boy but [C. W.] Lapses into His Vicious Habits," *Detroit Free Press,* October 18, 1908.

57. "Operations to Prevent Crime?" Two years later, the boy appeared again before the court and was sent to prison. "Surgery 'Cures' Bad Boy."

58. His MD was from the University of Louisiana. MS C 142 Association of Military Surgeons of the United States Records, c. 1901–41, box 4, National Library of Medicine, Bethesda, MD. His military record, which he filled out in 1909, elaborates several "contributions to medical and surgical literature": "the treatment of external aneurysms by direct compression," an antiseptic solution, an operation for hemorrhoids, and one for gastroptosis. These exhausted the space he had on the form; he did not mention the brain surgeries.

59. "Rare Skill at Clinic," *Washington Post,* October 31, 1913.

60. He trephined even if "there was no history of traumatism, but simply a functional disturbance very much on the general lines of so-called *idiopathic* disease." Ernest Laplace, "The Surgical Treatment of Insanity," *Medical and Surgical Reporter* 74, no. 26 (1896): 806, emphasis in the original.

61. Ernest Laplace, "Improvement of Brain Function by Surgical Interference," *Medical and Surgical Reporter* 74, no. 26 (1897): 801.

62. Ernest Laplace, "Improvement of Brain Function by Surgical Interference," *Journal of the American Medical Association* 29, no. 14 (1897): 682.

63. Ibid.

64. "Operations to Prevent Crime?," 17. In Philadelphia, the juvenile court judge James E. Gorman cited two cases of "pressure on the brain": "Brain Surgery Lessens Crime," *Springfield Republican*, October 7, 1906. Judge Norris S. Barratt sent another boy to Desiderio Roman, a homeopath, for surgery. On Roman's education, see Seward M. Transue, ed., *The Medic: The 1934 Yearbook of the Hahnemann Medical College* (Philadelphia: Hahnemann Medical College, 1934).

65. "News of the Week," *Medical Record* 78, no. 14 (1910): 588.

66. "Surgeon Gives Boy a New Soul," *St. Louis Post-Dispatch*, April 13, 1906.

67. "Science Cures Crime," *Los Angeles Times*, May 25, 1906.

68. "Relation of Physical Well Being to Moral Degeneracy Is Being Determined by Interesting Operation on a Boy at Toledo," *Cincinnati Enquirer*, May 25, 1906. "To the Knife," *Detroit Free Press*, June 3, 1906.

69. "Reforming Bad Boys with Surgeon's Knife," *San Antonio Gazette*, September 15, 1906.

70. "Surgery for Moral Depravity," *Baltimore Sun*, March 29, 1903; "Knife Used to Remove Thieving Tendencies," *San Francisco Call*, September 17, 1900.

71. See, for instance, "[Q.] May Be Made New Man," *Los Angeles Herald*, February 15, 1909; "Physical Ailment Forces Youth to Annex Property," *Los Angeles Herald*, August 10, 1908; "Blind Man Pleads Guilty, Is Put on Probation," *Los Angeles Herald*, September 29, 1907. For some of these cases the surgical procedure is not specified.

72. "Making Bad Boys Good," *The San Diego Union and Daily Bee*, May 13, 1907.

73. Curtis D. Wilbur, "The Delinquent Child; [Read] before the Fifth California State Conference of Charities and Corrections, 1908," in *Report and Manual for Probation Officers of the Superior Court Acting as Juvenile Court, Los Angeles County, California* (Los Angeles: Commercial Printing House, 1912), 53–54.

74. Alexandra Minna Stern, "Sterilized in the Name of Public Health: Race, Immigration, and Reproductive Control in Modern California," *American Journal of Public Health* 95, no. 7 (2005).

75. David J. Rothman, *Conscience and Convenience: The Asylum and Its Alternatives in Progressive America*, rev. ed. (New York: Aldine de Gruyter, 2002), 56.

76. Ibid., 59.

77. See the example of vagrancy, which was deemed to be a particularly pressing social problem in France in the late nineteenth century, and whose visibility mediated the emergence of the diagnostic category of "fugue" or "ambulatory automatism." Ian Hacking, *Mad Travelers: Reflections on the Reality of Transient Mental Illnesses* (Charlottesville: University Press of Virginia, 1998).

78. Daniel J. Kevles, *In the Name of Eugenics: Genetics and the Uses of Human Heredity* (New York: Knopf, 1985), 72. Victoria Getis, *The Juvenile Court and the Progressives* (Urbana: University of Illinois Press, 2000), esp. chaps. 4 and 5. Hans Pols, "Beyond Clinical Frontiers: The American Mental Hygiene Movement, 1910–1945," in *International Relations in Psychiatry: Britain, Germany, and the United States to World War I*, ed. Volker Roelcke, Paul Weindling, and Louise Westwood (Rochester, NY: University of Rochester Press, 2010); Ian Robert Dowbiggin, *Keeping America Sane: Psychiatry and Eugenics in the United States and Canada, 1880–1940*, (Ithaca, NY: Cornell University Press, 1997).

79. Edward F. Waite, "The Physical Bases of Crime: From the Standpoint of the Judge of a Juvenile Court," in *Physical Bases of Crime, a Symposium: Papers and Discussion*

Contributed to the Twenty-Eighth Annual Meeting of the American Academy of Medicine, Minneapolis, June 14, 1913 (Easton, PA: American Academy of Medicine Press, 1914), 107–8.

80. Milton Fraser Percival, *Notes on Medical Subjects: From His Student Days at Medico-Chirurgical College, Philadelphia, 1891–1905*, vol. 2., College of Physicians of Philadelphia.

81. "Adenoids Cause Juvenile Crime," *San Francisco Call*, August 10, 1908.

82. The Pennsylvania Society to Protect Children from Cruelty, *Thirteenth Annual Report* (1906), p. 19, PSPC Acc. 150, box 1A. Urban Archives, Temple University Archives, Temple University.

83. Ibid., appendix A, p. 53.

84. "10,000 Little Criminals to Be Made Good by Surgery," *Indianapolis Morning Star*, August 26, 1906; "The Surgeon's Knife as a Check to Crime," *New York Times*, August 12, 1906.

85. "May Remedy Crime in Young," *Chicago Daily Tribune*, February 1, 1910.

86. "To the Knife."

87. "Brain Surgery Lessens Crime"; "Making Bad Boys Good by Surgery," *Sunday Oregonian*, August 26, 1906. This widespread publicity and the conflation of brain surgery with other types of surgery prompted one of the doctors in Philadelphia to declare that no brain surgeries for "feebleminded persons" had been performed and that brain surgery was useful only in cases of tumor or fracture that had resulted in pressure on the brain. "The Surgeon's Knife as a Check to Crime."

88. John Kolmer, "Surgery, a Promoter of Morals," in *Annual Congress of the National Prison Association of the United States* (Lincoln, NE: Press of William B. Burford, 1905), 291–92.

89. "Would Try Brain Surgery on Convicts," *Tucson Citizen*, September 21, 1906; "Surgery on Crooks Doctor Suggests," *Meriden Daily Journal*, September 18, 1906.

90. "Interview with John D. Holstrom—Vollmer as a Man: Memories of a Close Friend and Colleague," in *The August Vollmer Oral History Project* (Berkeley: The Regents of the University of California, 1972), 37.

91. Rowell quoted in "Girl to Risk Life for Reform," *San Francisco Call*, March 28, 1911.

92. Jacob Piatt Dunn, *Greater Indianapolis: The History, the Industries, the Institutions, and the People of a City of Homes*, vol. 2 (Chicago: The Lewis Publishing Company, 1910), 932–33; "Dr. John Kolmer, Pioneer in Trephining Surgery, Is Dead."

93. "Union State Hospital," *Indianapolis News*, July 15, 1901.

94. Ibid.

95. "Surgeon's Knife Makes an Incorrigible Boy Obedient."

96. They also included practitioners like E. H. Pratt, a proponent of "orificial surgery," in which bodily orifices were assailed for all manner of conditions. E. H. Pratt, "A Brief Chapter in the History of Orificial Surgery," in *Orificial Surgery, Its Philosophy, Application and Technique*, ed. Benjamin Elisha Dawson et al. (Newark, NJ: Physicians Drug News Co., 1912), 26–39; "Knife Cures Moral Defect," *Washington Post*, October 24, 1913.

97. Martin S. Pernick, *The Black Stork: Eugenics and the Death of "Defective" Babies in American Medicine and Motion Pictures since 1915* (New York: Oxford University Press, 1996), 83.

98. Ibid., chap. 3; Nathaniel C. Comfort, *The Science of Human Perfection: How Genes Became the Heart of American Medicine* (New Haven, CT: Yale University Press, 2012).

99. Kolmer, "Surgery, a Promoter of Morals," 292.

100. Miller, "Cut Out 'Bad Spots' in Boy's Brain."

101. "Boy Soon to Leave Hospital," *Indianapolis Star*, July 22, 1905.

102. "Reform by Surgery," *New York Times*, May 13, 1903.

103. Engel, "Mental Improvement." Engel described the boy's behavior in starkly adult terms that betray the kind of essentialist thinking that some applied to the concepts of "criminality" and "criminal tendency" at this time: when scolded, the boy "put out his tongue and acted like a *hardened criminal*"; he hit his mother and destroyed furniture. My emphasis.

104. "The Criminal Brain Not Necessarily Degenerate," *Journal of the American Medical Association* 25, no. 21 (1895). Laplace participated in a debate in 1895 at the Philadelphia Academy of Natural Sciences on the subject of Lombroso's theories of degeneration and the "born criminal," and though the audience seemed to be divided on that theory, it is unclear exactly what Laplace's position was. He recounted his examination of Léon Gambetta's brain after the French statesman's death, and declared it to be very small and "strongly developed in the region of the speech centers, which corresponded with his great oratorical ability during life."

105. "Surgeon's Knife Makes an Incorrigible Boy Obedient."

106. Kolmer noted that one boy's scalp on the left side of the head was very tight, which indicated to him that "a greater injury was received during one of his falls than was ever appreciated by those about him." Kolmer, "Surgery, a Promoter of Morals," 296. In another boy's case, it was the probation officer and "others of the court [who] conceived the idea that a physical defect was responsible for the lad's mental attitude. The mother and sister then remembered a fall received by the boy when 3 years old." "Bad Boy Is Made Good by a Surgical Operation."

107. "Use Knife to Make a Cure: Surgeons Think Criminal Tendencies Due to Pressure on the Brain," *Lincoln Daily News*, January 3, 1916.

108. "Reforming Bad Boys with Surgeon's Knife."

109. "Knife Lets Virtue Loose"; Engel, "Mental Improvement."

110. "Bad Boy Ran to Jail from Surgeon's Knives," *Philadelphia Inquirer*, April 26, 1914.

111. "Accidents Cause Criminal Instinct," *The Indianapolis Morning Star*, April 26, 1905.

112. "Brain Surgery Ends in a Poor Hair Cut," *Kalamazoo Gazette*, October 27, 1906.

113. "Science Cures Crime."

114. See for instance, "Asleep at the State House," *Indianapolis Morning Star*, September 30, 1905; "Falls from Grace Again," *Detroit Free Press*, March 3, 1907.

115. "Hold Youth Made Moral by Knife," *Plain Dealer*, October 15, 1908.

116. James B. Morrow, "Prisoners Treated as Human Beings," *Daily Tribune*, August 16, 1908; Robert H. Bremmer, "The Civic Revival in Ohio: Harris R. Cooley and Cooley Farms," *American Journal of Economics and Sociology* 14, no. 1 (1954).

117. Harris R. Cooley, "The Farm Colony: Our Experiment in Cleveland; What It Has Demonstrated, What Are the Limitations of Colony Treatment," in *Proceedings of the National Conference of Charities and Correction at the Thirty-Ninth Annual Session*

Held in Cleveland, Ohio, June 12–19, ed. Alexander Johnson (Fort Wayne: Indiana Fort Wayne Printing Company, 1912), 192.

118. "Still Has Faith in Use of Knife," *Plain Dealer*, March 3, 1907.

119. "Head Repairing," *Salt Lake Weekly Tribune*, April 14, 1892.

120. "Possibilities of Surgery," *Daily Herald*, May 31, 1893.

121. "'Unfortunate' Criminals," *San Francisco Chronicle*, April 23, 1911.

122. Clara Newman Murray, "Correspondence," *Health* (April 1908): 249.

123. "Surgery to Prevent Crime," *The American Lawyer* 14, no. 9 (1906).

124. In the case of smallpox vaccination, see Michael Willrich, *Pox: An American History* (London: Penguin Books, 2011). For medical experimentation, see Susan E. Lederer, *Subjected to Science: Human Experimentation in America before the Second World War* (Baltimore: Johns Hopkins University Press, 1995).

125. Susan E. Lederer, *Flesh and Blood: Organ Transplantation and Blood Transfusion in Twentieth-Century America* (Oxford: Oxford University Press, 2008), 5.

126. "Magicians of Surgery Making Over Man," *San Francisco Sunday Call*, November 21, 1909.

127. "Adenoids Cause Stir," *Washington Post*, November 29, 1909. In this case the father refused adenoid surgery for his son because family circumstances made it impossible to nurse the boy post operation.

128. "Denies He Ordered Surgical Operation," *Indianapolis Morning Star*, November 22, 1905.

129. On Cushing, see Michael Bliss, *Harvey Cushing: A Life in Surgery* (New York: Oxford University Press, 2005).

130. Harvey Cushing, "The Special Field of Neurological Surgery after Another Interval," *Archives of Neurology and Psychiatry* 4, no. 6 (1920): 609; Harvey Cushing, "Surgery of the Head," in *Surgery: Its Principles and Practice*, ed. William W. Keen (Philadelphia: W. B. Saunders, 1908), 233–37.

131. "Kleptomaniac Cured," *Princeton Union*, June 8, 1911.

132. Rosemary Stevens, *In Sickness and in Wealth: American Hospitals in the Twentieth Century* (New York: Basic Books, 1989), 90; Joel D. Howell, *Technology in the Hospital: Transforming Patient Care in the Early Twentieth Century* (Baltimore: Johns Hopkins University Press, 1995), 66–67. For a condemnation of unnecessary surgeries, see William Mayo, "Presidential Address: American College of Surgeons 1919 Annual Meeting," *Surgery, Gynecology and Obstetrics* 30 (1920).

133. Cushing, "Surgery of the Head," 256.

134. Cushing and Sachs did sideline, for complex reasons, one surgeon who performed decompressions on children with "spastic paralysis" and at least one procedure on someone with a criminal conviction. See Delia Gavrus, "Skill, Judgement and Conduct for the First Generation of Neurosurgeons, 1900–1930," *Medical History* 59, no. 3 (2015).

135. Andrew T. Scull, *Madhouse: A Tragic Tale of Megalomania and Modern Medicine* (New Haven, CT: Yale University Press, 2004).

136. Ian Hacking, "Degeneracy, Criminal Behavior, and Looping," in *Genetics and Criminal Behavior*, ed. David Wasserman and Robert Wachbroit (Cambridge: Cambridge University Press, 2001).

137. On race, see Khalil Gibran Muhammad, *The Condemnation of Blackness: Race, Crime, and the Making of Modern Urban America* (Cambridge, MA: Harvard University Press, 2010).

138. Tamara Myers, "Embodying Delinquency: Boys' Bodies, Sexuality, and Juvenile Justice History in Early Twentieth-Century Quebec," *Journal of the History of Sexuality* 14, no. 4 (2006).

139. Delia Gavrus, "Men of Dreams and Men of Action: Neurologists, Neurosurgeons, and the Performance of Professional Identity, 1920–1950," *Bulletin of the History of Medicine* 85, no. 1 (2011); Delia Gavrus, "Men of Strong Opinions: Identity, Self-Representation, and the Performance of Neurosurgery, 1919–1950" (PhD diss., University of Toronto, 2011).

140. On the public controversy that resulted from attempts to apply psychosurgery to "violent behavior" in the 1970s, see Brian P. Casey, "The Surgical Elimination of Violence? Conflicting Attitudes Towards Technology and Science during the Psychosurgery Controversy of the 1970s," *Science in Context* 28, no. 1 (2015).

141. Edward E. Mayer, "Prefrontal Lobotomy and the Courts," *Journal of Criminal Law and Criminology* 38, no. 6 (1948).

Chapter Five

Prosthetic Imaginaries

Spinal Surgery and Innovation from the Patient's Perspective

Beth Linker

In November 1960, *Time* magazine ran a splashy medical news report with the rather futuristic title "Spines of Steel."[1] The article featured the work of the orthopedic surgeon Paul H. Harrington (1911–80), who had devised a method of straightening scoliotic spines using a series of implantable metal rods and hooks embedded in the vertebral column. So as to visualize the sleekness of Harrington's instrumentation, *Time* included a black-and-white photograph of the physically imposing surgeon, his large hands gracefully clutching one of his metal rods, slender as a soda straw. Although Harrington did not have a definitive cure—or a method to prevent the occurrence of spinal curvatures caused by scoliosis—his rods promised a new era in scoliosis treatment, with traditional and seemingly more cumbersome modes of medical intervention left behind (figs. 5.1–5.2).[2]

To many surgeons today, Harrington's innovation is seen as a pivotal moment in the surgical management of severe scoliosis.[3] From the 1960s onward, Harrington's instrumentation would become the standard method of scoliosis correction and fusion throughout the world for more than a quarter of the

Parts of this essay were published in Beth Linker, "Spines of Steel: A Case of Surgical Enthusiasm in Cold War America," *Bulletin of the History of Medicine* 90, no. 2 (2016): 222–23, 226–32, 234–49.

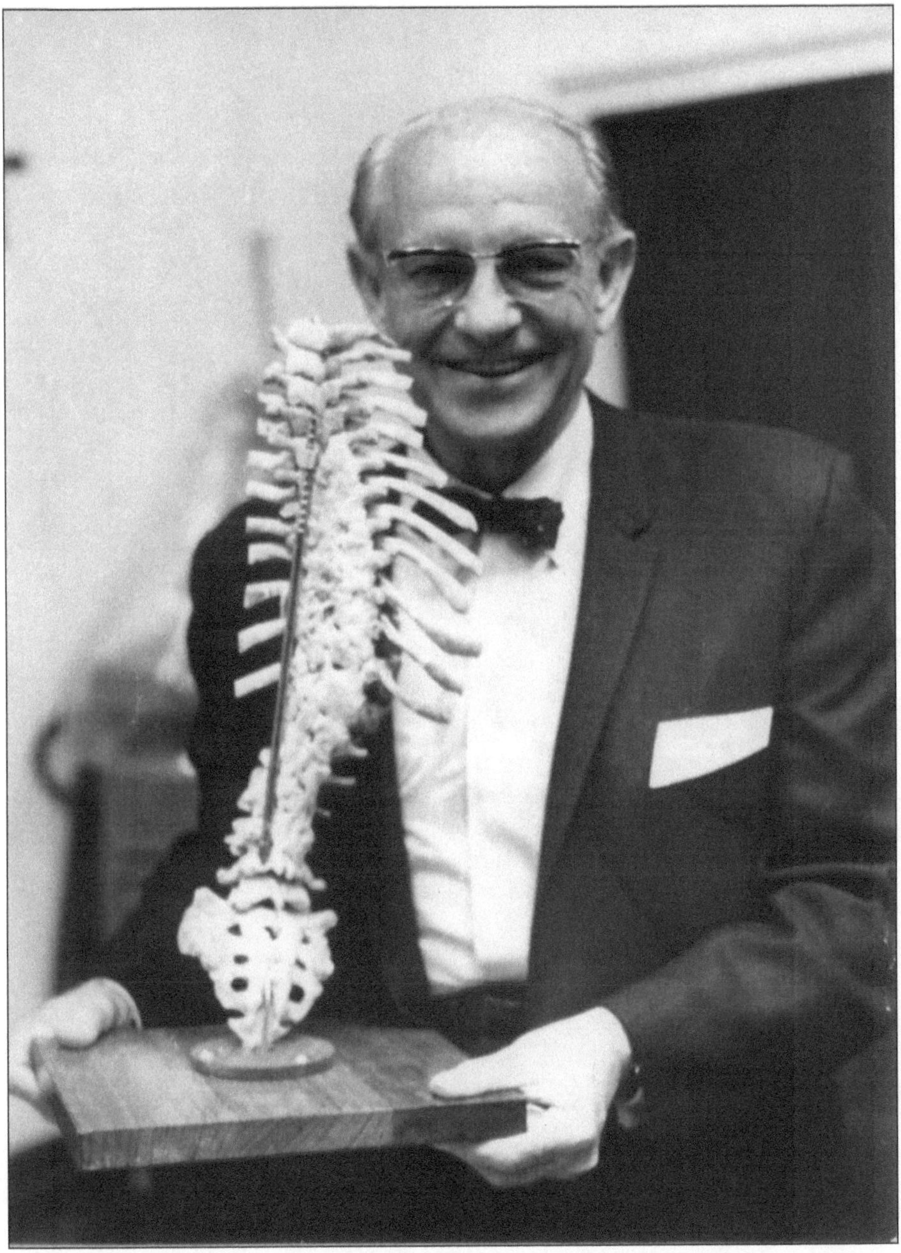

Figure 5.1. Harrington in attendance at the 1971 Scoliosis Research Society meeting in Nijmegen, Holland, shown holding an autopsy specimen using the Harrington rods in the Netherlands. Courtesy of Paul Randall Harrington, MD, Archives, University of Kansas Medical Center, Kansas City, Kansas. Photograph by Pierre Stagnara.

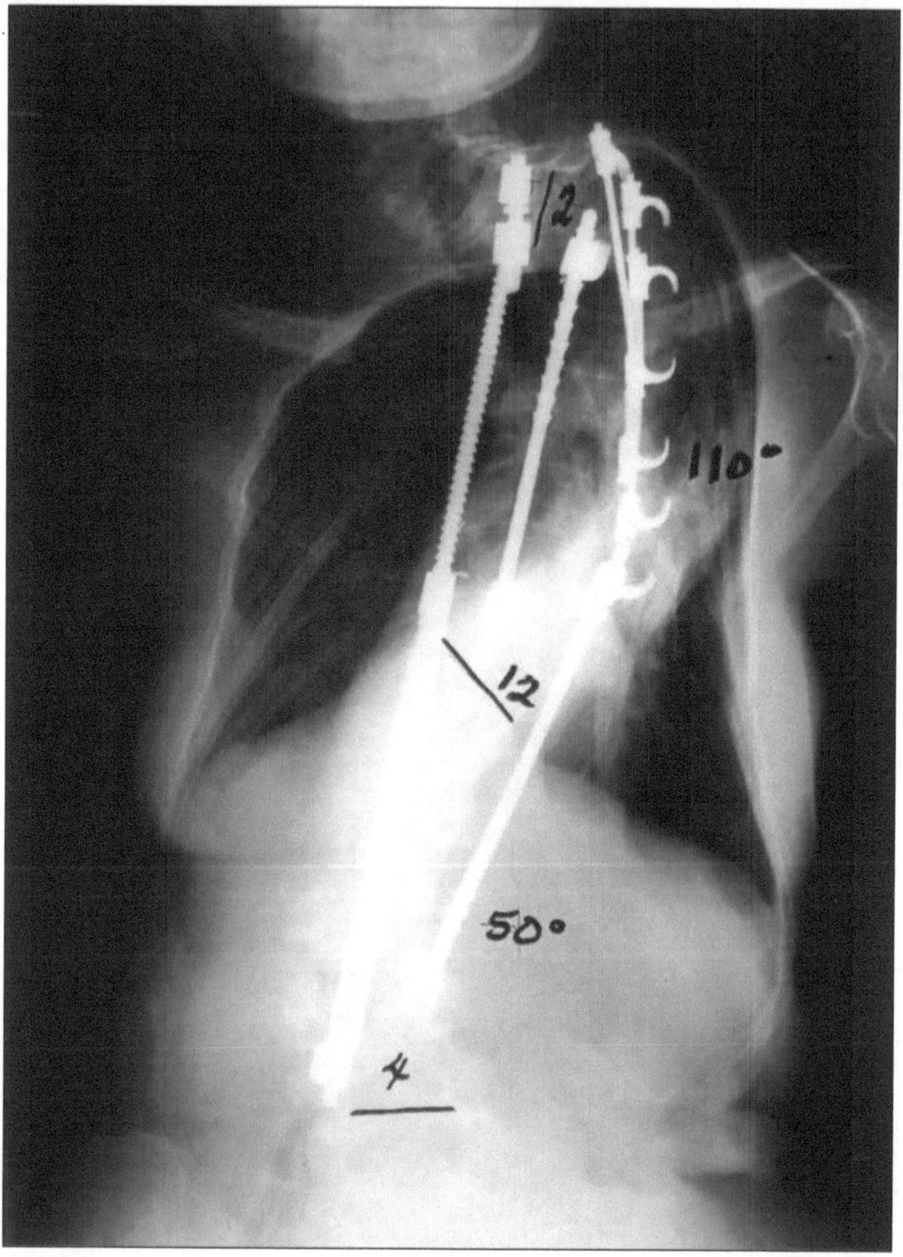

Figure 5.2. An x-ray image of Harrington Rods being used to correct severe scoliosis. Courtesy of Paul Randall Harrington, MD, Archives, University of Kansas Medical Center, Kansas City, Kansas.

century.[4] In the words of two orthopedic surgeons writing in 1999, Harrington's "instrumentation was a clear milestone in scoliosis surgery providing for the first time, a reliable means of obtaining and maintaining maximal deformity correction." The advantages of Harrington's system, they write, "were obvious."[5]

Whereas the success of Harrington's surgery may seem obvious to orthopedists practicing now, the advantage of metal implantation was not at all clear to his contemporaries. In the mid-twentieth century, leading practitioners in the field endorsed various forms of scoliosis treatment. According to a 1941 study of sixteen US orthopedic clinics in prominent university research centers, postural exercise was one of the most commonly prescribed modalities of treatment, even though many orthopedists doubted its efficacy.[6] Other popular forms of treatment included body casts, bone fusions, or a combination of the two. Of the sixteen clinics surveyed, thirteen used the Risser turnbuckle cast, named after the inventor-orthopedist Joseph C. Risser (1892–1982).[7] In the 1930s, Risser devised a two-part plaster cast with a turnbuckle that surgeons would twist daily for several weeks to forcibly correct a patient's curvature. Once the curve had been reduced, many surgeons would then perform an open operation to surgically fuse the vertebrae into a straightened position, using an autologous bone graft to reinforce arthodesis (fixation).[8]

By the time that Harrington began experimenting with his rod technique, the casting-fusion method of correction appeared to be the best method of treatment both in terms of efficacy and patient safety. The reported mortality rate for spinal fusions was around 1.6 percent during the pre–World War II years, a low percentage compared with operations performed in other emerging surgical specialties.[9] Treatment success and efficacy had long been points of contention among scoliosis experts, for medical intervention rarely, if ever, resulted in complete correction of the curve. Reports coming from surgeons performing casting and fusions during the 1940s indicated that the average patient could experience anywhere from 27 to 65 percent curve correction. Later, when researchers measured the success of Harrington's instrumentation, they found that patients could attain a 61 percent correction, but with four times the rate of infection and instrument breakage compared with previous surgical measures.[10]

What, then, persuaded orthopedic surgeons in the 1960s and thereafter to gradually adopt a riskier method of scoliosis treatment and abandon the conventional forms of casting and fusion? What did Harrington's rod system—and subsequent metal implantation systems—have to offer that more conventional methods did not? These questions are all the more compelling when one considers the fact that the prevalence of scoliosis declined during the first half of the twentieth century, from 50 percent of the population in 1922 to an estimated 2 percent of the population in 1955.[11] As diseases that commonly caused scoliosis in the first half of the twentieth century began to recede (e.g., rickets, bone tuberculosis, and polio), so too did disease-based scoliosis. The rise of the Harrington Rod System thus occurred at the same time that orthopedists increasingly focused their attention on "idiopathic scoliosis," a relatively obscure disease category that received little attention until the postwar years when scoliosis specialists mounted a widespread public-health campaign educating Americans about the danger of unexplainable back curvatures and encouraged surgical intervention when detected.[12]

To understand how a seemingly more invasive and riskier surgical approach to scoliosis correction would be adopted just at the point when the prevalence of disease-based scoliosis drastically decreased, this paper examines not only Harrington's efforts to innovate and recruit other surgeons to his system, but also—and most important—the central role that everyday people with scoliosis played in legitimizing Harrington's system. As Thomas Schlich and Christopher Crenner make clear in the introduction to this volume, surgical innovation and success must be understood not just in terms of technological novelty but also in the context of the prevailing social, political, and economic conditions that make a new technique "effective, useful, and practicable." This scholarly approach is particularly conducive to understanding the history of scoliosis and its orthopedic interventions, for scoliosis treatment is a unique medico-surgical intervention that relies on the utilization of various body technologies, ranging from exercise and braces to internal hardware.

More than other areas of medicine, surgery is a technological intervention that involves a two-tiered category of users, with surgeons as the users of tools and techniques and patients as end-users, embodying and interacting with various permanent and semipermanent body technologies that alter a person's physicality.[13] As body technologies that are both applied and worn/embodied, scoliosis therapy engages both kinds of users in a dynamic interplay whereby efficacy, practicability, and success are mutually constitutive and reinforced by social, cultural, and economic concerns.[14]

Using patient correspondence from the Paul R. Harrington Archives, this essay examines over six hundred letters that Harrington received between 1960 and 1965 in response to *Time*'s announcement of his surgical innovation.[15] In a strict sense, the people writing to Harrington are not patients per se, for at the time of their writing, they are not under his care (though they are sometimes patients under the care of other surgeons). What makes this kind of archival documentation particularly fruitful is that, unlike patients who have already committed themselves to a particular surgeon, these letter writers are in the *process* of making a decision, deliberating over various medical and surgical interventions concerning scoliosis treatment. It is this process of weighing options—of deciding to seek medical intervention or not, of deciding whether Harrington's regime seems better than someone else's—that makes these letters particularly useful in demonstrating how those with scoliosis affected clinical notions of "surgical success," and in turn helped to determine which kind of surgical interventions would go on to succeed and which would not.[16] These letters also offer a window into the culture and representation of scoliosis, showing how the media offered its own version of medical knowledge and progress, and how Harrington's rods tapped into the midcentury cultural allure of steel and cybernetics.[17]

In the end, the correspondence between Harrington and his *Time* readers reveals that while the surgeon labored to perfect his rod technique throughout the 1950s and into the 1960s—constantly modifying and recalibrating so as to overcome inherent flaws with the system—he also held out a surgical imaginary, a promise that spines could be dramatically and permanently straightened with negligible casting and immobilization. Though this imaginary was never fully realized, it nonetheless attracted journalists looking for stories of medical "miracles" and certain people with scoliosis, particularly those who felt physically, socially, financially, and psychologically disabled by their curved backs. Living at a time of heightened body surveillance and stigma against all kinds of physical "deformities," mid-twentieth-century Americans with scoliosis faced persistent discrimination in both their personal and professional lives. Inherent to the story of Harrington's success, then, is how scoliosis—and especially idiopathic scoliosis—came to be defined as a disability and how certain surgeons and patients came to see metal rod implantation as a viable and agreeable tool to alter one's biology, making so-called deformed spines conform to contingent standards of beauty and health.

* * *

When the thirty-four-year-old Harrington first arrived in Houston, Texas, to begin his career as an orthopedic surgeon in 1945, he probably could not have predicted that his work in the Lone Star State would mimic the military service he has just completed as part of the Seventy-Seventh Evacuation Hospital in World War II. To Harrington's surprise, Houston would become a city devastated by the deadliest and most disabling polio epidemics in the country, with the worst outbreak occurring in the year 1952. Polio migrated to the US South during the 1940s. During the outbreaks in the 1950s, many Texans exhibited symptoms of bulbo-spinal polio, a type of polio that left individuals—usually children—unable to swallow or breathe without artificial support.[18] Certain observers likened the scene in Houston to a military field hospital, with physicians and nurses working around the clock attending to patients and their families. During the height of the epidemic, certain hospitals promised "combat pay" to its medical personnel.[19]

In 1950, Harrington became part of one of the leading polio rehabilitation centers in Texas, known as the Southwestern Poliomyelitis Respiratory

Center (later named the Southwestern Poliomyelitis Research and Rehabilitation Center).[20] With steady funding from the National Foundation for Infantile Paralysis, academic backing from Baylor University College of Medicine, and institutional support from Houston's Jefferson-Davis Hospital, the center became a premiere teaching and research institute dedicated to the rehabilitation of respiratory-involved polio patients. The primary mission of Southwestern was to keep bulbo-spinal polio patients from becoming dependent on artificial respiratory devices (such as the iron lung) and to get the most severally affected reintegrated back into society, avoiding lives of institutionalization, seclusion, and immobility.[21]

Catalyzed by rising death rates and ever-increasing incidence of paralytic, respiratory-dependent polio, Southwestern and its team of medical specialists readily adopted new technologies and aggressive therapies to push their patients—and the largely marginalized field of rehabilitative medicine—forward in order to bring about more efficacious and scientifically grounded treatment regimes. Leading the Southwestern rehabilitation team since its 1950 opening, Dr. William A. Spencer (a pediatrician trained at Johns Hopkins) championed the integration of new technologies, especially computer technologies, into rehabilitative medicine. Rejecting the older notion of rehabilitation as "after care," Spencer insisted that rehabilitation become a first responder in medicine by relying on physiological data gained from mathematical modeling and computer analysis. Spencer referred to rehabilitation as "medical humanetics," which he defined as "a union of medicine, psychology, social science, mathematics, and computer technology."[22] The team at Southwestern—which consisted of several orthopedic specialists (including Harrington), a physiologist, an Otolaryngologist, as well as a team of nurses, physical therapists, and occupational therapists—compiled data on a patient's diet, pulse, blood pressure, EKG, subjective complaints, and psychological tests and fed it into a computerized medical record system.[23] With this data, Spencer's team calculated when it was safe for paralytic patients to sit and stand upright without overstressing the heart and other vital systems of the human body.

If there was one unifying goal shared by Southwestern's eclectic team of rehabilitation specialists, it was that patients, no matter the severity of paralysis, would stand upright again as soon as possible, with or without assistive devices. The ever-present goal of standing—and more important, walking again—was a relatively new development in the history of rehabilitation. In earlier periods, when one's gait was socially paramount, this goal was not of primary interest since walking imperfectly was seen as worse than not walking at all.[24] But uprightness became a moral and physiological imperative in post–World War II America, especially in polio care. The iron lung—in which a person was consigned to live a life as a permanent "horizontal"—symbolized the ultimate failure of rehabilitation. With the assistance of

Harrington and a team of physiotherapists, the Southwestern team developed and researched "standing beds," vertical wooden gurneys with footboards and body straps that could simulate a standing position for severely paralyzed patients.[25]

It was in this context that Harrington first began his research into the surgical management of spinal scoliosis, a condition that many polio patients with severe paralysis acquired. Achieving spinal stability and verticality for patients with scoliosis was paramount to the goal of ambulation. Harrington and the Southwestern team conducted several studies that showed how assisted weight bearing helped otherwise immobile patients maintain bone density, muscular tone, vascular regularity, and pulmonary health.[26]

At first, Harrington relied on more conventional methods of surgical management to assist with spinal stability, performing casting and bone grafting. This method had been perfected by Risser, a California orthopedist who contended that to properly correct scoliosis, the patient had to first undergo prolonged cast wear so as to bring about spinal alignment before a surgeon could attempt arthrodesis (the technical term for surgically induced bone fusion). Very few surgeons who wanted to see the profession of orthopedic surgery modernize—that is, shed the old "strap and buckle" image of their specialty by becoming skilled at an array of specialized open operations—dissented from Risser. Having interned with Russell A. Hibbs (the man who still today is seen as the father of spinal fusion surgery) at the New York Orthopedic Hospital in the 1920s, Risser earned a reputation for being a Hibbs's protégée, and thus a leading voice in spinal surgery.[27] After setting up his own practice in the Los Angeles area during the 1930s, Risser spent his early career both promoting and improving on Hibbs's technique by incorporating the turnbuckle cast as part of the surgical system. By 1955, Risser created a new ambulatory casting system, known as the Risser Localizer Jacket, which meant that patients did not have to spend as much time immobilized in bed as they had with the earlier turnbuckle system. Nonetheless, Risser's "walking cast" and fusion method still necessitated up to three years of hospitalization in specialized rehabilitation units.[28]

Although Risser insisted that his technique was the best option for surgically managing polio scoliosis, Harrington found traditional methods of fixation lacking both from a surgical and rehabilitative perspective. In his initial attempts at spinal fusion in patients with severe paralytic polio, Harrington discovered that the technique often failed, with spinal curvatures reappearing and becoming even more severe within months after operating.[29] The reappearance of curvatures, or "failed fusions," was a common outcome in spinal surgery at the time, and a reason why Risser and other orthopedic surgeons insisted on prolonged casting, so that lasting ossification would occur. In addition to being dissatisfied with the efficacy of the technique, Harrington, like his Southwestern counterparts, found prolonged bedrest to be at odds with the more ambitious rehabilitation goals of standing and walking.

Harrington thus began experimenting with different surgical techniques that would bring about quicker and more lasting spinal correction and stability. His ultimate goal was to do away with spinal fusion altogether and to bring cast wear to a minimum. Already in 1949, Harrington began testing the use of metal hooks and rods that, when placed along the vertebral column, created a "dynamic correction system" that did not necessitate traditional fixation.[30]

The historical record does not reveal what initially inspired Harrington to attempt a nonfusion metal implantation operation. To the uninitiated, Harrington likened the principles of his system to an automobile tire jack, and perhaps car repair is one place where he drew insight.[31] Although many orthopedists writing about Harrington's invention make it seem as if he was the first surgeon to use mental implants for spinal correction, published sources indicate otherwise. With a similar intent of bringing about a "quicker and more effective [spinal] correction," Dr. Francis Glen Allan at the Royal Orthopaedic Hospital in England developed an "Allan Jack" in the early 1950s. Like Harrington's instrumentation, the Allen Jack was an instrument used to forcibly correct spinal concavities.[32] The 1950s was also a time when orthopedic surgeons increasingly relied on metal implants and devices to make musculoskeletal repairs. Just as the military favored steel-structured aircrafts over wood-based ones during the interwar period because the former signified modernity, orthopedic surgeons saw steel as a way to modernize their own profession and thus began performing open operations using man-made metals to replace hips and fortify fractured bones.[33]

Harrington conducted an initial set of experimental surgeries with his hook and rod system between the years 1949 to 1954. He relied on nineteen patients, fourteen of whom had polio scoliosis, the majority female.[34] Being part of an experimental surgical group in which prototypes were constantly be tested and redesigned, most of the initial nineteen patients underwent multiple operations. From the outset, Harrington relied, at least in part, on the subjective reports of his patients in order to determine efficacy and success. Eight out of the nineteen original patients reported feeling the "same" or "worse" after undergoing as many as eleven separate operative procedures along the way.[35] Harrington made as many as thirty-five modifications to the rod system during the five years of initial experimentation. He found that one of the most serious problems was instrument breakage. Bars and rods broke in eleven of the original nineteen patients.

Despite these rather discouraging results, Harrington forged ahead with his research and by 1955 won two NFIP grants. He also gained an esteemed colleague, the orthotist Thorkild Engen, who had extensive experience as a brace maker for polio patients in Warm Springs, Georgia. From 1955 to

1960, Harrington applied his instrumentation to forty-two patients with polio scoliosis. The instrumentation continued to evolve slowly over time. After one surgery took place, Harrington and Engen would "modify the design for the next patient, according to how the operation on the previous patient went."[36] It was during this second phase of product development that Harrington realized that his idea for a "dynamic correction system" was untenable. Patients from phase 1 of the experimentation who had received instrumentation without fusion or casting experienced improvement for only six months to one year, and then most of them required what surgeons rather euphemistically called "reinstrumentation." By contrast, during this second phase of experimentation, Harrington admitted that he used fusion "extensively to accomplish better results."[37]

Despite his hopes of doing away with fusion and casting altogether, Harrington's method ended up being a *modification* of an already well-established approach to scoliosis surgery, not a radical departure from it. Despite latter-day tales of a "Harrington rod revolution," Harrington knew his technique was not as different from conventional surgical methods as he had hoped. And he was disappointed by this fact. As late as 1959, a year before the *Time* magazine article appeared, Harrington reported that he found "many discouraging facets to the study" of spinal correction through mental implantation.[38]

Another surgeon might have given up, might have considered the "dynamic correction system" a failure and resorted to the tried and true methods employed by an older generation of orthopedists. But Harrington persisted despite the initial setbacks. He continued to tinker with his system, attempting to make modifications that would decrease the amount of time patients had to be in casts without sacrificing lasting spinal correction. The question, then, is: What kept him going? Why did Harrington persevere in the face of rather disappointing results?

According to his own account, Harrington attributed his perseverance to the financial support of the NFIP and to the professional encouragement that he got from his colleagues at Southwestern as well as a handful of orthopedic colleagues from other university research centers.[39] Additionally, Zimmer Manufacture, a leading US orthopedic device company, began taking an interest in Harrington's instrumentation. At first the relationship between Harrington and Zimmer was that of buyer and seller. Upon completing the initial phase of his experimentation in 1954, Harrington began sending his device blueprints to engineers at Zimmer, who would fill Harrington orders. By the late 1950s, demand for Harrington's instrumentation steadily increased, owing, in large part, to Harrington's tireless travel and demonstration schedule, where other surgeons were introduced and encouraged to buy his products. In response to this uptick in sales, Zimmer requested exclusive rights to manufacture and market the product, as well as the exclusive right to use Paul R. Harrington's name to sell the product.[40] It was a contractual agreement that served Harrington, who was worried that other surgeons might steal his intellectual property, and Zimmer, who wanted to reap the financial benefits of an ostensibly growing market.[41]

But there was another crucial factor that helped Harrington sustain his belief in the hook and rod system: namely, he was spurred on by patients who urged him to find a better way to manage their condition. Beginning in 1959, Harrington received a deluge of letters after local newspapers began to cover his medical success stories. In the summer of 1960 the *Houston Post* medical news reporter, Jean Walsh, wrote a glowing feature story about Harrington and the strides he had made in scoliosis surgery. Walsh deemed Harrington's approach a "new and happier method" of scoliosis care, emphasizing the relatively short hospital stays and immediate results.[42] As soon as the *Houston Post* story hit the wire, the Associated Press picked it up, and versions of the report fanned out across the United States. Harrington reached national recognition in November 1960 when *Time* magazine ran a version of the AP article with the glitzy "Spines of Steel" title.

In response to the media making Harrington's surgical imaginary seem like a reality, families of children with scoliosis, young teenagers diagnosed with spinal curvature, and middle-aged Americans who had already lived with the condition for decades wrote to Harrington to celebrate his invention and to ask if they, too, could get their spines "jacked" into place.[43] Many of those writing to Harrington shared their struggles and frustrations with other doctors, some of whom deemed scoliosis an untreatable condition, and others of whom believed that the deformity required years of medical attention. These letters bolstered Harrington's conviction that conventional methods of scoliosis management needed to be abandoned and that a new surgical system had to be established.

* * *

"I have always marveled at the great medical strides made in recent years," wrote Wanda, a thirty-nine-year-old Californian, in a November 1960 letter to Harrington, "but never once dreamed or even hoped that someone has been doing something that might help me."[44] Born in 1921, Wanda did indeed witness many changes in medical and surgical care. From her perspective, many deadly diseases and infections of her childhood were now managed by antibiotics and vaccines, with Salk's 1954 polio vaccine trial being the latest medical accomplishment that made everyday life feel more secure. When her curved back was detected during her high school years, she was told that nothing much could be done, and that, since it was not deadly, she would manage to live with it. Despite being told to keep a stiff upper lip, Wanda admitted to Harrington that her back "always bothered me—probably to this point more aesthetically than physically. But now as I'm older it lets me down more frequently physically."[45]

The letters contained in the Harrington Archives—a correspondence that includes over six hundred handwritten and typed notes—make clear that patients with scoliosis and their family members were fairly well versed in what biomedicine had to offer, and they did not hesitate to seek out a second opinion when a particular plan of treatment did not suit them. Those who wrote to Harrington tended to be white and working class, and they hailed from all regions of the country. They were the kind of people who had enough means and education to subscribe to and read their local newspapers and *Time*. Of particular note is that those with polio scoliosis constituted only a fraction of patient inquiries, even though Harrington first developed his instrumentation explicitly for that particular patient group. Although a good majority of prospective patients writing to Harrington had idiopathic scoliosis, most letter writers did not emphasize their diagnostic category but rather focused on the lived experience of having a curved back—and what treatment, if any, they were willing to undertake.

Most of the people writing to Harrington were in search of better medical options concerning scoliosis care. Many who sought out Harrington had already received treatment from other orthopedic surgeons, including leading experts such as Dr. John Robert Cobb of New York and Dr. Risser in California, as well as teams of orthopedic surgeons at Boston Children's Hospital and Henry Ford Hospital. These letters put Harrington, who was not yet considered a scoliosis expert, in a tricky position: his new technique was winning the hearts of prospective patients before it had persuaded the minds of scoliosis experts. Although Harrington became a darling of the media in 1960, he had not yet published the results of his surgical experimentation in a peer-reviewed journal (he would not do this until 1962). So although Harrington slowly gained the support of certain influential scoliosis experts during the late 1950s and early 1960s, he and his technique would not reach full professional acceptance until the mid-1960s, if not later.

Whereas peer-review publications and presentations at professional meetings carried weight in the world of orthopedics, patients felt that they had more pressing matters concerning their health and well-being and did not find it necessary to wait for the professional vetting process. This was especially true among the patients who had been consulting Dr. Cobb, who adopted a wait-and-see approach to scoliosis care. Known for his strict noninterventionist stance toward scoliosis care, Cobb would often monitor scoliosis curvatures for years before prescribing treatment. (Ever the diagnostician, Cobb developed a way to measure spinal curvatures using a geometrical technique known as the "Cobb angle," which is still used today.) Cobb rarely prescribed exercise, bracing, or surgery, for he believed that too many surgeons rushed into treatment, mostly in order to convince patients and parents that "something could be done" or to "improve an x-ray shadow."[46] Taking the long view on the history of scoliosis treatment, Cobb observed that over the course of hundreds of years "there had been great enthusiasm for certain plaster casts, frames, beds, corsets, exercises and operations." But, he continued, "most of these have been discarded after arousing much hope in some patient only to have it end in despair."[47] Urging for a better understanding of the natural history of the disease, Cobb wanted surgeons to resist the temptation to intervene since, in many cases, curves spontaneously stopped growing, and in others, the curve progressed even after bracing and fusion were complete. "Parents are usually relieved to know that many scoliosis patients need no treatment," Cobb insisted. He advised that "a little sensible reassurance to the patients and her parents is better than a lot of unnecessary, inadequate, and expensive so-called treatment."[48]

Not all patients seemed convinced by Cobb's reassurances. In one 1961 letter, the parents of an eighteen-year-old girl from Trenton, New Jersey, recounted how ever since their daughter Judy was twelve years old, they were told that nothing could be done except to monitor the curve. When Judy turned fifteen, her parents took her to see Dr. Cobb, who agreed that close observation was the best course of action. Cobb maintained that Judy's curve was not severe enough for surgery (the correspondence does not reveal the numerical degree of her curvature) and that since Judy had already achieved full skeletal maturation, the curve would not worsen. But a year and a half later, Judy grew taller and the curve increased. Most worrisome, she began to complain of back pain. Judy's parents severed ties with Dr. Cobb and their local doctor (who was following Cobb's advice) and began seeking out other opinions. "My Husband and I know now," wrote her mother Lillian, "from all the things the doctors didn't say, that Judy should have been operated on when she was fifteen."[49] Having determined that their daughter was undertreated, Judy's parents believed that she needed surgery. About Harrington's procedure, they wrote: "We are interested in your operation because to the laymen's minds it sounds logical and right."[50]

Although Judy's mom said that she did not intend to "criticize any of the physicians" who had treated her daughter, she put Harrington in a difficult spot.[51] Harrington's initial response to Judy and her parents was tentative. "Your daughter, Judy," he opened in his letter, "presents a problem."[52] Namely, her case pit the more junior Dr. Harrington against the more senior Dr. Cobb. Harrington admitted to Judy and her parents that it would be several years before his procedure was considered a viable option within the orthopedic community. With all the caveats, however, Harrington closed the letter by saying that Judy's condition sounded significant enough "to indicate [surgical] stabilization of the spine."[53] In less than a week, Judy's mother replied to Harrington with great enthusiasm, saying that although Harrington's was "comparatively new," it was "not a deterrent."[54]

More letters expressing dissatisfaction with Dr. Cobb followed. In the spring of 1961, a twenty-three-year-old speech therapist from Brooklyn, New York, wrote Harrington to tell him that while she had been going to Dr. Cobb since the age of eleven (when her thoracic curve was first noticed), she wondered if something more could be done.[55] Cobb never prescribed exercises or braces, even when, at the age of twenty-two, she consulted him owing to new symptoms of "numbness and heaviness" in one arm. She asked Cobb about the possibility of performing a spine fusion. He did not recommend surgery, partly because of the length of time that such a treatment required and also because he did not feel the curvature was severe enough. Never really accepting Cobb's recommendation, the speech therapist reached out to Harrington to express "great interest" in his work. "I do not take the thought of an operation lightly," she wrote to Harrington, proving to him that she respected Cobb's noninterventionist stance, "but I am quite serious about undergoing your procedure," she admitted.[56]

Cobb was not the only orthopedic surgeon who believed that nonintervention was often the best course of action. Other physicians in New York City and beyond believed that the treatment for scoliosis was often worse than the condition itself, and that little could be gained from surgery, bracing, or casting.[57] Many scoliosis experts believed that the wait-and-see approach was a kinder and gentler medicine that avoided harmful consequences, even if curvatures became worse. Cobb, in particular, was concerned about the psychological troubles brought about by the "misuse" of braces, casts, devices, and surgery. "When a child is forced to [undergo] treatment of scoliosis," he wrote, "and then does not note any improvement, and is even told that the curve is worse, it may be doing more psychiatric harm than orthopedic good."[58]

But surgeons like Cobb were fast becoming the minority in midcentury America. More and more surgeons became convinced that scoliosis had to be aggressively managed, otherwise the curve would progress and lead to problems of pain and fatigue later in life. Despite a general consensus that curves would progressively worsen, orthopedic surgeons vehemently disagreed about how best to control such a fate. Some experts advocated exercise, whereas others preferred plaster casts. Some insisted on metal braces, and others on surgery. In 1948, when the American Academy of Orthopaedic Surgeons (AAOS) formed a Committee to Study Scoliosis, the committee of experts could not agree on even the most basic of standardized protocols of care. One informant recounted an AAOS scoliosis meeting the following way: "After meeting for some 18 hours, no agreement was reached on any one of the ten major factors in the treatment of scoliosis and only partial agreement was reached in 17 minor issues." Tensions mounted, and at one point the chairman of the committee had to "break up two fist fights before the meeting was adjourned."[59]

Surgeons new to the field of scoliosis complained of mass "confusion" and wondered how they were supposed to provide quality care if even "those who have worked with scoliosis . . . don't agree."[60] This sense of confusion and frustration was felt most, though, by patients and their families who had to negotiate a minefield of inflated egos and conflicting medical advice. One frustrated Indiana father of a fourteen-year-old girl with a 55 degree "S" curve wrote to Harrington about how he and his wife had taken their daughter to three orthopedic specialists in Chicago, but none of them could agree on a course of treatment.[61] Another mother of three young children wrote to Harrington telling him that she had consulted her family doctor, an orthopedist, and her children's pediatrician, seeking each physician's advice on how she should manage her curve. "My family doctor says wait," she wrote to Harrington, "my orthopedic surgeon says waiting will make it worse. "My children's doctor," she continued, "says to do what is best for them and myself and to use my own judgment." Exasperated by the differing opinions, she made a plea to Harrington: "I feel in the middle of a cross-fire. I don't know what to do. . . . Help me."[62]

For every letter that expressed frustrations with undertreatment and bewilderment at differing medical opinions, Harrington received numerous more objecting to overtreatment. Take, for example, the case of eleven-year-old Gregory from New York. In 1955 when Gregory was six, he was taken to Dr. Risser for consultation. At Risser's recommendation, Gregory underwent a fusion operation at Boston Children's Hospital. But the fusion failed. From the time Gregory was eight years old until he was ten, his mother describes how he had spent year after year trying one cast after another, first a Risser jacket, then a "leather brace," and finally a Milwaukee brace. None of it "proved successful," she wrote despairingly. "All this time," she told Harrington, "we received no encouragement about his condition, except that he was not getting worse."[63]

Gregory and his family were not alone. Theresa from Oregon told of her son's treatment for scoliosis, which started when he was two years old, in a full body cast and traction. He remained hospitalized for two years, during which time he was put in a "series of turnbuckle casts." Once his curvature reached 60 degrees when he was nine years old, Theresa was told that the "only thing that could be done was a series of fusions." "Each operation," she writes, "was followed by a year in a body plaster, at the end of which time it would be determined whether or not the fusion had been successful." Eventually when her son reached his teen years, Theresa refused further treatment. "All the plasters . . . had caused serious breakdown of tissue on his back," so that even when her son was prescribed to wear a cast for a year, he could only tolerate it for more than six months.[64]

By the time Theresa read an article in the *Oregonian* newspaper about Harrington, her son was nearing eighteen years of age. "I may never know if my decision to refuse the proposed surgeries was right or wrong," she wrote to Harrington, with a twinge of guilt. But news of Harrington's work, she said, had "given re-birth to a lost hope" that a remedy existed for her son's "very badly twisted spine."[65]

As the Harrington correspondence makes clear, certain people with scoliosis and their families did not oppose operative procedures per se. Barely any of the letters contained in the Harrington correspondence expresses any real fear or resistance concerning anesthesia, mechanical manipulation, or the knife. What patients and their families worried about most was the duration, discomfort, and hardships that came along with the mandatory pre- and postoperative casting and bed rest. Several patients who wrote to Harrington told him that they had foregone surgery when they were young because they (or their parents) found the treatment more punishing than the condition itself. Mary from Maryland wrote, "When my condition was first diagnosed, surgeons told me it would necessitate a year in a New York City hospital." The surgery, Mary recounted, "consisted of three separate stages to move the spine and would mean full-length casts holding [me] in an uncomfortable position between operations." Because of "the expense, discomfort, and unsureness [*sic*] involved," Mary and her family opted out of surgery.[66]

When twenty-year-old Bonnie was told that she needed surgery at the age of fifteen, she felt she had a "vague idea" of what it entailed. But when her family physician took her to the Children's Hospital in Pittsburg to see the orthopedic ward where those who underwent spinal surgery recovered, Bonnie "walked out of there in hysterics." "After seeing the casts and thinking of the 9 months in it," Bonnie told Harrington, "I wouldn't listen to any talk of an operation." She refused treatment, feeling that "the operation would one day be perfected," and that she could wait.[67]

Sixteen-year-old Judy recounted a similar story. Although she had been admitted to the Hospital for Special Surgery in New York City a year prior to her 1961 letter to Harrington, she only "remained in the hospital for one night and then left." "I was always a very athletic person," she told Harrington, "and I didn't think that I could bear the thought of being on my back for a year." "My emotional and psychological state could not have lasted," she admitted.[68]

While some patients expressed concerns about the physical and mental demands that fusion and casting would require, others pointed to the extreme economic burden. The letter that most bluntly addresses this issue is one from Betty, a young twenty-five-year-old housewife from Alabama.[69] Having worn a brace for six years with no correction or relief, Betty's doctor encouraged her to have surgery. She refused for several reasons. Although Betty had medical insurance and knew that the surgeon's fee and hospital bill would be covered, she told Harrington that she could not take six months off (as the Alabama surgeon recommended) from her normal duties as a housewife. A mother of three young children—the oldest four years old and the youngest twelve weeks old—Betty would have had to pay for a housekeeper as well as someone to watch her children during her recovery, costs she could not afford. Moreover, she told Harrington that she did not feel that her children would survive "emotionally" for six months without her.[70]

Whereas Betty worried about the economy of her household, working-class men felt that spinal surgery would jeopardize their employability. Peter, a civil-service employee from New Mexico, told Harrington in a letter that despite having Blue Cross insurance, he could not take off more than two months of work without running the risk of losing his job. Harrington's proposed surgery with its two-to-six weeks convalescence plan seemed a more viable and conducive way for Peter to hold down his job.[71]

Harrington's operative procedure thus appealed to patients who had, up until learning of his metal rod procedure through the media, refused spinal surgery. Patients like Bonnie, Betty, and Paul wrote to Harrington because they believed his type of surgery promised a shorter and more feasible recovery period, which would enable them to maintain their current lifestyles without too much interruption. Harrington felt a deep affinity with these patients. Although in professional publications he made little comment on the bracing systems used by Risser, in his private correspondence he referred to casting as an unnecessary "punishment."[72] In response to Bonnie's description of the scoliosis ward at the Pittsburgh Children's Hospital, Harrington wrote, "It was rather amusing to have you say you looked at the patients and then you walked out in hysterics. This is the usual reaction in people of your age, . . . [it] must have been rather traumatic." Seeing wards of children in full body casts himself, he wrote Bonnie, was "one of the drives that has pushed me to attempt some other type of correction that would be acceptable to patients."[73]

The media picked up on Harrington's anticasting sentiments. Journalistic reports of Harrington's procedure made it seem as if cast wear had become a thing of the past. For example, the opening line of *Time*'s "Spines of Steel" article reads: "Capable of correcting spinal curvature in people up to the age of 40, Dr. Harrington's technique frees patients from the confines of a cast, permits them to lead normal lives during treatment."[74] Although, as I demonstrate above, Harrington had not yet attained his goal of creating a "dynamic correction system," he still held out hope that one day he would.

But scoliosis patients were looking for more than just a quick—or at least a quicker—fix. They were also looking for a medical intervention that could assure good outcomes, since many of the surgical modalities and therapies up to that point often led to disappointing results. When Diane from Ohio asked Harrington, "What percentage of the operations fail?" he responded not with numbers but with a qualification on what surgical success in scoliosis care meant. "There are failures in your sense of the word; that is, they are not as good as we would like to have them and [the curves] do settle [back into place] some."[75] "As far as total failure," he wrote to Diane, "there have been none."[76]

In scoliosis care, though, efficacy was not a universally agreed-on concept among surgeons or patients. Scoliosis specialists knew that complete correction of a spinal curvature was, for the most part, impossible, especially for patients with moderate-to-severe curvatures. This led certain surgeons, such as Cobb, to take a more nihilist stance when it came to therapeutic intervention. Other surgeons felt that they needed to combat curve progression; if they could halt curve progression, then they considered surgery a success. Harrington set his sights slightly higher than most of his colleagues, believing that he could attain, in most cases, a certain measure of correction.

Although Harrington was careful not to boast about the potential efficacy of his procedure in his early professional publications, he freely conveyed great optimism to the patients with whom he corresponded. On public record Harrington insisted that his early studies from the 1950s and early 1960s did "not attempt to study the results [or efficacy] of the instrumentation." Nor, he insisted, were his research findings enough to show when rod surgery was indicated. "Clinical indications for therapy," he wrote in 1962, "are still being worked out."[77] But such caution was rarely articulated when he penned letters to prospective patients. In 1963, Harrington wrote to one patient that the results of his instrumentation for mild back curvatures—curves that would measure up to 20 degrees—were "almost perfect." In moderate curvatures (25–40 degrees), Harrington wrote, the results were "quite good."[78] In yet another letter, Harrington told a potential patient that "all spines that we operate on are better and very rarely are they unsuccessful"[79]

* * *

Harrington's promise of a noticeable and lasting correction appealed to many people with scoliosis, particularly those who wished for cosmetic improvement. The desire to look better—or, as some patients put it, to look "normal" (as was billed in the *Time* article)—was something shared by a majority of the people writing to Harrington. Ted, a thirty-year-old coal miner from Pennsylvania, told Harrington that although his scoliosis "did not give him pain" or preclude him from work, the back curvature nevertheless made him "self-conscious." Ted, in fact, was more the norm than the exception. Early clinical studies demonstrated that 85 percent of those with idiopathic scoliosis did not experience back pain and could engage in the same everyday activities as those without back curvatures.[80] And yet, Ted wrote told Harrington, "I do not go swimming anymore because of how my back looks." Showing his willingness to do anything, no matter the chance of bad results, Ted concluded his letter by saying, "I would gladly take any chance there is if there is any risk in the operation. I would wholeheartedly take any risk whatsoever."[81]

The Harrington correspondence reveals the lengths to which some scoliotics would go to in order to mask their deformity. In an age when ready-to-wear clothing was the norm, many women with curved spines tailored their own clothing, adjusting sleeve and skirt hem lengths, purposely making their clothes uneven so as to correspond to—and thus hide—the bodily asymmetries that lay beneath the fabric. Others learned compensatory walking techniques to cover up lurching leg-length differences or sloping shoulders. Cathy from Los Angeles boasted that after twelve years of back exercises and consciously "walking like a queen," she was now "often taken for a [beauty] model," despite her scoliosis.[82]

Regardless of their ability to pass as "normal," many who had scoliosis thought of themselves as inherently deformed. "*I* know my spine is still shaped like an 'S,'" Cathy from Los Angeles wrote to Harrington, underlining the "I" three times so as to emphasize the highly personal—and painful—truth of her lived experience.[83] With equal clarity, Cathy made her expectations concerning surgery plain to Harrington. "Since there is a minimum of pain involved in my case," she wrote, "and since I have, after a great struggle risen high above the psychological torments that besieged me in my teens, the operation would be useless unless its cosmetic effect were clearly evident."[84]

Even though Harrington did not develop his instrumentation for the explicit purpose of cosmetic correction, many patients came to him for that reason alone.[85] Orthopedic surgeons were ostensibly aware of such patient concerns, for a 1941 study headed up the American Orthopedic Association found that the primary complaint of most scoliosis patients was dissatisfaction with physical appearances. Out of 425 case histories examined, 391 patients—or 92 percent—reported that they sought out medical treatment for the exclusive purpose of cosmetically remedying their curvatures.[86]

At first, Harrington expressed ambivalence about the idea of his instrumentation being used for cosmesis only. In response to an early patient inquiry, Harrington wrote, "my indication for doing this procedure are not for cosmetic results, but for reestablishing stability to the spine in the paralyzed or scoliotic spine."[87] As time went on and he received more and more letters from patients expressing desires for cosmetic improvement, Harrington began to relent. Though as late as 1972 Harrington insisted in print that "the cosmetic effects to be gained by instrumentation of the scoliotic spine must be considered as secondary" and that cosmesis "should not take precedence in the responsible surgeon's judgment," he did not always follow his own advice in practice.[88]

Additionally, from a product viability standpoint, Harrington knew that the patient population for whom he had originally designed his instruments was dwindling. By the mid-1950s, the initial Salk vaccine trails seemed to portend that polio—and thus paralytic scoliosis—would be a disease of the past. Accordingly, polio research funding tapered off during the late 1950s; Harrington received his last year of NFIP funds in 1960. Harrington thus knew that in order for this system to have a chance at becoming a clinical standard of treatment, he would need to apply it to a new, disease-free patient population, one primarily concerned about cosmetic appearance.

Concern for cosmetics should not be taken as merely superficial complaints, nor should Harrington's move to treat this population be seen as simple opportunism. Certain patients conveyed very real worries and psychic pain from their experiences with back curvatures, and Harrington seems to have offered a sympathetic and understanding ear. "I'm becoming a monster to my children," Darlene from Pennsylvania wrote about her physical form.[89] Joanne, who also experienced great shame in her appearance, wanted medical doctors to put as much emphasis on psychic pain as they did physical pain. After a visit to her local orthopedists in Oregon, Joanne wrote Harrington this: "Dr. Chuinard asked me if my condition caused me any great physical pain, and I said that although it does cause me some pain, it wouldn't be described as great." Having a sense that surgeons saw physical pain as a more legitimate complaint than psychological suffering, Joanne proceeded: "However, I wondered why he didn't ask me about emotional distress. I believe this is just as important, if not more important." Recounting her years as a teenager with a curved back, Joanne reminded Harrington that "young people can be cruel . . . you can imagine the comments they had about me."[90]

Women like Joanne—and men like Ted—would have no doubt been routinely physically scrutinized, not just by their peers but also by school, military, and work officials. In midcentury America, posture exams were commonplace. In the nation's elite universities, physical education departments took nude posture photographs of all incoming freshman as part a general health assessment. The military and life insurance agencies also used posture screens to evaluate an individual's level of fitness and assess potential risk for disease and disability. These screens, in turn, bred prejudice and fear of "defective" bodies. To the examiners in charge of such screening, a curve spine raised suspicions of an underlying infectious disease process or, if that was disproven, an innate weakness in an otherwise perfectly healthy population of people.[91] According to one letter, UCLA's teacher program refused to admit a thirty-one-year-old woman after a posture screen revealed her scoliosis.[92] Other patients wrote to Harrington with concerns about losing their jobs, fearing that an employer (or fellow employees) might detect the curvature and deem them—and their bodies—unreliable for the workplace.

Once Harrington made the switch in his practice to operating almost full time on patients with idiopathic scoliosis (rather than polio-induced paralytic scoliosis), and receiving increased media coverage for it, his procedure came to be seen as a way to make deformed spines—and the people with such curvatures—beautiful, straight, and "normal" again. Though he originally devised his instrumentation for severe curvatures in order to stabilize the spines of those with disease-based scoliosis, he decided by the mid-1960s that his instruments had their most "specific application" in mild-to-moderate forms of adolescent idiopathic scoliosis.[93] At the same time, he refused to operate on curvatures of 90 degrees or over, since "above 90 degrees was felt to be in the nature of a salvage, rather than a treatment, procedure."[94] Operating on a younger, healthy, and less-effected population of scoliotics, Harrington began to get, rather predictably, better surgical success rates, with curvature corrections of up to 50 percent and more. With numbers like these, even the most skeptical colleagues began to see the virtues of Harrington's rod technique.

* * *

The Harrington correspondence offers a window into how those with scoliosis sought out information concerning risk, compared different surgical options, and assessed the value of what Harrington had to offer, especially regarding the emotional and financial costs that one incurs when undergoing surgery. Looking at the process of surgical innovation through letters such as these demonstrates how patients can play a critical role in the diffusion, adoption, and success of certain surgical technologies over other alternatives.

Of course surgical systems cannot be understood without first understanding the contingencies of how and why certain somatic aberrations become defined as surgical problems in the first place. The nature of scoliosis changed dramatically over the course of the first three-quarters of the twentieth century, shifting from a second-order, disease-based condition (a sequale of various acute disease processes) to a first-order disability, a physical "defect" according to the socially constructed norms that equated symmetry, physical uprightness, and alignment with beauty and health. As cosmesis became the primary motive for the medical management of scoliosis in postwar America, surgical success became defined more and more by patients. In her book on the history of cosmetic surgery, Elizabeth Haiken rightly points out that when it comes to the surgical management of beauty, "authority derives as much from the patient . . . and consumer culture . . . as from the surgeon."[95] Whereas surgeons tended to trust x-ray images to determine progress, patients measured success by nonquantitative and highly personalized metrics, such as how well the surgery improved one's self-image or the ability to mask the curvature from the gaze of others.

In the decades following his *Time* magazine debut, Harrington went on to enjoy a career of professional accolades and awards, despite perennial glitches in his surgical system and reports of disgruntled patients who had undergone the procedure only to regret it.[96] The resistance to his system (among other surgeons as well as among patients) never gained much traction, for Harrington's procedure complemented changes already happening on various levels of American culture and the healthcare system. Harrington's promise of a speedy recovery satisfied hospital administrators and insurance companies who urged shorter hospital stays, as well as leaders in the orthopedic profession who wanted to finally shed the old "strap and buckle" bracemaker identity of the field.

Harrington's technique also fit into a growing willingness among Americans to undergo open operations to cure, fix, and ameliorate a whole host of diseases and so-called defects, despite the inherent risks associated with surgery.[97] Health-policy analysts began to take note of America's culture of "surgical enthusiasm" in the late 1960s when operation rates in the United States exceeded those in most European countries.[98] Why America's surgical culture differs from that of other countries requires further study. Although it is tempting to fall back on the trope of "knife-happy" Americans as a possible explanation, this paper demonstrates that patients had more nuanced views when it came to surgical options. The Harrington correspondence shows, perhaps counterintuitively, that certain people with scoliosis found open operations less invasive and more conservative—in terms of money, time, and physical energy—than closed operations such as casting and other medico-surgical alternatives.

A few lone voices challenged the need to medically manage scoliosis in postwar America. Based on preliminary studies on the natural history of the condition—research that was, and still is, not readily funded or encouraged—a handful of orthopedists claimed that a curved back did not significantly compromise one's morbidity or mortality, which, in effect undermined the assumption that scoliosis was a disability requiring a surgical fix in the first place.[99] These early natural history studies relied, of course, on a small population of people with scoliosis who refused medical interventions such as Harrington's surgery. Although a few pockets of resistance against operative management of scoliosis existed, "modern" scoliosis treatment in postwar America became ever more synonymous with Harrington's rod technique as the century progressed. Billed as a "spines of steel" system, Harrington offered a vision in which orthopedic surgeons could straighten backs with steel so as to ameliorate a new population of scoliosis patients, many of whom, though disease free, felt unwell and deeply stigmatized.

Notes

Research for this article was generously funded by the Pearce Fellowship in the History of Medicine at the University of Kansas Medical Center (KUMC), where the Paul R. Harrington Archives are housed. I wish to thank the KUMC faculty and staff, especially Dr. Marc A. Asher, Nancy Hulston, Dr. Christopher Crenner, and Dr. Douglas C. Burton for their guidance and support. This article also benefited from the feedback of the fellow participants of the Asher Symposium on Innovation in Surgery. Nathan Ensmenger, Naomi Rogers, and Dominique Tobbell provided invaluable comments and research tips. Elaine LaFay offered shrewd research assistance in the final stages of the piece.

1. "Spines of Steel," *Time*, November 14, 1960, 56.

2. The secondary-source literature on Harrington is scant. Dr. Marc Asher at the University of Kansas, who helps oversee the Paul R. Harrington Archives (HA), has the most comprehensive understanding of the man and his work. See Asher, *Dogged Persistence: Harrington, Post-Polio Scoliosis, and the Origin of Spinal Instrumentation* (Traverse City, MI: Chandler Lake Books, 2015). See also Marc A. Asher and Douglas C. Burton, "Reflection: Paul Randall Harrington (1911–1980)," *Journal of Bone & Joint Surgery* 93, no. 24 (2011): e151.

3. The clinical definition of "severe" scoliosis is not a static concept, as it is dependent on who is doing the defining (patient or physician) and which, if any, diagnostic technologies are deployed. In the 1940s, the American Orthopedic Association defined severe scoliosis as any curve greater than 45 degrees (the angle of curvature is usually determined through a basic geometric measure using x-ray imagery), with mild defined as any curve up to 20 degrees, and moderate as a 25–45 degree angle. Today severe scoliosis is customarily defined as any curvature over 60 degrees. For the importance of diagnostic visuals to twentieth-century surgery, see David S. Jones, "Visions of a Cure: Visualization, Clinical Trials, and Controversies in Cardiac Therapeutics, 1968–1998," *Isis* 91, no. 3 (2000): 504–41.

4. John Dove, "Evolution of Spinal Surgery," in *The Evolution of Orthopaedic Surgery*, ed. Leslie Klenerman (Boca Roton, FL: CRC Press, 2002): 159–66.

5. Kathleen Y. Moen and Alf L. Nachemson, "Treatment of Scoliosis: An Historical Perspective," *Spine* 24, no. 24 (1999): 2572.

6. A. R. Shands et al., "End-Result Study of the Treatment of Idiopathic Scoliosis: Report of the Research Committee of the American Orthopaedic Association," *Journal of Bone & Joint Surgery* 23, no. 4 (1941): 964.

7. Ibid., 970.

8. Carmelita Calderwood, "Structural Scoliosis: Nursing Care," *The American Journal of Nursing* 41, no. 12 (1941): 1403–10.

9. Russel A. Hibbs, Joseph C. Risser, and Albert B. Ferguson, "Scoliosis Treated by the Fusion Operations: An End-Result Study of Three Hundred and Sixty Cases," *Journal of Bone & Joint Surgery* 13, no. 1 (1931): 91–104. For risks of cardiac surgery early in the twentieth century, see David S. Jones, *Broken Hearts: The Tangled History of Cardiac Care* (Baltimore: Johns Hopkins University Press, 2013). During the 1960s, Jones writes, the "operative morality rate of 15–35 percent remained common and tolerated" (123).

10. Moen and Nachemson, "Treatment of Scoliosis," 2572.

11. Robert J. Cook, "Report of the Orthopædic Examination of 1393 Freshmen at Yale University," *Journal of Bone & Joint Surgery* 4, no. 2 (1922): 247–65. A. R. Shands, Jr. and Harry B. Eisberg, "The Incidence of Scoliosis in the State of Delaware: A Study of 50,000 Minifilms of the Chest Made during a Survey for Tuberculosis," *Journal of Bone & Joint Surgery* 37 (1955): 1243–49.

12. Beth Linker, "A Dangerous Curve: The Role of History in America's Scoliosis Screening Programs," *American Journal of Public Health* 102, no. 4 (2012): 606–16.

13. In recent years, historians of technology have urged a more user-centered approach to understanding innovation. One of the most ambitious works that exemplifies this approach is David Edgerton, *The Shock of the Old: Technology and Global History since 1900* (London: Profile Books, 2006). A handful of medical historians have also been attentive to the role that patients play in technological innovation, specifically in the history of pharmaceuticals. For only a few examples, see Andrea Tone, *The Age of Anxiety: A History of America's Turbulent Affair with Tranquilizers* (New York: Basic Books, 2008); Elizabeth Siegel Watkins, *On the Pill: A Social History of Oral Contraceptives, 1950–1970* (Baltimore: Johns Hopkins University Press, 2011); and Dominique Tobbell, "Charitable Innovations: The Political Economy of Thalassemia Research and Drug Development in the United States, 1960–2000," in *Perspectives on Twentieth Century Pharmaceuticals*, ed. Judy Slinn and Vivianne Quirke (Bern: Peter Lang, 2009).

14. Bruno Latour, *Reassembling the Social: An Introduction to Actor-Network-Theory* (Oxford: Oxford University Press, 2005). For more examples in realtion to surgery, see Thomas Schlich, *Surgery, Science and Industry: A Revolution in Fracture Care, 1950s–1990s* (New York: Palgrave MacMillan, 2002); Alex Faulkner, "Casing the Joint: The Material Development of Artificial Hips," in *Artificial Parts, Practical Lives: Modern History of Prosthetics*, ed. Katherine Ott, David Serlin, and Stephen Mihm (New York: New York University Press, 2002), 199–226; and Julie Anderson, Francis Neary, and John V. Pickstone, *Surgeons, Manufacturers and Patients: A Transatlantic History of Total Hip Replacement* (New York: Palgrave Macmillan, 2007).

15. For privacy and protection, I have de-identified letter writers throughout this essay. In citations I also removed the letter writers' cities of origin, but retained the state of origin.

16. On the historical process of how patients became "consumers" during the first half of the twentieth century, see Nancy Tomes, "Merchants of Health: Medicine and Consumer Culture in the United States, 1900–1940," *Journal of American History* (2001): 519–47.

17. Eric Schatzberg's study on the shift from wood-based to steel-structure aircraft during the interwar period demonstrates that although steel aircraft were not demonstrably "better," given the accepted metrics of the time, Air Corp leaders nevertheless preferred steel because it signified modernity. Harrington's use of steel demonstrates similar cultural work, as evidenced by *Time*'s coverage and other media reports. See Schatzberg, *Wings of Wood, Wings of Metal: Culture and Technical Choice in American Airplane Materials, 1914–1945* (Princeton, NJ: Princeton University Press, 1999). Of course, steel spines also touches on the fascination with cybernetics in postwar America. See Ronald Kline, "Where are the Cyborgs in Cybernetics?," *Social Studies of Science* 39, no. 3 (2009): 331–62; Donna J. Haraway, *Simians, Cyborgs, and Women: The Reinvention of Nature* (New York: Routledge, 2013); and David Serlin,

Replaceable You: Engineering the Body in Postwar America (Chicago: University of Chicago Press, 2004).

18. There are several good twentieth-century histories of polio in the United States. See, for example, Naomi Rogers, *Polio Wars: Sister Elizabeth Kenny and the Golden Age of American Medicine* (New York: Oxford University Press, 2014); Naomi Rogers, *Dirt and Disease: Polio before FDR* (New Brunswick, NJ: Rutgers University Press, 1992); and Daniel J. Wilson, *Living with Polio: The Epidemic and Its Survivors* (Chicago: University of Chicago Press, 2005).

19. Heather Green Wooten, *The Polio Years in Texas: Battling a Terrifying Unknown* (College Station: Texas A&M University Press, 2009), 76.

20. Southwestern would later be renamed again to become the Texas Institute for Rehabilitation and Research.

21. Wooten, *Polio Years in Texas,* 110.

22. "Time in Hospital Cut by Computers," *New York Times,* July 21, 1963, 49.

23. William A. Spencer and Carlos Vallbona, "Applications of Computers in Clinical Practice," *Journal of the American Medical Association* 191, no. 11 (1965): 917–21.

24. Daniel J. Wilson, "And They Shall Walk: Ideal versus Reality in Polio Rehabilitation in the United States," *Asclepio* 61, no. 1 (2009): 175–92. Bess Williamson also makes this point about the importance of standing and ambulation in "Electric Moms and Quad Drivers: People with Disabilities Buying, Making, and Using Technology in Postwar America," *American Studies* 52, no. 1 (2012): 12.

25. Paul R. Harrington, "Standing Bed in Poliomyelitis," *The Physical Therapy Review* 32, no. 13 (1952): 1–3.

26. Ibid.

27. Joseph C. Risser, "Treatment of Scoliosis during the Past 50 Years," *Clinical Orthopaedics and Related Research* 44 (February 1966): 109–13; M. M. Manring and Jason Calhoun, "Joseph C. Risser Sr., 1892–1982," *Clinical Orthopaedics and Related Research* 468, no. 3 (2010): 643–45.

28. See "Happy Girl," *Los Angeles Times,* November 5, 1955; and "Months in Casts," *Los Angeles Times,* October 3, 1952, 32.

29. Wooten, *Polio Years in Texas,* 122. Southwestern became a leader in research studies concerning the physiology of respiration and heart function—the medical team was responsible for developing the physiograph, a heart and lung monitor that would go on to become a commonplace device at every hospital bedside.

30. Paul R. Harrington, "The History and Development of Harrington Instrumentation," *Clinical Orthopaedics and Related Research* 227 (1988): 3; and Asher, *Dogged Persistence,* 238.

31. For tire jack imagery, see Dr. Andrew J. Ryan, Houston, Texas, to D.K.B., New York, November 4, 1960, in "Time Article, 1960, Patient Inquiries," Paul R. Harrington Archives (HA), University of Kansas Medical Center, Kansas City, Kansas (hereafter TPI/HA).

32. F. G. Allan, "Scoliosis: Operative Correction of Fixed Curves," *Journal of Bone & Joint Surgery* 37, no. 1 (1955): 92–96.

33. Schatzberg, *Wings of Wood.* Postwar orthopedic surgery can be seen as participating in the technological rationalization of social life. Indeed, orthopedic surgery's midcentury attempt to fortify all parts of the body with steel could be seen

as one of the best examples of Weber's *stahlhartes Gehäuse* (shell as hard as steel) reified, an idea turned into material reality. Peter Baehr, "The 'Iron Cage' and the 'Shell as Hard as Steel': Parsons, Weber, and the Stahlhartes Gehäuse Metaphor in the Protestant Ethic and the Spirit of Capitalism," *History and Theory* 40, no. 2 (2001): 153–69. For more on the history of hip replacements and internal fixations of fractures, see Anderson, Neary, and Pickstone, *Surgeons, Manufacturers and Patient*; Faulkner, "Casing the Joint"; and Schlich, *Surgery, Science and Industry*.

34. Paul R. Harrington, "Treatment of Scoliosis: Correction and Internal Fixation by Spinal Instrumentation," *Journal of Bone & Joint Surgery* [*Am*] 44 (1962): 592–610.

35. Ibid.

36. "Harrington, Paul Randall," *Who's Who in Orthopedics*, ed. Seyed Behrooz Mostofi (London: Springer, 2005), 124–25. See also Harrington, "History and Development," 110.

37. Harrington, "Treatment of Scoliosis," 592. Despite improved results from the instrumentation, Harrington encountered other complications including "disengagement of the purchasing hooks" and bone erosion at the site where the hooks gained purchase. Harrington admitted that the distraction hook is "the weakest feature of the whole procedure" (604).

38. Harrington, "History and Development," 111.

39. Ibid., 110.

40. At Zimmer's encouragement, Harrington crafted pamphlets and wrote an entire script for a film that was used to instruct surgeons step-by-ste, through the process of applying his hook and rod system. Part of the agreement that Harrington struck with Zimmer was that no surgeon was "permitted to purchase instruments or to use them without first having observed a demonstration of the procedure, a prerequisite that was carried on for approximately two years" (Harrington, "History and Development," 112). Harrington sealed lasting relationships and product loyalty among fellow orthopedists across the country by making personalized visits to demonstrate his operative technique.

41. In one 1957 letter that he penned to Zimmer Manufacturing, Harrington recounted how, when he attended the Fourth International Poliomyelitis Congress in Geneva, Switzerland, to present his work, his blueprints along with a full prototype set of instruments were stolen. Showing how Cold War politics insinuated itself into even the most obscure medical specialties, Harrington wrote that he was "suspicious of the Russians." Paul R. Harrington, Baylor University, to Mr. James P. Keeton, Chief Engineer, Zimmer Manufacturing Company, Warsaw, Indiana, September 12, 1957, box HA 124, file 1/10/1957–11/18/1957, TPI/HA.

42. This article is referenced in several letters to Harrington. I have yet to find the original article. Some of what Walsh said can be deduced from the various Associated Press versions of the story. See, for instance, "Houston Surgeon Now Corrects Curved Spines with Steel Rods," *Corsicana Daily Sun*, October 20, 1960, 26, www.newspapers.com/image/12749819 (accessed August 9, 2014).

43. "How I would love to have my spine jacked into place," wrote "Wanda" G.M.C, California, to P. R. Harrington, Houston, Texas, November 9, 1960, in "Time Article, 1960, Patient Inquiries," TPI/HA.

44. Ibid.

45. Ibid.

46. John R. Cobb, "Scoliosis—Quo Vadis?," *Journal of Bone & Joint Surgery* 40, no. 3 (1958): 507–10.

47. Ibid., 507.

48. Ibid., 510.

49. L.G.R., New Jersey, to P. R. Harrington, Houston, Texas, January 15, 1961, TPI/HA.

50. Ibid.

51. Ibid.

52. P. R. Harrington to L.G.R, New Jersey, February 2, 1961, TPI/HA.

53. And after seeing Judy's x-rays, Harrington told the mother that he could "straighten [Judy's] spine considerably by using his spine instrumentation procedure." Ibid.

54. L.G.R., New Jersey, to P. R. Harrington, Houston, Texas, February, 8, 1961, TPI/HA. Emphasis in the original.

55. L.W.D., New York, to P. R. Harrington, Houston, Texas, n.d., TPI/HA. See also a letter from Dr. Frederick R. Thompson concerning a thirty-four-year-old Long Island man (clerical worker) who had been under Cobb's medical supervision since he was thirteen years old and sought out Dr. Thomspon for surgical treatment. Dr. Frederick R. Thompson, New York, New York, to P. R. Harrington, February 18, 1961, TPI/HA.

56. L.W.D., New York, to P. R. Harrington, Houston, Texas, n.d.

57. See, for example, Dennis K. Collis and Ignacio V. Ponseti, "Long-Term Follow-Up of Patients with Idiopathic Scoliosis Not Treated Surgically," *Journal of Bone & Joint Surgery (Am)* 51, no. 3 (1969): 425–45. Henry O. Kendall and Florence P. Kendall, "Developing and Maintaining Good Posture," *Physical Therapy* 48, no. 4 (1968): 319; and Moen and Nachemson, "Treatment of Scoliosis," 2574.

58. Cobb, "Scoliosis—Quo Vadis?," 510.

59. Asher, *Dogged Persistence*, 17–18.

60. Cobb, "Scoliosis—Quo Vadis?," 507.

61. C. D. W., Indiana, to P. R. Harrington, Houston, Texas, October 23, 1960, TPI/HA.

62. B.F.D., Alabama, to P. R. Harrington, Houston, Texas, n.d., TPI/HA.

63. M.E.U, New York, to P. R. Harrington, Houston, Texas, October 18, 1960, TPI/HA.

64. T.R.T, Oregon, to P. R. Harrington, Houston, Texas, May 7, 1965, TPI/HA.

65. Ibid.

66. M.W.R, Maryland, to P. R. Harrington, Houston Texas, January 4, 1961, TPI/HA. Mary also tells Harrington that she has "no pain or discomfort." But that "naturally being female and comparatively young, I would give almost everything I have to be like other women, and could enjoy the wearing of stylish clothes."

67. M.B.A., Pennsylvania, to P. R. Harrington, Houston, Texas, October 24, 1960, TPI/HA.

68. J.F., New York, to P. R. Harrington, Houston, Texas, September 25, 1961, TPI/HA.

69. B.F.D., Alabama, to P. R. Harrington, Houston, Texas, n.d., TPI/HA.

70. Ibid.

71. M.P.M, Texas, to P. R. Harrington, Houston, Texas, November 14, 1960, TPI/HA.

72. W.W., New York, to P. R. Harrington, Houston, Texas, November 22, 1960, TPI/HA.

73. Paul R. Harrington, Houston, Texas, to M.B.A., Pennsylvania, December 23, 1960, TPI/HA.

74. "Spines of Steel," 56.

75. P. R. Harrington, Houston, Texas, to A.C.H., Ohio, April 9, 1963, TPI/HA.

76. Ibid.

77. Harrington, "Treatment of Scoliosis," 607, 599.

78. Paul R. Harrington, Houston, Texas, to L.W.B., California, November 2, 1960, TPI/HA. For more on how clinicians at the time defined mild, moderate, and severe, see note 3 above.

79. Paul R. Harrington, Houston, Texas, to B.W., Texas, November 7, 1963, TPI/HA.

80. Shands et al., "End-Result Study," 977.

81. E.S., Pennslyvania, to Paul R. Harrington, Houston, Texas, October 23, 1960, TPI/HA.

82. C.R., California, to Paul R. Harrington, Houston, Texas, n.d., TPI/HA.

83. Ibid.

84. Ibid.

85. In her book *Venus Envy*, the historian Elizabeth Haiken shows that the psychological condition known as the "inferiority complex" was discussed quite frequently in women's magazines at the time and fueled the medicalization of cosmetic sugery. See Haiken, *Venus Envy: A History of Cosmetic Surgery* (Baltimore: Johns Hopkins University Press, 1997).

86. Shands et al., "End-Result Study," 964.

87. Paul R. Harrington, Houston, Texas, to A.M.C., Florida, October 31, 1960, TPI/HA.

88. Paul R. Harrington, "Technical Details in Relation to the Successful Use of Instrumentation in Scoliosis," *Orthopedic Clinics of North America* 3 (1972): 50.

89. D. K., Pennsylvania, to P. R. Harrington, Houston, Texas, December 3, 1960, TPI/HA.

90. J. K., Oregon, to P. R. Harrington, Houston, Texas, July 28, 1965, TPI/HA.

91. For more on heighten body surveillance practices in the twentieth century, see Linker, "Dangerous Curve."

92. M.L.B., California, to P. R. Harrington, Houston, Texas, November 4, 1960, TPI/HA.

93. Harrington, "Spinal Fusion," 470.

94. P. R. Harrington and J. H. Dickson, "An Eleven-Year Clinical Investigation of Harrington Instrumentation: A Preliminary Report of 578 Cases," *Clinical Orthopaedics and Related Research* 93 (1973): 113–30, 114.

95. Haiken, *Venus Envy*, 7.

96. In 1973, the Association for Bone and Joint Surgeons awarded Harrington the Nicolas Andry Award, an honor named after an eighteenth-century French physician who coined the term *orthopaedia* (a word that combines the Greek roots *orthos*—"straight," and *pais*—"a child"). For patient complaints about the rod system, see Edmund J. Sass, *Polio's Legacy: An Oral History* (Lanham, MD: University Press of America, 1996).

97. See Haiken, *Venus Envy*; as well as Robert A. Aronowitz, *Unnatural History: Breast Cancer and American Society* (New York: Cambridge University Press, 2007); and Barron H. Lerner, *The Breast Cancer Wars: Hope, Fear, and the Pursuit of a Cure in Twentieth-Century America* (New York: Oxford University Press, 2001).

98. John, R., C. Pearson, Björn Smedby, Ragnar Berfenstam, Robert F. L. Logan, Alex M. Burgess, and Osler L. Peterson, "Hospital Caseloads In Liverpool, New England, and Uppsala," *Lancet* 292, no. 7567 (1968): 559–66.

99. Collis and Ponseti, "Long-Term Follow-Up of Patients."

Chapter Six

Disruptive Potential

The "Landmark" REMATCH Trial, Left Ventricular Assist Device (LVAD) Technology, and the Surgical Treatment of Heart Failure in the United States

SHELLEY MCKELLAR

> "The [REMATCH] trial was analogous to randomizing Titanic patients to a lifeboat or the sea."
>
> —Cardiac surgeon Stephen Westaby

Heart failure is a progressive, life-threatening condition that affects an estimated twenty-six million people worldwide, including 5.8 million Americans.[1] For the patient in heart failure, their heart is simply not pumping blood as it should, and most die within five years after diagnosis owing to complications arising from poor or inadequate blood flow (such as organ failure) or from contracting infections in their weakened condition (such as pneumonia).[2] The problem may be a case of left-sided heart failure (most common), right-sided heart failure, or both. The heart-failure patient may feel extreme fatigue, a shortness of breath, and possibly an increased heart rate, which will make everyday activities like walking and climbing stairs increasingly difficult. As the condition worsens, the patient experiences a buildup of fluid in the feet, ankles, and legs (edema), a congestion of blood in the lungs, perhaps memory problems, and even impaired thinking.[3] There is no cure for heart failure. As one physician commented, "Heart failure is a lethal disease with a worse life expectancy than many types of cancer."[4]

In the United States, heart failure is among the most costly cardiovascular disorders owing to its intensive use of medical resources, including lengthy hospital stays and expensive medications. The number of new cases of heart failure increases with patient age, and with the rising number of elderly people in the United States, a greater proportion of the American population suffers from heart failure each decade. In 2013, the direct and indirect costs of caring for the heart-failure patient in the United States, including hospitalization and medications, is about $31 billion, and this number is expected to more than double by 2030.[5] More people are surviving heart attacks and other cardiac conditions, perhaps because of more successful therapies or better education about heart disease. This means that people are living longer with damaged hearts and thus carry the risk of heart failure. To be clear, mortality rates from coronary heart disease have been declining since the 1960s yet it still remains the leading cause of death in many developed countries.[6] Various medical and epidemiological studies report that heart failure in the United States is most common in older people (age sixty-five and older), African Americans, overweight individuals, and previous heart attack patients. As well, more men than women battle this condition.[7] Medical researchers point to coronary artery disease, high blood pressure, and diabetes as the common causes leading to heart failure.[8] Medical practitioners thus aim to treat these underlying causes toward relieving symptoms and improving the quality of life for their heart-failure patients.

The two primary treatment options for heart-failure patients are drug therapy, to arrest disease progression and treat symptoms, and cardiac transplantation, to replace the failing and damaged heart. For those patients in severe heart failure, cardiac transplantation remains the gold-standard treatment when medications no longer adequately manage their condition. But with roughly 2,200 heart transplants performed each year in the United States, there are not enough donor hearts available for the estimated 100,000 transplant-eligible patients.[9] Other surgical options for mild-to-moderate heart failure include coronary revascularization, valve surgery, intra-aortic balloon counterpulsation, or various cardiac remodeling procedures to stop further cardiac damage and to improve heart function. Initially heart-failure patients treat their condition with multiple medications, with vasodilator drugs and angiotension-converting enzyme (ACE) inhibitors as the cornerstone of medical therapy for this condition.[10] Inotropic drugs to increase heart muscle contractions, beta-adrenergic blocking agents to improve blood flow, as well as some antiarrhythmic agents to suppress irregular heart rhythms are additional medications used in the treatment of heart failure.[11] Designed to arrest disease progression and treat heart failure symptoms, most cardiac drugs are much less effective in advanced heart failure cases. For patients facing imminent death, a replacement of badly damaged hearts can be done either through cardiac transplantation or mechanical means. Some cardiac surgeons have declared cardiac transplantation as "epidemiologically trivial" because of the limited availability of donor hearts.[12] During the 1990s, mechanical circulatory support, notably left ventricular assist device (LVAD) technology, emerged as a viable alternative therapy to address both the donor shortage for heart-failure patients on waiting lists as well as the desire to treat those patients ineligible for cardiac transplantation.

The development of LVAD technology for long-term mechanical circulatory support began in the 1970s when the US National Heart, Lung and Blood Institute (NHLBI) funded collaborative university-industry teams with large, renewable research contracts. The NHLBI's decision to fund this targeted research emerged from the aim of the US Artificial Heart Program, established in 1964, to build a range of mechanical circulatory support systems (MCSS) for different heart-failure patient needs. In the 1960s, the cardiac surgeon Michael DeBakey's clinical success with the short-term use of mechanical pumps in patients suffering from acute heart failure after cardiac surgery encouraged MCSS researchers to improve device function and reliability for longer-term use.[13] In the 1970s, LVAD technology was intentionally conceptualized as a long-term and permanent, rather than short-term and temporary, therapy to combat heart failure. NHLBI funding supported the development of implantable LVADs designed for a two-year lifetime.[14] Dismal outcomes with heart transplantation at the time bolstered the development of LVAD technology as an alternative to biological replacement of the heart owing to the inherent problems of cardiac transplantation, namely, organ rejection risks, complications of immunosuppression, and poor donor heart supply.[15]

During the 1980s, the introduction of the immunosuppressive drug cyclosporine contributed to improved cardiac transplant outcomes, establishing heart transplantation as the best treatment for end-stage heart failure. This development forged a new role for LVAD technology as a bridge-to-transplantation device for patients waiting for a donor heart. By the early 1990s, the US Food and Drug Administration (FDA) and US Centers for Medicare and Medicaid Services (CMS) awarded regulatory approval and reimbursement for LVADs as bridge-to-transplantation devices. The success and limitations of cardiac transplantation stimulated research on LVAD technology as a permanent therapy for heart-failure patients. The success of transplantation forged scientific legitimacy and public enthusiasm for heart replacement overall. In this period, as David Jones describes with myocardial revascularization elsewhere in this volume, the ambitious pursuit of surgical reengineering and rebuilding the body, which included tinkering with the once-deemed "off-limits" heart, held widespread appeal. The limited supply of donor organs supported the alternative approach of "off-the-shelf" mechanical circulatory support devices for heart replacement. Could LVAD implants secure a "therapeutic niche" in the treatment of heart failure similar to the case of coronary revascularization, as argued by Jones?[16] The positive outcomes of patients using LVADs as bridge-to-transplantation devices encouraged LVAD researchers to promote the longer-term use of these devices, targeting those heart-failure patients ineligible for cardiac transplantation. Driven by the clinical promise of these devices and the need to provide convincing pro-device data, LVAD investigators proposed comparing the use of LVADs against the optimal drug therapy (not cardiac transplantation) in transplant-ineligible heart-failure patients through a clinical trial, named the Randomized Evaluation of Mechanical Assistance for the Treatment of Congestive Heart Failure (REMATCH) study.

This paper focuses on the much-lauded "landmark" REMATCH study and its results, published in 2001 in the prestigious *New England Journal of Medicine*, as a key turning point in the scientific and technological achievement of LVADs and the validity of permanently implanting mechanical pumps as "destination therapy," a distinction marked by certain ominous implications within the guise of reassuring assessment. It focuses exclusively on discussions and debates aired in the medical literature among device researchers and clinicians involved in the management of heart-failure patients. This paper examines the reporting of the REMATCH study results by its investigators and the "landmark" praise and rhetoric assigned to the clinical trial within the medical community. It reveals the extent to which the REMATCH study results positioned LVADs as a desirable therapy for heart-failure patients, which then fueled support for extending the clinical indications for implanting LVADs.[17] It seemed poised to be a legitimizing moment for LVAD technology. On the one hand, the REMATCH study demonstrated that large randomized, controlled trials in cardiac surgery were doable, rigorous, and convincing. This was important for LVAD technology specifically and cardiac surgery in general. Long relegated as somewhat fanciful devices, mechanical circulatory support technology sought clinical acceptance alongside pacemakers, stents, and other cardiac devices as a transformative means by which to restore heart function. Positive clinical trial results promised to offer greater legitimacy to these devices, as well as to surgical innovations more broadly. On the other hand, LVAD technology was seductive and extraordinary: could a mechanical heart truly replace or assist a dying native heart? The REMATCH study results appeared to bolster the allure of technological fixes in Western medicine, while also adding to the quandaries raised in deciding to use new technologies, as described by Renee C. Fox and Judith P. Swazey, Stuart Blume, and David Jones, among others.[18] It contributed to the transplant imaginary surrounding organ replacement, as described by the scholars Susan Lederer, Thomas Schlich, and Lesley Sharp.[19] REMATCH study results that supported LVAD implantation promised to stabilize the use of this device for an evidence-based medical community and technology-enamored society.

As momentum in support of these devices grew, LVADs appeared poised as a possible "disruptive technology," a concept introduced by the Harvard Business School professor Clayton M. Christensen in the mid-1990s to describe innovative but imperfect new technology that displaces an established procedure.[20] In reality, LVAD technology evoked a "disruptive potential" rather than complete disruption after the initial reporting of study results and the "landmark" rhetoric that followed. In the medical community, the REMATCH study situated LVAD technology much more convincingly as a legitimate alternative to the conventional medical and surgical treatment for end-stage heart-failure patients, but clinical uptake was sluggish at best. The "landmark" rhetoric was not employed by all physicians, some of whom advocated a more tempered, cautious view of the REMATCH study results. In the end, LVADs did not displace optimal drug therapy or cardiac transplantation for end-stage heart-failure patients at this time. Certainly the results of the REMATCH study muddled, if not outwardly challenged, traditional medical views of LVAD technology as "last resort" therapy or limited temporary devices. But the technological limitations of LVADs still lingered, which sustained the more prudent course for its use.

RCTs in Surgery: The REMATCH Study

The randomized clinical trial (RCT) is the revered standard in evidence-based medicine for evaluating new therapies. It is an experimental study conducted on clinical patients, where the investigator controls an intervention through random assignment while blinding the physician or patient or both to the assigned treatment to eliminate biased measurement. This experimental design is meant to offer clinically meaningful results; that is, offer strong cause-and-effect conclusions about the safety and efficacy of new therapies, often in direct comparison with older treatments. Dating from antibiotic research during World War II, RCTs aimed to replace traditional methods of evaluation, such as retrospective case studies, by producing objective, rigorous data of therapeutic efficacy of new drugs, devices, or procedures in medicine. Was a new treatment better than an older one? Could RCT evidence change conventional knowledge and improve clinical practice with the adoption of new therapies? The RCT sought to remove uncertainty surrounding novel treatments; however, as the medical historian Harry Marks and others have demonstrated, RCTs did not always provide convincing data or resolve therapeutic controversy.[21]

But is the use of RCTs to evaluate surgical interventions even feasible or arguably better than other experimental and observational studies? In this volume, Christopher Crenner shows how postwar use of controlled clinical trials in surgery emerged out of the field's interest in evaluating new procedures and their therapeutic effects beyond the traditional case series study. Focusing on the controversial use of sham surgery, Crenner shows how placebo-controlled studies exposed subjective patient experiences and the flawed value of two popular surgical procedures: internal mammary artery ligation and gastric freezing. Measuring surgical success beyond the conventional case series to the broader-sanctioned clinical trial in medical research suggested progress, less bias, and more accurate evidence of therapeutic value, according to RCT proponents. But as Crenner states, it is not "a straightforward history" of clinical trial data supplanting traditional case series evidence in surgery; the use of RCTs in surgery was "contested and slow."[22]

Many surgical-researchers resisted clinical trials for good reasons.[23] They were expensive, difficult to conduct, and as some surgeons argued, there are fundamental differences between testing drugs and evaluating new surgical procedures or technology. In surgery, there were simply too many variables to control in order to offer objective results. Surgeons held varying skills, operated in various institutional centers, and faced unique patient cases despite similar diagnoses. Double-blinding the surgeon and patient was not always feasible, and any random assignment might possibly be unethical when assigning experimental treatments to life-threatening illnesses. Unlike drug trials, surgical procedures or technologies tend to undergo refinement during the course of a study, resulting in improved outcomes in the later operations in comparison with early operations. When comparing a surgical intervention with a nonsurgical treatment, both surgeon and patient will likely know the treatment assignment, and this in turn may shape outcome expectations and perhaps bias results. When it comes to heart surgery specifically, the life-threatening and urgent situations of cardiac patients may challenge cooperation, as very ill patients may not wish their treatment to be decided by chance or be comfortable with the irreversibility of some surgical options.

Debates about the best cardiac therapies—both surgical and medical treatments—abounded in the 1970s and 1980s. The medical historian David Jones describes the fierce controversy among physicians over the efficacy of coronary artery bypass grafting (CABG) that was not settled by RCTs in these decades.[24] Still RCTs in surgery need not be dismissed, according to Jones, who acknowledges the entrenchment of the traditional surgical research methods of animal experiments, case reports, and case series to evaluate new procedures.[25] Yet as regulatory bodies tasked with granting market approval and reimbursement of new medical devices, such as the FDA and

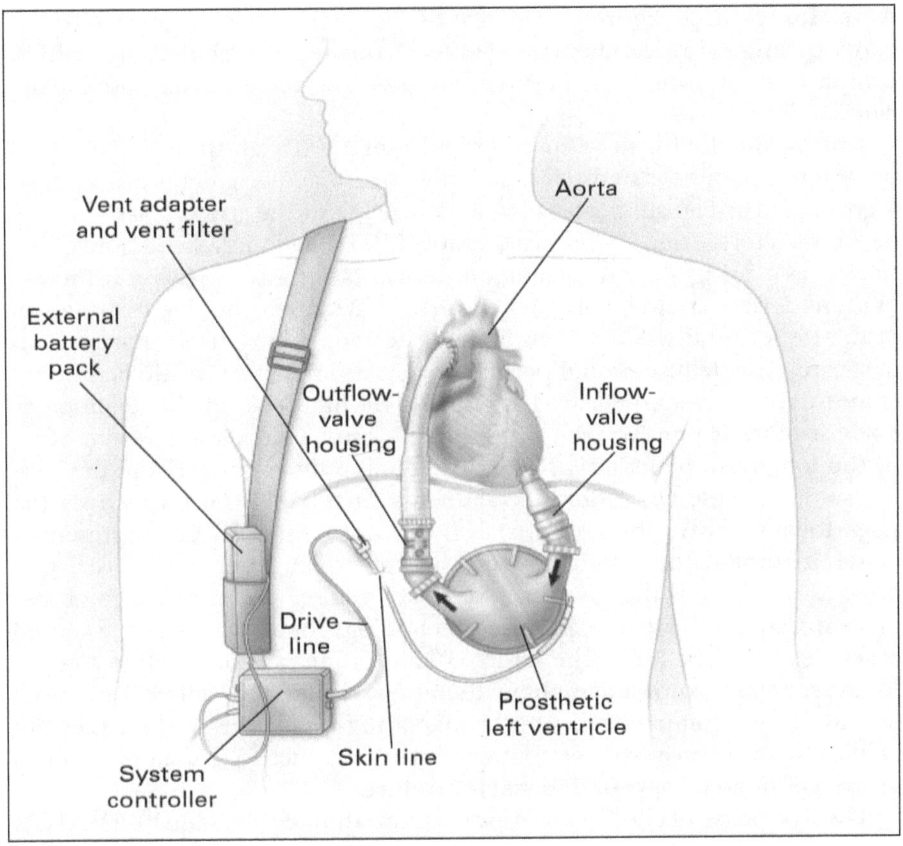

Figure 6.1. Components of the Left Ventricular Assist Device. In this system, there are two main parts: (1) the implanted mechanical pump (prosthetic left ventricle), and (2) the external system controller and power source (battery pack). In the body, blood returns from the lungs into the left side of the heart and exits through the left ventricular apex into the prosthetic left ventricle via an inflow-valve cannula. Blood is then actively pumped through an outflow-valve cannula into the ascending aorta for circulation through the body. The prosthetic left ventricle is placed inside the body's peritoneal cavity. Connected to the prosthetic left ventricle is a drive line that penetrates the skin to provide an air vent and an electrical cable to the external system controller and battery pack. Eric A. Rose et al., "Long-Term Use of a Left Ventricular Assist Device for End-Stage Heart Failure," *New England Journal of Medicine* 345, no. 20 (2001): 1437. Copyright © 2001 by the Massachusetts Medical Society.

the CMS, required rigorous evidence of therapeutic benefits over risks for patients, surgical researchers needed to reconcile the technical and ethical complexities of using RCTs in surgery to fit within the evidence-based medicine model.[26]

During the 1990s, the clinical promise of LVADs and the limitation of treatment options for transplant-ineligible heart-failure patients encouraged a group of cardiac surgical-researchers to expand the use of these devices beyond a short-term, temporary therapy. LVADs had already demonstrated success as a bridge-to-transplantation device, but it was uncertain if the use of these devices could be broadened further. What was the "life expectancy" of the device, and was it safe to implant in people long term? For patients in severe heart failure, would permanent LVAD implants provide better outcomes than conventional drug therapy? The high cost of this technology made it more expensive than drug therapy, but would these costs be offset by the long-term benefits?[27] There was genuine uncertainty about the relative value of these two different treatments among clinicians, which set the stage for an active comparison trial. It was not clear if LVADs represented better treatment than optimal drug therapy, which inferred clinical equipoise and bolstered the case for a RCT. As Crenner points out, a "high bar in testing" might serve to legitimize a technology for a wary audience should outcomes favor the use of the device. While Crenner acknowledges a grand "quest for exact knowledge about therapeutic effects" in clinical research overall, device companies bound by increasing regulation in the American medical marketplace had economic motives to gather RCT data in order to secure commercial approval for their product.[28]

The first phase of clinical testing was a pilot study, dubbed the PREMATCH trial, which yielded valuable and necessary information to move forward with a large-scale clinical trial. Between April 1996 and April 1998, twenty-one patients were randomized to receive either a HeartMate LVAD implant or drug therapy in five medical centers. The value of this trial was the collection of preliminary data on patient outcomes and device reliability. Could this older, sicker, and transplant-ineligible group of patients withstand the LVAD implant surgery? Yes. Did LVAD patients fare significantly better or worse than those treated with medications? It remained uncertain. At three months, each treatment group had an almost 30 percent mortality rate, which substantiated clinical equipoise for a definitive, larger clinical trial.[29] Was the LVAD technology reliable? Yes. The HeartMate vented electric device, developed by the Thoratec Corporation, was still undergoing major modifications but the pilot study provided sufficient safety and efficacy data to secure premarket approval (PMA) of this device from the FDA in 1998 as well as furthered the experience of surgeons with the device.[30]

The pilot study also prompted investigators to refine certain aspects of the study. Most significantly, researchers tightened the comparative focus on their study. Instead of comparing LVAD technology with standard community heart-failure care, investigators chose to test device implant outcomes against optimal drug therapy for severe heart therapy. What would that "optimal" protocol look like? This necessitated the development of standards for both the medical treatment and surgical treatment of patients in the absence of explicit guidelines for optimal medical management and long-term LVAD implants. As a result of the pilot study, investigators finalized the REMATCH protocol design and consolidated support for the second phase of clinical testing—a definitive multicenter RCT.[31]

The REMATCH clinical trial, conducted from May 1998 to July 2001, remains the only RCT to compare the permanent implantation of an LVAD with conventional drug therapy in transplant-ineligible heart-failure patients. It was an investigator-initiated study collaboratively conducted between Columbia University, the National Institutes of Health (NIH), and the Thoratec Corporation. The trial was led by the cardiac surgeon Eric Rose, who was chair of surgery at Columbia University and surgeon-in-chief at Columbia Presbyterian Medical Center. The NIH provided financial support for the costs of data collection and analysis as well as operation costs, as did the Thoratec Corporation, which also donated the LVADs and related equipment for the trial.[32] The CMS paid for all treatment costs, except for the implant hospitalization, which was covered by participating hospitals. Some medical centers did not participate in the trial owing to the financial burden of the implant hospitalization. No RCT patients were charged for any study costs owing to the unethical nature of financially exploiting vulnerable patients with a life-threatening condition. The REMATCH trial took place in twenty experienced US cardiac transplantation centers with expertise in the treatment of severe heart failure. The clinical trial was supervised by a steering committee and carried out by an operations committee with an independent coordinating center. Institutional Review Boards at each of the participating medical centers approved the study protocol and all patients signed written informed consent forms.[33]

The REMATCH study enrolled a total of 129 patients in severe heart failure, and none were eligible for cardiac transplantation. Various clinical conditions deemed a patient ineligible for cardiac transplantation, including peripheral vascular disease, pulmonary hypertension, obesity, substance abuse, psychosocial factors, renal problems, or pulmonary dysfunction. Most commonly, the age of patients kept them from organ donor waiting lists. Given these contraindications for transplantation, patients in the REMATCH study were older individuals (average age was sixty-six) with severe left ventricular dysfunction as well as other medical problems. These were quite sick people, with complex medical issues, looking to extend their lives. Through random assignment, sixty-eight patients received an LVAD—Thoratec's HeartMate XVE LVAD—and sixty-one patients followed a drug treatment regimen, including angiotension-converting-enzyme (ACE) inhibitors, which focused on optimizing organ perfusion and minimizing symptoms of congestive heart failure. Individual investigators at each medical site determined the eligibility of patients for the study, and a gatekeeper at the coordinating center ensured all candidates met strict trial patient criteria. The REMATCH study was not a double-blind trial owing to the surgical risk associated with the LVAD operation and the obvious nature of its implantation. The patients, surgeons, and other investigators were not blinded to the treatment assignment but most were blinded to interim outcomes. Statisticians recorded interim outcomes for both groups. Also, Thoratec investigators monitored LVAD patient data for device safety reasons, but they were blinded to all outcomes from the medical-therapy patient group. The study was designed with patient death from any cause as the primary end point, and after the predetermined number of ninety-two deaths had occurred, enrollment in the trial ended.[34]

Given the uncertainty surrounding LVAD technology as a long-term therapy in an older, sicker population, the results of the study surprised many in the medical community. REMATCH investigators reported that LVAD patients lived significantly longer than medical-therapy patients. After one year of treatment, 52 percent of LVAD patients compared with 25 percent of medical-therapy patients were living; after two years, the survival rate was 23 percent for LVAD patients compared with 8 percent of medical-therapy patients.[35] LVAD patients stayed in hospital longer (median number of days was eighty-eight) compared with the drug therapy group (median number of days was twenty-four). For those who died during the study, medical-therapy patients succumbed to heart failure, whereas LVAD patients tended to die of infection or mechanical failure of the device.[36] The REMATCH study confirmed conventional knowledge that available cardiac drugs managed mild-to-moderate heart failure much more successfully than end-stage heart failure.

Still the REMATCH results also pointed to significant LVAD complications and adverse events for LVAD patients, including problems of bleeding, neurological dysfunction, infections, thromboembolic complications, and renal failure. The percutaneous line that connected the implanted LVAD with external power and controller units was often infected, which contributed to sepsis as the most common cause of death in the device group. Device reliability continued to be an issue. During the course of the trial, seventeen devices in fifty-two patients needed replacement, usually due to mechanical pump failure or inflow valve incompetence, prompting device modifications by the Thoratec Corporation and the implementation of infection management guidelines by REMATCH investigators.[37] The number of adverse events experienced by LVAD patients reportedly declined thereafter.[38]

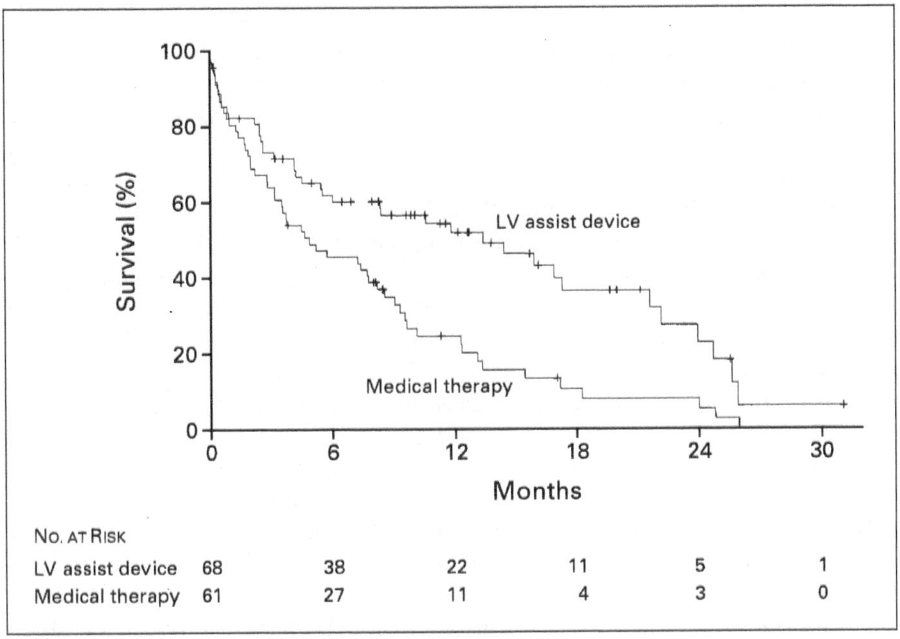

Figure 6.2. Higher Survival Rate of LVAD implant patients in comparison to medical therapy patients, as per Kaplan-Meier Analysis of Survival. Rose et al, "Long-Term Use of a Left Ventricular Assist Device for End-Stage Heart Failure," 1439. Copyright © 2001 by the Massachusetts Medical Society.

Even with these occurrences, LVAD patients reported a better quality of life and functionality than the medical-therapy patients, according to the REMATCH study. Did this represent an acceptable tradeoff for LVAD patients given the natural history of advanced heart failure? REMATCH trial investigators stated that it did.[39] It was clear that the survival rate for heart-failure patients with medical therapy was poor, and that LVAD implantations improved on that survival rate. When the trial ended in June 2001, three out of the five surviving patients in the medical therapy arm of the study crossed over for an LVAD implant.[40] Still, the overall two-year LVAD patient survival rate of 23 percent was hardly cause to rejoice, and reported LVAD-related complications strongly called for device improvement.[41]

REMATCH Results Generate Varied Responses

The REMATCH trial results were significant, no doubt surprising many cardiac specialists who had been watching from the sidelines. The REMATCH study demonstrated that long-term support with an LVAD was not only feasible but it also provided higher survival rates than optimal drug therapy for severe heart-failure patients who were not candidates for cardiac transplantation. The device was not a cure for heart failure. Indeed REMATCH investigators agreed that cardiac transplantation far exceeded the survival rate of LVAD-implanted patients in their study.[42] Still the REMATCH results suggested a promising role for LVADs as a life-extending device—a "lifeboat," according to Stephen Westaby—for some heart-failure patients, notably those who were transplant-ineligible. Westaby further commented: "The clear survival advantage for patients receiving LVADs now justifies the use of circulatory support well beyond the transplant setting."[43] The medical community appeared united in its description of the REMATCH trial as a "remarkable," "unprecedented," and "landmark" study for moving the potential clinical use of LVAD technology forward in a way that past case studies had not.[44]

Yet there were undeniable practical and economic concerns with this technology, which several members of the medical community raised in response to the REMATCH study. The cardiologist Lynne Stevenson, a nationally renowned leader in heart failure and director of the Cardiomyopathy and Heart Failure Program at the Brigham and Women's Hospital in Boston, acknowledged the "exciting new option" of LVADs but promoted a cautious view of its use.[45] For clinicians, end-stage heart-failure management emphasizes individual care; physicians seek to relieve patient symptoms and to decrease disease progression in mild-to-moderate stages, and in advanced heart-failure cases, they concentrate on prolonging function and quality of life for their patients. As a therapy for end-stage heart-failure patients, Stevenson stated that device durability was the predominant limiting factor against the widespread clinical use of LVADs.[46] Indeed, the most obvious issue was that these devices were far from perfect.

Stevenson and other cardiologists worked in a rapidly changing medical landscape and acknowledged that the field of heart failure management was progressing quickly in this period.[47] Cardiologists did not sound an anti-LVAD technology horn, but they were restrained in its clinical uptake. The complexity of therapeutic options was increasing, which, as pointed out by Stevenson and her colleagues at the American Heart Association, made shared decision making more crucial and challenging in the management of advanced heart failure.[48] For the most part, cardiologists acknowledged LVADs as an evolving technology, to which they advocated for better devices and patient care practices to improve outcomes. Arguably, this would help lower the high rate of complications associated with LVAD implants, a necessary factor if this technology had any hope of widespread adoption. Clinical information about device implantation, performance, and patient care management had been built on knowledge gained in the laboratory through bench testing and animal experiments with these devices. Described by some surgeons as "learning-by-using" experiences, any clinical shortcomings or potential new applications of the technology will necessarily lead to more bench research and design modifications, which would in turn loop back to improved patient outcomes.[49]

REMATCH investigators anticipated and adjusted for such a learning curve scenario with implantation of the Heartmate LVAD. In the early stages of the REMATCH trial, surgeons reported an inflow valve incompetence problem with the LVAD that negatively affected blood flow through the device. During the second half of the study, several device modifications were made, specifically (1) the screw ring connectors on the inflow and outflow grafts were now locking to avert disconnection, and (2) the outflow graft had added "bend relief" to prevent kinking.[50] Similar "learning-by-using" changes related to postimplant patient care also took place. The problem of sepsis in LVAD patients declined after: (1) specific infection management guidelines, which defined the choice of antimicrobial prophylaxis, were written; and (2) postoperative patients were fitted with abdominal binders which immobilized the exiting driveline, reducing trauma and deterring infection.[51] LVAD patients who enrolled later in the study benefited from these changes, an improved-outcome trend that continued post-REMATCH trial.[52] REMATCH investigators monitored device performance carefully to ensure than any redesign made to address one problem did not introduce the possibility of another problem. Still, the cardiac surgeon Matthias Loebe stated: "If we want to consider mechanical assist devices as a real alternative . . . we definitely have to improve their technical performance."[53] Understandably, persistent reports of device malfunctions made clinicians wary.

Would the introduction of LVADs as destination therapy lead to an indication "creep" with pressure to implant VADs in less ill patients? The University of California cardiologist Barry Massie warned that "this is a treacherous path to follow."[54] Granted, the patients enrolled in the REMATCH study were extremely ill. As Massie points out, many of these patients were "too far gone" at the start of the trial to realistically recover from any operation or device complications. As Stevenson pointed out, the field was learning to identify those patients who were "sick enough" to warrant an LVAD implant and yet "well enough" to survive the surgery.[55] Arguably a less-ill group of heart-failure patients would have responded better to an LVAD implant in the REMATCH study. But then this same group might have also improved considerably with optimal drug therapy without device and implantation risks. Massie reminded others that individual cases of patients being "delisted" from transplant lists after responding well to drug treatment were known in the field. Given the present state of LVAD technology, he argued that the complications associated with the device outweighed the potential benefit for less-ill heart-failure patients.[56]

Wrapped up in the discussion of device durability and patient outcomes was the issue of cost. The University of Pennsylvania cardiologist Mariell Jessup stated the obvious: "We now know that ventricular assist devices prolong life; we do not yet know for how long and at what cost."[57] LVAD technology and its management was very expensive and labor intensive. REMATCH investigators reported that the mean total cost for the LVAD patient in the study was $210,187, which included the $60,000 cost for the device and other direct medical costs related to surgery and recovery. (At approximately $200,000, the average cost of cardiac transplantation is roughly the same in this period.) This was significantly more expensive than treating the patient in the drug therapy group, which was directly related to the lengthy stay in hospital for the LVAD patient. On average, LVAD patients stayed eighty-eight days in hospital compared with only twenty-four days spent in hospital by patients in the drug therapy group. The cost of taking care of these LVAD patients was roughly $4,000 a day, which elicited considerable negative reactions from hospital administrators.[58] The pressure for cost reduction was evident if greater adoption of LVADs as destination therapy was to take place.

The REMATCH study results prompted other device clinical trials, in large part initiated by other device companies seeking entry into the medical marketplace.[59] Between 2000 and 2003, the Investigation of Nontransplant-Eligible Patients Who Are Inotrope Dependent (INTrEPID) clinical trial took place in thirteen medical centers in the United States and Canada that had experience implanting the Novacor LVAS as a bridge-to-transplantation device. Like the REMATCH trial, the INTrEPID study sought to demonstrate mechanical device superiority over optimal medical management (OMM) of patients ineligible for heart transplantation, but this time the device to be implanted permanently was the Novacor LVAS. The INTrEPID study was a prospective, nonrandomized clinical trial with fewer patients who were younger, but otherwise had similar patient characteristics to those in the REMATCH trial.[60] The results of the INTrEPID study reinforced the REMATCH data by demonstrating that LVAD patients survived longer with improved functional capacity and quality of life than OMM patients.[61] Together these two studies provided a "proof-of-concept" that prolonged (permanent) LVAD support for heart-failure patients was promising.[62] But the Novacor LVAS patients had the ghastly mortality rate of almost 75 percent at one year, hardly enough for the "fledgling field" of mechanical circulatory support systems to trounce competing heart failure treatments, according to Stevenson.[63] Although the trials demonstrated that LVADs could provide longer-term support for a critically ill patient population (Class IV heart-failure criteria for inclusion), issues of device durability and function remained. No one disputed the fact that incidences of device failure and adverse medical events needed to be lowered. In addition, patient selection was important—could patients not so critically ill benefit more from this technology? As Stevenson admitted, the REMATCH study included "the sickest group of heart-failure patients ever to enter a clinical trial."[64] As well, improved postoperative and longer-term patient management strategies needed to be defined. In any case, the results of the INTrEPID trial supported yet another trial of the Novacor LVAS, but this time comparing it with its prime competitor.

The Randomized Evaluation of Novacor LVAS in a Non-Transplant Population (RELIANT) trial, which began in 2004, was a randomized patient study to compare morbidity and mortality outcomes in patients implanted with Novacor LVAS compared with patients implanted with the HeartMate LVAD. Both devices were electrically actuated, "wearable" pulsatile LVADs with comparable patient results from single-device studies. The pulsatile Novacor LVAS was larger and heavier than the HeartMate LVAD. Although the Novacor LVAS had comparable mechanical reliability and durability, Novacor LVAS patients experienced a higher rate of thromboembolic events leading to stroke, and subsequently, clinicians tended to favor the HeartMate LVAD. Still, the researchers behind the Novacor system argued that their device was the better LVAD, and wanted RCT results to prove this. Corporate bidding trumped biomedical research wishes to answer this question. The Novacor LVAS was phased out of investigational use before the completion of the RELIANT study, and no reports of this study were ever published.[65] The manufacturer, WorldHeart Corporation, pulled its support of the study to redirect funding to the development of a different technology platform in late 2006.[66] Although the industry-academic alliances were necessary to develop this technology, their relationship was not always smooth and noncontroversial, and corporate bottom lines tended to dominate over loftier research pursuits.

Like the WorldHeart Corporation, other industrial-academic teams also pursued multiple technology platforms that led to the emergence of next-generation ventricular assist devices. New biomaterials, miniaturization, and improved pump designs promised to resolve problems of thromboembolism, infection, and patient mobility that challenged the older pulsatile LVADs (Thoratec PVAD, HeartMate LVAD, and Novacor LVAS). At the same time that new LVAD technology was emerging, the distinction between temporary or permanent use of these devices became blurred once again. Back in the 1980s, bioethicists first raised this issue after numerous "temporary" Jarvik-7 total artificial heart (TAH) implant patients experienced complications that removed them from the transplant list. These cases of temporary-turned-permanent bridges meant that patients unintentionally found themselves spending their remaining days tethered to a machine.[67] Would LVAD-implant patients be more willing to accept these risks? Owing to long waiting lists, LVAD-supported patients waiting for a heart transplant might well be implanted with their device for a year or longer, during which time they may lose their transplant status.[68] Were LVADs better than TAH technology and thus this was only a remote risk? Conversely, patients initially ineligible for transplantation may improve on LVAD support to resolve their previous contraindications and thereafter become transplant eligible. These categories for use were merging clinically as the distinction of temporary or permanent therapy became less relevant for patients and clinicians. As stated by the cardiac surgeon James Kirklin, "the clinical reality is that few therapies are exclusively 'either/or' for the duration of the heart failure patient's life."[69] The ambiguous nature of transplant status for many patients led surgeons to employ a strategy of "bridge-to-candidacy" or "bridge-to-decision," an emerging gray zone between "bridge-to-transplantation" and "destination therapy" indications for the clinical use of LVAD technology.

Conclusion: A "Landmark" Study?

The REMATCH trial was a "landmark" study for several reasons. First, it demonstrated that large randomized, controlled trials in cardiac device surgery were doable, rigorous, and convincing. The RCT protocol employed in the REMATCH study quelled skepticism that unique surgical variables such as the surgeon's skill or specialized institutional care environments prevented the rigorous testing and comparison of new surgically implanted devices. Favorable LVAD data gathered through a clinical trial provided reassuring assessment for both regulatory and medical evaluation. Second, the REMATCH study marked a key turning point in the technological achievement of LVADs. It demonstrated the efficacy and reliability of the HeartMate LVAD as permanent or destination therapy, extending clinical indications for LVAD technology beyond bridge-to-transplantation to a new patient subset. For this older, sicker patient population who were not eligible for cardiac transplantation, LVAD treatment produced better survival outcomes than conventional drug therapy, according to REMATCH results, which secured device approval from medical technology regulators and payers. As the physician Muriel Gillick commented, it was "virtually a foregone conclusion" that regulatory bodies interested in device safety more than clinical effectiveness would approve LVAD use based on the "high-quality data" gathered in the RCT.[70] In 2002, the FDA approved the HeartMate LVAD as a long-term destination therapy for transplant-ineligible patients in advanced heart failure. Not long after, the CMS approved reimbursement for the use of these devices as destination therapy in October 2003. Third, the REMATCH trial provided a benchmark for heart-failure devices as destination therapy. The INTrEPID trial, the RELIANT study, and others sought to repeat favorable patient results with their device or directly tested their device against the HeartMate LVAD used in the REMATCH study.

The influence of the REMATCH study on the broader adoption or clinical uptake of LVAD technology as destination therapy is more ambiguous. The REMATCH study provided proof of concept of LVADs as destination therapy but faltered in the transition to broad clinical utilization. On the one hand, the REMATCH study reported that patient survival outcomes with LVADs were higher than those who were treated with optimal drug therapy, and thus this realized the clinical promise of this technology and fueled further research and development. On the other hand, the quality of the REMATCH results was simply not strong enough to lead to widespread adoption of the technology in its current state. As the cardiologist Sharon Hunt commented, it was "new data [but] old problems." In terms of LVAD patient mortality and device malfunction rates, the REMATCH study reported better results, but "not much," according to Hunt.[71] The REMATCH study and the subsequent device trials that it inspired immediately thereafter underscored the inherent limitations of these pulsatile pumps, referred to as first-generation LVAD technology. Survival outcomes of LVAD patients were better than those treated with optimal medical therapy; however, it was still poor.[72] In addition to the device limitations, it was costly; approved reimbursement did not fully cover hospital expenses.[73] Nonetheless, the REMATCH results suggested that LVAD implantation should be added to the treatment options for this patient population. The debate whether coronary artery disease was focal or diffuse or both remains ongoing, in part, as argued by Jones, because persistent therapeutic competition sustains coexistence of different approaches.[74] Cardiologists and cardiac surgeons support multiple treatments in their toolbox to serve individualized patient scenarios. LVADs were an imperfect and expensive technology that, rather than directly displace other treatments, settled on being recognized as a justifiable alternative option for some heart-failure patients.

According to the International Registry for Mechanically Assisted Circulatory Support (INTERMACS), a nationally mandated database of all patients implanted with a mechanical circulatory support device, few pulsatile pumps were implanted as destination therapy.[75] Between 2006 and 2009, less than 10 percent of LVADs had been implanted permanently.[76] There was no significant clinical uptake of LVAD technology as destination therapy in the immediate post-REMATCH era. Many cardiologists did not believe that the risk-benefit ratio for LVADs as destination therapy was favorable enough for most of their heart-failure patients. The REMATCH results were hardly compelling with a 23 percent LVAD patient survival outcome at two years and a high incidence of device replacement at eighteen months.[77] Formed to assess current LVAD technology challenges and opportunities, the NHLBI Working Group recommended that the next-generation devices aim to deliver a 50 percent survival outcome at two years, with minimal time in the hospital after implantation, for LVAD patients. It was their hope that improved technology would become an attractive therapy to treat patients with less advanced but progressive heart failure.[78] A less-ill patient population boded well for the device and it contributed to the blurring of indications for the use of this device. Heart-failure patients who improved with LVAD therapy often became the bridge-to-decision or bridge-to-candidacy group as their transplant eligibility status fluctuated.

The next generation LVAD that would dominate the post-REMATCH era was the nonpulsatile device or axial-design, continuous-flow rotary pump. This second-generation technology demonstrated improved patient survival and device performance over the older pulsatile systems. The quieter, smaller, and more durable HeartMate II rotary pump represented the new technology. In 2008, the FDA gave market approval to the continuous-flow Heart Mate II LVAD as a bridge-to-transplantation device.[79] Two years later, the FDA approved the HeartMate II pump for permanent or destination therapy after a clinical trial reported a 58 percent survival rate of HeartMate II-implanted patients at two years compared with a 24 percent survival rate of patients implanted with the older pulsatile LVAD.[80] Clinical uptake of the new HeartMate II device, for both bridge-to-transplantation and destination therapy, was significant and almost immediate. According to the INTERMACS database, there was a marked increase in the number of LVADs implanted as destination therapy—more than 30 percent of total implants—in 2010 and 2011; this surge coincided with FDA approval of the HeartMate II pump for destination therapy in January 2010.[81] In 2011, the Thoratec Corporation discontinued sale of the older HeartMate XVE LVAD (that had been used in the REMATCH trial).[82] In 2016, LVADs are implanted permanently in transplant-ineligible heart-failure patients, but some clinicians are advocating consideration of LVADs as a "transplant alternative" for heart-failure patients who may decline transplantation owing to its common serious complications of graft failure, rejection, and infection.[83] According to many heart-failure clinicians, the expansion of LVAD use is both needed and warranted.[84]

The REMATCH study demonstrated the viability of LVAD technology as a life-extending device and promoted more RCTs with less sick patients. The cardiac surgeon Stephen Westaby dubbed the REMATCH participants as "Titanic patients" who were facing imminent death, and the device served as a lifeboat for some individuals. Given the advanced stage of heart failure in these patients, another cardiac surgeon, O. Howard Frazier, stated that it "was a miraculous thing that any of them survived."[85] Westaby and others call for implanting LVADs in patients before terminal decline, before the ship hits the iceberg. It became evident soon after the REMATCH trial that real clinical uptake would necessitate improved devices and better patient outcomes, thus requiring more surgical RCTs. The REMATCH trial had established a precedent from which the development of future devices would have difficulty ignoring. Certainly there were many relevant dissenting views in health policy, public health, palliative medicine, and bioethics about high-cost and complex new technologies, such as LVADs, expressed outside the medical literature that have not been addressed in this paper. The discussion surrounding the REMATCH study results is a specific moment in cardiac surgical innovation that captures both the excitement alongside the cautious optimism of medical practitioners regarding the meaning and impact of LVAD technology, RCTs in surgery, and the adoption of new devices in surgery.

Notes

Epigraph. Soon J. Park et al., "Left Ventricular Assist Devices as Destination Therapy: A New Look at Survival," *Journal of Thoracic and Cardiovascular Surgery* 129, no. 1 (2005): 16, "Discussion." See also Stephen Westaby, "Ventricular Assist Devices as Destination Therapy," *Surgical Clinics of North America* 84, no. 1 (2004): 91–123.

1. José Lopez-Sendon, "The Heart Failure Epidemic," *Medicographia* 33, no. 4 (2011): 363–69, http://www.medicographia.com/2012/02/the-heart-failure-epidemic/ (accessed November 3, 2013).

2. V. L. Roger et al., "Heart Disease and Stroke Statistics—2012 Update: A Report from the American Heart Association," *Circulation* 125, no. 1 (2012): e2–220; William T. Abraham and Henry Krum, *Heart Failure: A Practical Approach to Treatment* (New York: McGraw-Hill Medical, 2007), 15–17; Paul Dudley White, *Heart Disease*, 3rd ed. (New York: Macmillan, 1944), 763.

3. American Heart Association, "Classes of Heart Failure," http://www.heart.org/HEARTORG/Conditions/HeartFailure/AboutHeartFailure/Classes-of-Heart-Failure_UCM_306328_Article.jsp (accessed November 3, 2013).

4. American Heart Association, "Heart Failure Patients Living Longer, but Long-Term Survival Still Low," May 15, 2013, http://newsroom.heart.org/news/heart-failure-patients-living-longer-but-long-term-survival-still-low (accessed November 3, 2013). See also Samuel W. Joffe, Kristy T. Webster, David D. McManus, Michael S. Kiernan, Darleen M. Lessard, Jorge L. Yarzebski, Chad E. Darling, Joel M. Gore, and Robert J. Goldberg, "Improved Survival after Heart Failure: A Community-Based Perspective," *Journal of the American Heart Association* 2, no. 3 (2013): 1–9.

5. Salynn Boyles, "AHA: Heart Failure Costs Likely to Soar," MedPage Today (April 25, 2013), http://www.medpagetoday.com/Cardiology/CHF/38678 (accessed November 5, 2013); CDC, Heart Failure Fact Sheet, http://www.cdc.gov/dhdsp/data_statistics/fact_sheets/fs_heart_failure.htm (accessed November 5, 2013); Abraham and Krum, *Heart Failure*, 13–15.

6. David S. Jones and Jeremy A. Greene, "The Decline and Rise of Coronary Heart Disease," *American Journal of Public Health* 103, no. 7 (2013): 1207–18; David S. Jones, *Broken Hearts: The Tangled History of Cardiac Care* (Baltimore: Johns Hopkins University Press, 2013).

7. National Heart, Lung and Blood Institute, "Who Is at Risk of Heart Failure?," http://www.nhlbi.nih.gov/health/health-topics/topics/hf/atrisk.html (accessed November 3, 2013).

8. National Heart, Lung and Blood Institute, "What Causes Heart Failure?," http://www.nhlbi.nih.gov/health/health-topics/topics/hf/causes.html (accessed November 5, 2013).

9. Lynne Warner Stevenson and Eric A. Rose, "Left Ventricular Assist Devices: Bridges to Transplantation, Recovery and Destination for Whom?," *Circulation* 108 (2003): 3060. US Department of Health and Human Services, "Annual Report of the US Organ Procurement and Transplantation Network (OPTN) and the Scientific Registry of Transplant Recipients (SRTR), Chapter 6—Heart Transplantation in the United States, 1999–2008," http://www.ustransplant.org/annual_reports/current/chapter_vi_AR_cd.htm?cp=7 (accessed September 10, 2014).

10. Chana A. Sacks, John A. Jarcho, and Gergory D. Curfman, "Paradigm Shifts in Heart-Failure Therapy—A Timeline," *New England Journal of Medicine* 371, no. 11 (2014): 989–91.

11. Dennis M. McNarmara and Arthur M. Feldman, "Pharmacogenomics and Pharmacogentics in Heart Failure," in *Heart Failure: A Companion to Braunwald's Heart Disease*, ed. Douglas L. Mann (St. Louis, MS: Elsevier Saunders, 2011): 626–33; Lynne Warner Stevenson and Robert L. Kormos, "Mechanical Cardiac Support 2000: Current Applications and Future Trial Design," *Journal of the American College of Cardiology* 37, no. 1 (2001): 349.

12. Stevenson and Rose, "Left Ventricular Assist Devices," 3060.

13. See M. E. DeBakey, "Left Ventricular Bypass Pump for Cardiac Assistance," *American Journal of Cardiology* 27 (January 1971): 9–10; "Heart Pump Placed in Mexican Woman," *New York Times*, August 9, 1966, 15; "Heart Pump Removed from Houston Patient," *New York Times*, August 19, 1966, 35; "Heart Pump Patient Leaves Hospital in Houston," *New York Times*, September 7, 1966, 36.

14. By the 1990s, the NHBLI was supporting second-generation LVADs designed for a five-year lifetime. See John T. Watson, "Prospects for Implantable Circulatory Support," in *Heart Replacement—Artificial Heart*, ed. T. Akutsu and H. Koyanagi, 6th ed. (Tokyo: Springer-Verlage, 1998).

15. Institute of Medicine, *The Artificial Heart: Prototypes, Policies, and Patients* (Washington, DC: Institute of Medicine, 1991): 14–25. See also Shelley McKellar, "Negotiating Risk: The Failed Development of Atomic Hearts in America, 1967–77," *Technology and Culture* 54, no. 1 (2013): 1–39; Shelley McKellar, "Artificial Hearts: A Technological Fix More Monstrous than Miraculous?," in *The Technological Fix: How People Use Technology to Create and Solve Problems*, ed. Lisa Rosner (New York: Routledge University Press, 2004): 13–29.

16. See chapter 8 in this volume.

17. The discussion among bioethicists regarding destination therapy and the questions of patient quality of life and LVAD deactivation are not discussed in this paper. For a sample of this discussion see Aaron G. Rizzieri, Joseph L. Verheijde, Mohamed Y. Rady, and Joan L. McGregor, "Ethical Challenges with the Left Ventricular Assist Device as a Destination Therapy," *Philosophy, Ethics, and Humanities in Medicine* 3, no. 1 (2008): 1–15; K. A. Bramstedt and N. S. Wenger, "When Withdrawal of Life-Sustaining Care Does More Than Allow Death to Take Its Course: The Dilemma of

Left Ventricular Assist Devices," *Journal of Heart and Lung Transplantation* 20, no. 5 (2001): 544–48; K. A. Brandstedt, "Destination Nowhere: A Potential Dilemma with Ventricular Assist Devices," *ASAIO Journal* 54, no. 1 (2008): 1–2.

18. Renee C. Fox and Judith P. Swazey, *The Courage to Fail: A Social View of Organ Transplants and Dialysis* (Chicago: University of Chicago Press, 1978); Renee C. Fox and Judith P. Swazey, *Spare Parts: Organ Replacement in American Society* (New York: Oxford University Press, 1992); Stuart Blume, *The Artificial Ear: Cochlear Implants and the Culture of Deafness* (New Brunswick, NJ: Rutgers University Press, 2010); Jones, *Broken Hearts*. See also Stanley Joel Reiser, *Technological Medicine: The Changing World of Doctors and Patients* (New York: Cambridge University Press, 2009).

19. Susan Lederer, *Flesh and Blood: Organ Transplantation and Blood Transfusion in Twentieth-Century America* (New York: Oxford University Press, 2008); Thomas Schlich, *The Origins of Organ Transplantation* (Rochester, NY: University of Rochester Press, 2010); Lesley A. Sharp, *The Transplant Imaginary: Mechanical Hearts, Animal Parts and Moral Thinking in Highly Experimental Science* (Berkeley: University of California Press, 2014).

20. Clayton Christenson proposes two categories of new technologies: sustaining and disruptive. The first category refers to established technologies on which incremental changes are made. The second category refers to a new technology that, although unrefined or unclear in its purpose, threatens to disrupt established technologies. See Clayton Christensen, *The Innovator's Dilemma: The Revolutionary Book That Will Change the Way You Do Business* (New York: Harper Business, 1997; repr. 2011).

21. Harry M. Marks, *The Progress of Experiment: Science and Therapeutic Reform in the United States, 1900–1990* (New York: Cambridge University Press, 1997); Susan Lederer, *Subjected to Science: Human Experimentation in America before the Second World War* (Baltimore: Johns Hopkins, 1995); Kenneth Stanley, "Design of Randomized Controlled Trials," *Circulation* 115 (March 6, 2007): 1164–69; David S. Jones, "Visions of a Cure: Visualization, Clinical Trials, and Controversies in Cardiac Therapeutics, 1968–1998," *Isis* 91 (2000): 504–41; Marcia Meldrum, "Departures from the Design: The Randomized Clinical Trial in Historical Context, 1946–1970" (PhD diss., State University of New York at Stony Brook, 1994); Scott H. Podolsky, "Antibiotics and the Social History of the Controlled Clinical Trial, 1950–1970," *Journal of the History of Medicine and Allied Sciences* 65, no. 3 (2010): 327–67.

22. As Christopher Crenner states, the case series in surgery is "both practical and influential and remains, with subsequent refinements, a mainstay of the surgical scientific literature." Crenner, "Placebos and the Progress of Surgery," chapter 7 of this volume, p. 157.

23. The significance of RCTs in the evaluation of surgical interventions is discussed in the medical literature worldwide, as seen in R. S. McLeod, "Issues in Surgical Randomized Clinical Trials," *World Journal of Surgery* 23 (1999): 1210–14; N. S. Abraham, "Will the Dilemma of Evidence-Based Surgery Ever Be Resolved?," *Australian and New Zealand Journal of Surgery* 76 (2006): 855–60. Possible solutions to surgical RCT challenges are discussed in: Stevenson and Kormos, "Mechanical Cardiac Support 2000," 340–70; Forough Farrokhyar et al., "Randomized Clinical Trials of Surgical Interventions," *Annals of Surgery* 251, no. 3 (2010): 409–16; Jeffrey S. Barkun et al., "Evaluation and Stages of Surgical Innovations," *Lancet* 374

(September 26, 2009): 1089–96; Patrick L. Ergina et al., "Challenges in Evaluating Surgical Innovation," *Lancet* 374 (September 26, 2009): 1097–1104; Nuh N. Rahbari et al., "Development and Perspectives of Randomized Clinical Trials in Surgery," *American Journal of Surgery* 194 (Suppl. to October 2007): S148–S152.

24. Jones, *Broken Hearts.*

25. Jones, "Visions of a Cure," 523, 529; See also John H. Alexander and Eric D. Peterson, "Translating Trials to Clinical Practice in Cardiac Surgery," *Nature Reviews* 10 (June 2013): 306–7.

26. Stevenson and Kormos, "Mechanical Cardiac Support 2000," 343; Eric A. Rose et al., "The REMATCH Trial: Rationale, Design and End Points," *Annals of Thoracic Surgery* 67 (1999): 724.

27. See M. V. Badiwala, "Left Ventricular Device as Destination Therapy: Are We There Yet?," *Current Opinion in Cardiology* 24, no. 2 (2009): 184–89; M. G. McGee et al., "Extended Support with a Left Ventricular Assist Device as a Bridge to Heart Transplantation," *ASAIO Transactions* 37, no. 3 (1991): M425–26; K. R. Kanter et al., "Bridging to Cardiac Transplantation with Pulsatile Ventricular Assist Devices," *Annals of Thoracic Surgery* 46, no. 2 (1988): 134–40.

28. Crenner, "Placebos and the Progress of Surgery," 177.

29. Ursula Maria Schmidt-Ott et al., "Challenges in Conducting Implantable Device Trials: Left Ventricular Assist Devices in Destination Therapy," in *Clinical Evaluation of Medical Devices: Principles and Case Studies*, ed. K. M. Becker and J. Whyte, 2nd ed. (Totowa, NJ: Humana Press, Inc., 2006): 202–3.

30. In 1995, the US FDA granted IDE status to the HeartMate VE LVAS for use in transplant-ineligible patients as part of the REMATCH trial. In 1998, device safety and efficacy data from the pilot study (PREMATCH trial) secured PMA status from the FDA for longer-term bridge-to-transplant use. In 2003, an enhanced version of the HeartMate XVE LVAD received PMA approval from the FDA for permanent implantation in transplant-ineligible patients. See US FDA PMA Database, "HeartMate VE LVAS," http://www.accessdata.fda.gov/scripts/cdrh/cfdocs/cfpma/pma.cfm?id=21870 (accessed October 29, 2014); Rose et al., "REMATCH Trial," 725.

31. Schmidt-Ott et al., "Challenges in Conducting Implantable Device Trials," 202–3.

32. The cost of the REMATCH trial was approximately $25 million. The Thoratec Corporation as a partial sponsor contributed $3.6 million plus all necessary LVADs and related equipment (approximately $60,000 each). US Securities and Exchange Commission Form 10-K, submitted by the Thoratec Corporation for the fiscal year ended December 29, 2001, http://www.sec.gov/Archives/edgar/data/350907/000095014902000488/f79706e10-k405.htm (accessed November 3, 2014); Schmidt-Ott et al., "Challenges in Conducting Implantable Device Trials," 205; Eric A. Rose et al., "Long-Term Use of a Left Ventricular Assist Device for End-Stage Heart Failure," *New England Journal of Medicine* 345, no. 20 (2001): 1436.

33. For the original publication of the REMATCH results and full membership of the REMATCH Study Group, see Rose et al., "Long-Term Use of a Left Ventricular Assist Device," 1435–43.

34. Ibid., 1435–43.

35. In 2001, the ninety-second patient died in the trial, which had been the predetermined number at which to end the study. At the time of the final analysis,

ninety-five trial patients had died: fifty-four (of the sixty-one) OMM patients and forty-one (of the sixty-eight) LVAD patients. Rose et al., "Long-Term Use of a Left Ventricular Assist Device," 1438–39.

36. Ibid., 1440–41.

37. Schmidt-Ott et al., "Challenges in Conducting Implantable Device Trials," 212.

38. Four years after the publication of the REMATCH trial results, a group of cardiac surgeons implanting the HeartMate XVE LVAD as destination therapy in transplant-ineligible heart-failure patients reported a 40 percent lower rate of death and 2.1 times less likely patient experience with adverse events due to device improvements and better patient management at multiple medical centers. See J. W. Long, A. G. Kfoury, M. S. Slaughter, M. Silver, C. Milano, J. Rogers, R. Delgado, and O. H. Frazier, "Long-Term Destination Therapy with the HeartMate XVE Left Ventricular Assist Device: Improved Outcomes since the REMATCH Study," *Congestive Heart Failure* 11, no. 3 (2005): 133–38.

39. Rose et al., "Long-Term Use of a Left Ventricular Assist Device," 1442.

40. One patient continued with optimal medical management therapy, whereas another patient dropped out of the trial altogether, according to Schmidt-Ott et al., "Challenges in Conducting Implantable Device Trials," 211.

41. Rose et al., "Long-Term Use of a Left Ventricular Assist Device," 1435–43.

42. At this time, the one-year survival rate of cardiac transplant patients was more than 80 percent and the ten-year survival rate was nearly 50 percent. Taken from ibid., 1442.

43. Westaby's comments made publicly at the American Association for Thoracic Surgery meeting in Boston, Massachusetts, May 4–7, 2003, and cited in Park et al., "Left Ventricular Assist Devices as Destination Therapy," 16, "Discussion."

44. Robert O. Bonow, MD, Douglas L. Mann, MD, FACC, Douglas P. Zipes, MD, and Peter Libby, ed. *Braunwald's Heart Disease*, 9th ed. (Philadelphia, PA: Elsevier/Saunders, 2012), 619; Robert L. Kormos and Leslie W. Miller, eds. *Mechanical Circulatory Support: A Companion to Braunwald's Heart Disease* (Philadelphia, PA: Elsevier/Saunders, 2012), 272.

45. Lynne Warner Stevenson, "Left Ventricular Assist Devices as Destination Therapy for End-stage Heart Failure," *Current Treatment Options in Cardiovascular Medicine* 6 (2004): 471.

46. Ibid., 471; Lynne Warner Stevenson, "Ventricular Assist Devices for Durable Support," *Circulation* 112 (2005): e111–e115.

47. Anju Nohria, Eldrin Lewis, and Lynne Warner Stevenson, "Medical Management of Advanced Heart Failure," *Journal of the American Medical Association* 287, no. 5 (2002): 638; Stevenson, "Left Ventricular Assist Devices as Destination Therapy," 471.

48. Larry A. Allen, Lynne W. Stevenson et al., "Decision Making in Advanced Heart Failure: A Scientific Statement from the American Heart Association," *Circulation* 125 (2012): 1928–52.

49. Mehmet C. Oz et al., "Left Ventricular Assist Devices as Permanent Heart Failure Therapy: The Price of Progress," *Annals of Surgery* 238, no. 4 (2003): 275–76.

50. Ibid., 276; Walter P. Dembitsky et al., "Left Ventricular Assist Device Performance with Long-Term Circulatory Support: Lessons from the REMATCH Trial," *Annals of Thoracic Surgery* 78 (2004): 2128.

51. Oz et al., "Left Ventricular Assist Devices," 276.

52. Long et al., "Long-Term Destination Therapy," 138.

53. See discussion section following Dembitsky et al., "Left Ventricular Assist Device Performance," 2129.

54. Barry M. Massie, "Comment—LVADs as Long-Term Cardiac Replacement: Success but on What Terms and at What Cost?," *Journal of Cardiac Failure* 8, no. 2 (2002): 61.

55. Stevenson, "Left Ventricular Assist Devices as Destination Therapy," 471.

56. Massie, "Comment—LVADs," 61.

57. Mariell Jessup, "Mechanical Cardiac-Support Devices—Dreams and Devilish Details," *New England Journal of Medicine* 345, no. 20 (2001): 1490–93.

58. Oz et al., "Left Ventricular Assist Devices," 275, 278; Schmidt-Ott et al., "Challenges in Conducting Implantable Device Trials," 208; Rose et al., "Long-Term Use of a Left Ventricular Assist Device," 1442, table 6.

59. At this time in the United States, the two most popular LVAD systems used for BTT were the HeartMate LVAD and the Novacor LVAS, which were now being evaluated for DT in clinical trials. Almost simultaneously, another clinical trial in Europe was evaluating the Arrow LionHeart LVAD, a device developed by the Division of Artificial Organs at Penn State College of Medicine in conjunction with Arrow International Inc. of Reading, Pennsylvannia. Like the HeartMate LVAD and the Novacor LVAS, the LionHeart LVAD was also an implantable, pulsatile VAD. However, it differed owing to its transcutaneous energy transfer system (TETS) and compliance chamber to accommodate gas volume fluctuations, eliminating the need for a through-the-skin power and vent tube, thus reducing the threat of infection. The LionHeart LVAD became clinically available in the United States on an investigational-use basis when the FDA approved the Phase I clinical trial in 2001, but it has not achieved the next level of FDA commercial approval. See A. el-Banaysy et al., "Preliminary Experience with the LionHeart Left Ventricular Assist Device in Patients with End-Stage Heart Failure," *Annals of Thoracic Surgery* 75 (2003): 1469–75; W. E. Pae et al., "Does Total Implantability Reduce Infection with the Use of a Left Ventricular Assist Device? The LionHeart Experience in Europe," *Journal of Heart and Lung Transplantation* 26 (2007): 219–29; Katherine Lietz and Leslie W. Miller, "Will Left-Ventricular Assist Device Therapy Replace Transplantation in the Foreseeable Future?," *Current Opinion in Cardiology* 20 (2005): 133.

60. In the INTrEPID study, there were 55 patients (37 LVAD, 18 optimal medical therapy) with the mean age of 60 years compared with the REMATCH study of 129 patients (68 LVAD, 61 optimal medical therapy) with the mean age of 66 years. See Joseph G. Rogers and Francis D. Pagani, "Results of Clinical Trials to Date," in Kormos and Miller, *Mechanical Circulatory Support*, 286–87.

61. Joseph G. Rogers et al., "Chronic Mechanical Circulatory Support for Inotrope-Dependent Heart Failure Patients Who Are Not Transplant Candidates: Results of the INTrEPID Trial," *Journal of the American College of Cardiology* 50, no. 8 (2007): 741–47.

62. Rogers and Pagani, "Results of Clinical Trials to Date," 287.

63. Lynne Warner Stevenson and Gregory Cooper, "On the Fledgling Field of Mechanical Support," *Journal of the American College of Cardiology* 50, no. 8 (2007):

748–51. See also D. Checker, "Heart Failure: Issues and Guidelines—An Expert Interview with Lynne Warner Stevenson, MD," *Medscape Cardiology* 7, no. 2 (2003): http://www.medscape.org/viewarticle/462498 (accessed June 15, 2013).

64. Steve Stiles, "REMATCH: The Sickest Gain the Most from LVAD Destination Therapy," Medscape (August 16, 2004): http://www.medscape.com/viewarticle/783205 (accessed June 15, 2013).

65. P. M. Portner, "Permanent Mechanical Circulatory Assistance," in *Heart and Lung Transplantation,* ed. W. A. Baumgartner, B. Reitz, E. Kasper, and J. Theodore, 2nd ed. (Philadelphia: W. B. Saunders, 2002), 544; J. Jassawalla et al., "Next Generation Novacor LVAS: A Miniaturized Pulsatile Pump," *ASAIO Journal* 45 (2000): 157; Rogers and Pagani, "Results of Clinical Trials to Date," 287.

66. WorldHeart Corporation chose to focus its efforts on the next-generation Levacor VAD, technology rights that it had acquired from MedQuest Products, Inc. in 2005. On July 29, 2011, they announced the termination of their efforts to commercialize the Levacor VAD technology, stating that they felt it was no longer commercially competitive. The company switched its focus to developing and commercializing its smaller, next-generation MiFlow and Pedia Flow VADs. WorldHeart restructured its business and reduced its workforce by 42 percent. In 2012, the WorldHeart Corporation was acquired by Heart Ware International, Inc. See US Securities and Exchange Commission, Form 10-K submitted by the World Heart Corporation for the fiscal year ended December 31, 2011, http://www.sec.gov/Archives/edgar/data/1024520/000119312512143629/d281196d10k.htm (accessed November 3, 2014); WorldHeart Corporation Press Release, November 14, 2007, http://markets.financialcontent.com/stocks/news/read/3800876/WorldHeart_Reports_Third_Quarter_2007_Financial_Results (accessed July 27, 2012); WorldHeart Corporation Press Release, July 29, 2011, http://globenewswire.com/news-release/2011/07/29/452580/227966/en/WorldHeart-Will-End-Its-Levacor-R-VAD-Program-and-Will-Focus-on-Developing-Its-Next-Generation-MiFlow-TM-Miniature-Ventricular-Assist-Device.html (accessed July 27, 2012).

67. Gideon Gil, "The Artificial Heart Juggernaut," *Hastings Center Report* 19, no. 2 (1989): 29–30.

68. Stevenson and Cooper, "On the Fledgling Field of Mechanical Support," 750.

69. James K. Kirlin et al., "Long-Term Mechanical Circulatory Support (Destination Therapy): On Track to Compete with Heart Transplantation?," *Journal of Thoracic and Cardiovascular Surgery* 144, no. 3 (2012): 593–94. As reiterated by many clinicians, the status of "transplant ineligible" at one point in time is not necessarily a final judgment. See Sharon A. Hunt, "Mechanical Circulatory Support: New Data, Old Problems," *Circulation* 116 (2007): 462.

70. Muriel R. Gillick, "The Technological Imperative and the Battle for Hearts in America," *Perspectives in Biology and Medicine* 50, no. 2 (2007): 283.

71. Hunt, "Mechanical Circulatory Support," 461.

72. Rose et al., "Long-Term Use of a Left Ventricular Assist Device," 1438. See also Massie, "Comment—LVADs," 61.

73. To mediate these factors of device limitations and cost, the Thoratec Corporation paid for a mass marketing campaign of their HeartMate device to increase awareness of destination therapy for congestive heart failure as well as the REMATCH results to both the medical community and the public. But as the

physician Muriel R. Gillick states, "Despite the publicity blitz, the LVAD did not catch on." Gillick, "Technological Imperative," 286.

74. David S. Jones, "Surgical Practice and the Reconstruction of the Therapeutic Niche: The Case of Myocardial Revascularization," chapter 8 of this volume.

75. The INTERMACS database was established in 2005 by the NHLBI. It later inspired the launching of an international registry—the International Society for Heart and Lung Transplantation Registry for Mechanically Assisted Circulatory Support (IMACS)—in January 2013 that is similarly managed and directly connected to the American database. For more on INTERMACS and IMACS, see James B. Young and Lynne Warner Stevenson, "INTERMACS (Interagency Registry for Mechanically Assisted Circulatory Support) as a Tool to Track and Advance Clinical Practice," in Kormos and Miller, *Mechanical Circulatory Support*, 313–14; INTERMACS registry and website at www.INTERMACS.org (accessed June 12, 2013); IMACS registry and website at http://www.ishlt.org/registries/mcsdDatabase.asp and http://www.ishlt.org/ContentDocuments/2013FebLinks_IMACS.html# (accessed June 15, 2013).

76. Kirklin et al., "Long-Term Mechanical Circulatory Support," 593.

77. A total of twenty-nine devices were replaced in twenty-three patients. The reasons for device replacement included inflow valve incompetence (n=12), bearing failures (n=8), sepsis (n=3), diaphragm facture (n=2), outflow valve regurgitation or kinking (n=3), and fluid ingress (n=1). See table 7—Summary of LVAD Pump Replacements, in Dembitsky et al., "Left Ventricular Assist Device Performance with Long-Term Circulatory Support," 2127. See also F. Pagani et al., "Improved Device Durability with Continuous Flow LVADs," *Journal of American College of Cardiology* 54 (2009): 312–21; Leslie W. Miller, "Left Ventricular Assist Devices Are Underutilized," *Circulation* 123 (2011): 1552–58.

78. NHLBI Working Group, *Next Generation Ventricular Assist Devices for Destination Therapy* (2004), http://www.nhlbi.nih.gov/research/reports/2004-nextgen-vads.htm (accessed September 19, 2014).

79. In a prospective, multicenter study without a concurrent control group, 133 patients with end-stage heart failure awaiting heart transplantation received the new continuous-flow HeartMate II. At six months, 100 patients (75 percent) benefitted from the HeartMate II. This second-generation technology was deemed superior to the older pulsatile pumps. See L. W. Miller et al., "Use of a Continuous-Flow Device in Patients Awaiting Heart Transplantation," *New England Journal of Medicine* 357, no. 9 (2007): 885–96. For FDA approval, see http://www.accessdata.fda.gov/scripts/cdrh/cfdocs/cfpma/pma.cfm?id=20543 (accessed October 31, 2014).

80. This was a randomized, direct comparison clinical trial in which 134 transplant-ineligible patients received a continuous-flow device (new HeartMate II pump) and 66 transplant-ineligible patients were implanted with the pulsatile-flow device (older HeartMate LVAD). This older HeartMate LVAD was the device used in the earlier REMATCH study. See Mark S. Slaughter et al., "Advanced Heart Failure Treated with Continuous-Flow Left Ventricular Assist Device," *New England Journal of Medicine* 361, no. 23 (2009): 2241–51. For FDA approval see http://www.accessdata.fda.gov/scripts/cdrh/cfdocs/cfpma/pma.cfm?id=27606 (accessed October 31, 2014).

81. Kirklin et al., "Long-Term Mechanical Circulatory Support," 593.

82. US Securities and Exchange Commission Form 10-K, submitted by the Thoratec Corporation for the fiscal year ended December 28, 2013, http://www.

sec.gov/Archives/edgar/data/350907/000104746914000984/a2218290z10-k.htm (accessed November 3, 2014).

83. James K. Kirklin, "Terminal Heart Failure: Who Should Be Transplanted and Who Should Have Mechanical Circulatory Support?," *Current Opinion in Organ Transplantation* 19, no. 5 (2014), http://www.researchgate.net/publication/265345336_Terminal_heart_failure_who_should_be_transplanted_and_who_should_have_mechanical_circulatory_support (accessed September 19, 2014).

84. Miller, "Left Ventricular Assist Devices," 1556–57.

85. Park et al., "Left Ventricular Assist Devices," 16, "Discussion." See additional similar comments by the heart-failure specialist Dr. Reynolds Delgado of the Texas Heart Institute, cited in Gillick, "Technological Imperative," 287.

Chapter Seven

Placebos and the Progress of Surgery

CHRISTOPHER CRENNER

Introduction

What counts as progress in surgery? And how are the advances measured? In exploring innovation in surgery, it is necessary to ask how innovations are judged, and about the mechanisms for evaluation. This paper will consider the changing methods of evaluating surgical procedures in the later twentieth century by following the fortunes of one alternative and especially contentious method, the placebo-controlled clinical trial. On first consideration, the idea of a surgical placebo may seem odd, or even unsettling. A surgical placebo trial involves fooling some patients into thinking that they received a surgical procedure, with the goal to compare their outcomes to patients who did receive the procedure. The technique entered the modern experimental repertoire as an exciting, if controversial, method in the late 1950s. It subsequently dropped from sight and was considered for a time to be perhaps fundamentally unethical. In the 1980s, however, the placebo-controlled surgical trial reentered use. The surgical placebo—or the sham surgery—is now in the early 2000s an accepted part of the experimentalist's toolbox, if still controversial.

The fraught history of placebo surgery is interesting for what it reveals about the introduction in the late twentieth century of new methods for judging the effects of surgical procedures. In a conventional version of this story, surgery over the last few decades has witnessed a competition between two basic methods for building evidence of effect—the case series and the randomized clinical trial (RCT). For centuries surgeons measured the success of a new procedure in the accumulated experience of use and gradually formalized this process in the mechanism of the case series. Results from a single patient's case, if promising, led to further cases until a convincing series materialized, providing evidence of therapeutic effect or its absence.

Accumulating experience could lead to a registry of cases, creating a larger body of evidence. To generate a traditional case series, the surgeon had only to operate and collect results in a systematic, attentive way. The case series proved both practical and influential and remains, with subsequent refinements, a mainstay of the surgical scientific literature.[1] By the second half of the twentieth century, however, physicians recognized that even with stringent care they could not avoid the biases and indirect influences that distorted case series results. Medicine was also becoming increasingly familiar with the methods of the RCT, a more demanding form of evaluation. Whereas in a case series the requirements of surgical practice shaped the production of evidence, in the clinical trial this priority was reversed. Clinical trials sought to improve the quality of evidence through the reorganization of practice into a rigorously experimental format. The use of RCT methods promised to minimize bias and distortion, but mandated a new format to practice: randomizing patients to different treatments, at times concealing the nature of the treatment, and perhaps treating patients with placebo. Developed within medicine for the purposes of testing pharmaceutical treatment, the modern clinical trial came into use in surgery beginning in the 1950s. Although progress in the use of the RCT in surgery remains contested and slow even a half century later, the RCT has gradually assumed the status, as Shelley McKellar reminds us elsewhere in this volume, of a "gold standard" for surgical evaluation.[2]

Thus the career of the RCT looks at first glance like a straightforward history—describing how the innovative methods of clinical trials challenged and won acceptance among more traditional means of gathering evidence in surgery. But as other authors in this collection have shown, the model of diffusion and resistance to innovation misses important features of technical change.[3] Examining the career of placebo surgery helps to resolve the clinical trial into its constituent parts and exposes the alternatives and contingencies associated with its adaptation. Placebo controls in surgery—and the use of sham surgery as a placebo—followed an especially turbulent course. Resistance within surgery to the methods of placebo control was especially fierce and seemed to epitomize broader concerns over use of controlled trials. Tracing the path of placebo controls in surgery helps to open up a space between our examination of the changing means for surgical evaluation and the ideologically weighty story of the progressive advance of the RCT.

Support for placebo controls in surgery, for example, drew strength from a pair of developments in the later twentieth century that had little relevance for other methods in the RCT. The strongest impetus was an emerging suspicion that the perceived benefits of some surgical procedures relied heavily on nonspecific therapeutic benefits that could be identified as the placebo effect.[4] Only testing against placebos could expose the degree to which surgical effects derived from some nonspecific, therapeutic influence of surgical attention and manipulation. These concerns about unmeasured placebo effects derived in turn from a fundamental change in the expanding repertoire of surgical procedures. The surgeons' longstanding ambition to intervene in milder, chronic conditions inspired in the second half of the twentieth century a growing array of new, less risky, and less invasive procedures, as well as a host of new surgically implanted devices. Creating a placebo version of gallbladder surgery might exceed the capacity of even the best experimental stage management. But faking a minimally invasive procedure, or creating a placebo test for an implanted device, could require no more than a small incision or the flipping of a switch.

The resistance among surgeons to placebo trials was similarly complex and specific, embedded within a larger debate over the slow adaptation of RCTs generally. Advocates of controlled trials in surgery tended to treat the RCT as a single entity that set a unified, higher standard by displacing older assumptions and methods. And the RCT did forge a path by breaking down ingrained assumptions and displacing the surgeons' familiar methods. But the resistance to the RCT in surgery coalesced out of a variety of concerns, associated differently with its different elements. The problem, for example, of randomizing patients in surgical trials has generated a variety of different solutions over time. Was it advisable, or acceptable, to ask a single surgeon to perform different procedures for the same problem on a succession of different patients, determined perhaps by the flip of a coin? Resistance to placebo-surgical trials was expressed most commonly in terms of the ethics of risk and deception. As we will see, the return of placebo surgery to use after its early rejection required working out specific bioethical procedures that helped to moderate such ethical concerns.

The gradual acceptance of the RCT within surgery has been characterized as a progressive achievement, helping to promote the interests of public health over narrower and potentially biased interests of the surgical enterprise. The availability of a rigorous standard for therapeutic evidence could help to restrain the undue enthusiasm that might carry unproven new surgical procedures into widespread use.[5] But the availability of this new standard could also mean, as we shall see, legitimacy for a marginal surgical procedure that managed to clear the hurdle.[6] By singling out this one controversial method of experimental evaluation, this paper will explore the contingencies involved in introducing the clinical trial to surgery, without denying the satisfactions of a glimpse at the associated progressive goals.

Clinical Trials and Research Infrastructure

The placebo trial can be said to have entered modern surgery in a single moment in 1958 in an operating room of the Bell Memorial Hospital in

Kansas City, Kansas, as Dr. Fred Kittle made a shallow incision in the chest of his anesthetized patient. Kittle was involved in a clinical trial designed to test a popular new surgical procedure using ligation of the internal mammary arteries as a treatment for cardiac angina. In the conventional version of the procedure, a surgeon tied off the two arteries as they emerged into the superficial muscles of the chest wall, in an effort to redirect blood back toward a patient's ailing heart. On this occasion, however, Kittle left the two arteries alone, merely suturing closed his surgical wounds and sending the patient back to the recovery area. Kittle, along with the cardiologist E. Gray Dimond and a small academic medical team at the University of Kansas, had conceived of this sham surgery as a new and especially rigorous test of the mammary artery ligation procedure. Just before beginning the incisions, Kittle learned that his patient had been randomly assigned to receive a sham version of the procedure, whereas others would receive the convention procedure. Kittle's nontherapeutic incisions were intended to convince the patient that he had received the novel surgical treatment—when in fact he had not.[7] The procedure helped to mark a new era in the evaluation of surgical techniques.[8]

Kittle and his colleagues' use of placebos figured as part of a wave of new clinical experimentalism that swept into American medicine in the postwar period. The advantages of testing medical therapies through organized clinical trials, using a combination of randomization, prospective controls, and blinding, had been well established already in the 1930s by Ronald Fisher and Austin Bradford Hill. But applications in medicine were sporadic, with a few examples in pharmaceutical testing up through the 1940s.[9] In the postwar period, the growth of pharmaceutical testing and corresponding changes in academic medicine helped to expand use of clinical trials, along with "the evolving configurations of institutional, organizational, conceptual, human and material resources" that produced and sustained them.[10] Although the application of these experimental methods to surgery was not widely anticipated, the influence of the broader institutional changes was felt throughout medical institutions.

Rather remarkably, at the same time that Kittle and his group at the University of Kansas were conducting their clinical trial of internal mammary artery ligation, another group of physicians at the University of Washington were pursing an identical project.[11] Organized out of the academic section on cardiology at the university and led by a young medical researcher, Leonard Cobb, this other clinical trial of internal mammary artery ligation also used sham surgeries for the control group. The existence of two simultaneous, independent versions of the same experiment is surprising, but points to the emerging national support for such efforts. Changes at a federal level had established strong new sources of funding and guidance for clinical medical research. A major source was the National Institutes of Health (NIH), which was in the midst of extraordinary growth, with budgetary increases between 1950 and 1955 that more than doubled from $28 million to over $60 million.[12] The organizers of both the sham trials in Kansas City and in Seattle relied on funding from the National Heart Institute (now part of the National Heart, Lung and Blood Institute, or NHLBI), the first institute developed at the NIH. While supporting academic research at programs as far-flung as Seattle and Kansas City, the NIH was also building a stable infrastructure for clinical trials on its own campus. Programs like the intramural program for the development of chemotherapeutics at the National Cancer Institute became leaders in the application and refinement of clinical trials. In 1954, the National Cancer Institute established the national cooperative clinical groups and the Cancer Chemotherapy National Service Center, institutionalizing the creation of clinical trials. The NIH section on metabolic disease similarly initiated a large-scale clinical trial of new drugs for the treatment of diabetes.[13] The interest in clinical trials also gained ground in this period in the realm of regulation, for related reasons. With many new medications and treatments entering use, concern grew over the problems of safety and reliability. A group that Harry Marks has called the therapeutic reformers lent support to legislative initiatives that culminated in the passage in 1962 of the Kefauver-Harris Amendment, putting the force of the Food and Drug Administration (FDA) behind mandatory clinical testing of new drugs.[14] The act spelled out three phases for testing that drew on the methods of the clinical trial. These regulatory changes pushed pharmaceutical manufacturers to strengthen alliances with academic physicians to aid in the organization of clinical trials on a national scale. These systematic developments at the national level came hand in hand with rapid growth in the research infrastructure of academic medicine, as exemplified in the budding programs in academic cardiology and cardiothoracic surgery that supported Dimond, Kittle, and Cobb.[15]

Dimond and Cobb only serendipitously learned of each other's existence later at the annual meeting of the American Heart Association when they both showed up to present their parallel placebo-surgery studies. The two men were perhaps relieved to discover that their results agreed. Both experiments showed that internal mammary artery ligation, a widely popularized procedure, turned out to have about the same effect as a sham version. A majority of patients in both studies reported getting some relief from their cardiac angina—whether they received a real or a sham version. The two studies were understood to provide conclusive evidence that the widely reported benefits of the procedure were simply placebo effects. Sham surgery debuted as a clinical experimental method with power to deflate claims of promising new surgical procedures.

Publication of the two sham-surgery studies provoked a distinct reaction both within academic medicine and in the larger public media. What commentators found most striking was how susceptible patients were to the effects of the sham surgery. The surgical placebo effect was powerful, constituting a hidden and perhaps invalid influence of the surgeon's art. Set against a background of postwar anxieties over the sway of individual charismatic authority and the stark powers of new technologies, these trials generated eager attention. Intrigued by the results, Henry Beecher, a physician at Massachusetts General Hospital, brought sham surgery to the attention of a broad medical readership and provided a key interview for an article in the *Wall Street Journal* discussing the surgeries.[16] Beecher argued that the personal beliefs of an individual surgeon about the value of treatment could enhance the placebo effect—communicated through the surgeon's confident manner and reassuring advice. Cast in the setting of a deceptive sham operation, Beecher's characterization of surgical persuasiveness could not help but pick up an ominous tinge, reflected as well in the newspaper's coverage. The discussion of placebo surgery seemed to echo prevailing concerns during this Cold War period about the power and limits of authority. Scientific authority particularly came under scrutiny in the period. In the years between the publication of the Seattle groups' findings and Beecher's public discussions, Stanley Milgram published what became another notorious sham experiment with his psychological study on obedience. Milgram devised an experiment in which naïve subjects were instructed by a white-coated laboratory supervisor to administer apparently harmful electric shocks to another experimental subject. The arrangement was a sham: the lab-coated supervisor and the other subject were both collaborators, and the shock apparatus was a dummy device.[17] Such research projects hint at an ambivalent curiosity about the persuasive authority of science that provided context for the introduction of sham surgery to modern clinical trials.

Case Studies as Alternate Means of Therapeutic Evaluation

The path of the clinical trial in surgery was not a simple linear one, however. As in other instances explored in this volume, surgeons had alternative means at hand for evaluating treatments and continued to develop and refine the methods of the case series alongside the growing interest in surgical clinical trials. Before the midcentury in the United States, medicine and surgery shared the clinical case as a basic unit for the measure of therapeutic effect and the construction of therapeutic knowledge.[18] With the gradual adoption of the RCT in medical therapeutics, physicians in internal medicine came to relegate case reports largely to didactic purposes.[19] Even as surgeons in the postwar period began to try out the methods of the RCT, they continued to develop and strengthen the use of the traditional case series. Thomas Schlich provides evidence of these developments in his definitive study of the Swiss surgical group *Arbeitsgemeinschaft für Osteosynthesefragen* (AO). The AO began its work in the 1960s with the goal to establish and recursively improve the techniques of internal mechanical fixation of bone fractures. Their systematic approach built on and extended the methods of the conventional case series. In part to meet concerns about bias, the AO group enrolled patients systematically and sought long-term follow up on results without loss through dropout. In addition, they developed and shared standardized equipment and techniques and created a systematic classification of bony fractures, with orderly assignment of treatment protocols according to diagnosis. They further refined methods for large-scale data collection and analysis for the case series, creating a systematic registry of the group's surgical cases. In their first international reports, the members of the group could, for example, cite experience with four hundred cases of tibial fracture treated with bone screws by a standard method—no trivial series.[20] Through the production of such sophisticated and extensive case series data, the AO surgeons assembled a weight of evidence supporting their methods. Progress required strict attention to individual operative techniques with recurrent review and feedback. There was much in these methods to appeal to the surgeon. The craft nature of surgery with its emphasis on individual judgment and responsibility reinforced the value of case evidence.[21] Elsewhere in this volume David Jones charts the emergence of the widely successful procedure of coronary artery bypass surgery from among a welter of alternative techniques as a competition waged on the evidence of increasingly large series of successful reports.[22] In surgery, the cases series has remained a major form of therapeutic evidence; communications about new surgical treatments still appears today typically in the form of a case report and case series.[23]

Whereas the case series, backed up by laboratory demonstrations and the use of experimental animal models, continues to be a primary means for demonstrating surgical effects today, surgeons in the late twentieth century were increasingly being drawn into work with clinical trials. These efforts created hybrid paths of development as new treatments were pushed through different phases of refinement and evaluation. Observers began to assert that there was a hierarchy, or at least a sequence, of forms of evaluation, as a procedure moved from trials in individual cases and case series into evaluation in clinical trials.[24] The placebo-controlled surgical trial provided a stark demonstration of the rigor of the final stages of evaluation. This was the path followed by the internal mammary artery ligation procedure, for example, when many promising case studies culminated in a striking reversal with placebo-controlled clinical trials. It was a pattern followed also by what became a notorious example of the deflationary power of the placebo-controlled clinical trial when the innovative technique of gastric freezing met with a similar fate.[25]

Gastric Freezing and Placebo Controls

Gastric freezing, although not strictly a surgical procedure, had a distinguished surgical pedigree, invented and promoted out of the Department of Surgery at the University of Minnesota by the highly influential chair of the department, Owen Wangensteen. An international leader in academic surgery, the head of major organizations, and mentor to what seemed an entire generation of chairs of academic surgical departments across the United States, Wangensteen worked intensively through the midcentury on the surgical treatment of peptic ulcer disease. Peptic ulcers at this time, especially duodenal ulcers, were a major source of disability and death, accompanied unpredictably by intractable pain, perforation, and sudden hemorrhage. Wangensteen first conceived of gastric freezing during investigations into the use of lavage with freezing water to staunch sudden hemorrhages from ulcers. The early work from Wangensteen's surgical team reported results on experiments with rats, frogs, minnows, cats, and dogs, and concluded with details on a series of five patients successfully treated for massive gastrointestinal bleeding through cooling of the stomach lining. These experiments further suggested to Wangensteen that deep cooling of the interior of the stomach reduced acid production and digestive activity, with the promise to remove these stimuli to ulcers.[26]

Building on these experiments, Wangensteen became intrigued by the hypothesis that cooling to the point of actual temporary gastric freezing would prevent the subsequent return of ulcers by a longer reduction in digestive activity. The standard surgical treatments for the disease required partial surgical removal of stomach wall and might include resection of the stomach's nerves. Wangensteen saw promise in his less risky and invasive therapy. He began to enlist for his experiments a succession of patients coming to the university clinics for the surgical care of peptic ulcers. Wangensteen reflected on the popularity of the work in 1963, reporting to a colleague that "very few patients so far have defected from the study-program, reflecting the anxiety of patients to retain their stomachs."[27] Working with a local refrigeration company, Wangensteen devised a mechanism to pump freezing alcohol through a balloon that had been inserted on a tube and swallowed into the stomach. The publication of a case series documenting positive therapeutic results with the device secured considerable interest. In addition, Wangensteen was able to contrive dramatic laboratory demonstrations of the effect. He reported that a small spring frog with an oxygen line attached to its nose would survive intact for 20 hours in the stomach of a large Louisiana bullfrog if the stomach remained cooled to 4 degrees centigrade—although at room temperature "digestion of the inlying guest frog was quite complete in less than 10 hours."[28] Word of the therapeutic use of gastric freezing spread widely. By the mid-1960s thousands of patients had been treated, and gastric freezing devices from several competing manufacturers were being sold across the country.[29]

Although Wangensteen insisted that treatment with gastric freezing should be performed at the hospital, the procedure was relatively simple and caused few complications, at least from Wangensteen's team. As news of the procedure spread, physicians around the country replicated the procedure and began to report generally positive results, especially in the initial relief of ulcer pain. Wangensteen's first papers on gastric freezing referred to the procedure as a "physiological gastrectomy," emphasizing its ability to substitute for the conventional, aggressive surgical treatment of resection of the stomach. Wangensteen himself claimed to be diverting all patients arriving at his clinic at the University of Minnesota for surgical treatment of ulcers into treatment with freezing.[30]

The development of gastric freezing exemplified certain key aspirations of surgery during Wangensteen's career. Since the nineteenth century surgery had remained at its professional core a set of risky procedures designed to treat urgent, life-threatening problems, such as trauma, tumors, bleeding, and the rupture or obstruction of visceral organs. As the reach of surgery continued to grow under leadership from full-time academic surgeons such as Wangensteen, its principal accomplishments remained both invasive and bold, as exemplified by sporadic, stunning success in organ transplantation in the 1960s. But over the same period surgeons extended their efforts also toward milder, more chronic conditions. In a major lecture in 1936, Wangensteen announced the ambition to move surgery away from a limited focus on urgent rescue to target less dire conditions; and related aspirations were already evident in late-nineteenth-century efforts at prophylactic appendectomy, for example.[31] But it was the American surgeons in the second half of the twentieth century who might be said to have brought these goals to fruition. The Harvard surgeon Atul Gawande estimated that by 2010, when the repertoire of conventional surgery in the United States had reached over 2,500 different procedures, the average American would experience approximately nine surgical procedures in the course of a lifetime, choosing to go under the knife for such nonacute conditions as back pain, hernia, and obesity.[32]

The paired ambitions to tackle milder, chronic conditions and to develop less invasive surgical procedures would make increasingly clear both the feasibility and the value of placebo-controlled trials of surgery. Less risky, less invasive procedures such as internal mammary artery ligation and gastric freezing could be readily faked and replaced by sham contrivances. Surgeons were quick to point out, by contrast, that most major surgeries left little opportunity for successful shams. In addition, the treatment of milder, chronic discomforts and disabilities highlighted the importance of subjective outcomes. The placebo effect of surgery on patients thus weighed heavily in judging efficacy of such procedures.

The power of placebo evaluation was not lost on Wangensteen's colleagues. Surgical groups soon set out to test gastric freezing in rigorous, placebo-controlled trials. In 1964, surgeons at Bellevue Hospital, led by a young professor of surgery at Columbia Physicians and Surgeons, set in motion such a double-blinded, randomized, placebo-controlled trial of gastric freezing. Patients from Bellevue Hospital with stomach pain and confirmed gastric ulcers, who agreed to enter the study, were taken to the operating room for treatment. Half of the group, randomly selected, had sedation followed by the standard freezing treatment according to the process described by Wangensteen. The other half—referred to by the investigators as the "sham freezing" group—had the same preparation but received room-temperature water circulated through the balloon. The Bellevue team followed these patients for two years to assess the progress of their ulcers. On subsequent surveys, several patients reported "complete resolution" of their symptoms after one and two years. However, all the patients who had such a resolution were in the sham treatment group. Rigorous comparison of gastric freezing with placebo treatment offered convincing evidence of its transitory, and perhaps illusory, therapeutic effect.[33]

In 1969, a large, multicenter RCT comparing gastric freezing and sham-freezing published in the *New England Journal of Medicine* reached similar conclusions and effectively closed the book on Wangensteen's innovation.[34] Wangensteen, however, remained unpersuaded. He continued to defend the value of the procedure into the 1980s. In part, he seemed to reject the idea that the placebo-controlled RCTs provided evidence superior to his laboratory work, animal testing, and long case series of successful patient treatments. At the height of the controversy in 1967, the influential gastroenterologist Morton I. Grossman wrote to the editor of the *Journal of the American Medical Association* with a scathing indictment of Wangensteen's work on gastric freezing. The letter was forwarded to Wangensteen and apparently never published. Grossman accused Wangensteen of unethical conduct because he was continuing to experiment on patients with gastric freezing without first committing to perform blinded, controlled trials. Wangensteen wrote back directly to Grossman and initiated a series of lengthy letters. Grossman insisted that Wangensteen had insufficient evidence without controlled trials to justify human use of freezing, whereas Wangensteen countered that his long successful experience in the laboratory and with series of patients justified continued experimental development of the procedure. Wangensteen closed the correspondence with a final letter summarizing his position, saying "I do not believe it wise to try to codify all therapeutic research endeavors to conform to a standard pattern." There should be room, he continued, for "your philosophy and mine . . . to exist side by side." And he concluded, "You are keen for the controlled experiment. I am equally as enthusiastic over the sequence of observation, experiment, and experience."[35]

Both gastric freezing and internal mammary artery ligation inspired early attempts in surgery at placebo-controlled experiments—and in the latter case the use of sham surgery. These two momentarily popular, and subsequently debunked, procedures shared notable similarities that may have encouraged testing against placebo. Both were simple and minimally invasive procedures that aimed to replace complex and risky surgeries. Wangensteen promoted gastric freezing as a "physiological gastrectomy" that would obviate the need for surgical partial gastrectomy. The procedure of ligation of the mammary arteries similarly aimed to treat a condition otherwise amenable only to risky surgical work directly on the heart. Major placebo-controlled trials of both procedures developed within academic surgical units, where there may have been skepticism about the purported ease of these alternatives. In addition, these placebo-controlled trials involved physicians from academic departments where there was significant local familiarity with the use of clinical trials and placebo controls. E. Grey Dimond at Kansas City and Leonard Cobb at Seattle were both cardiologists, working in a field where placebo-controlled evaluation of medications was well established. Gastroenterologists from academic departments of internal medicine similarly contributed to the trials of gastric freezing.

The Contested Progress of the Surgical RCT in the 1970s

By the 1970s, the RCT had become a fundamental element of medical research and pharmaceutical regulation, but within academic surgery clinical trials followed a slow and rocky course. In 1968, the NCI published results on a randomized controlled trial of surgery and chemotherapy for gastric cancer, testing combinations of gastrectomy with adjuvant chemotherapy. In the initial phase, begun in 1957, the organizers limited the trial to a simple version of randomization, without blinding. Blinding was subsequently added along with placebo controls, with the aim to reduce bias. But even in the final design, the randomization, blinding and comparative controls were applied only to chemotherapeutic agents. Surgeons insisted on the need to determine the surgical procedure, whether total, partial, or distal gastrectomy, themselves at the time of the procedure—precluding the possibility of blinding or randomization.[36] With such hesitant starts, surgeons gradually became involved in a number of nationally prominent clinical trials of major surgical procedures, though these tended to generate considerable debate and controversy.

In 1971, Bernard Fischer began enrolling patients in a long-awaited, much discussed randomized surgical trial comparing radical mastectomy with the less destructive "total" mastectomy for breast cancer. Surgeons at the time criticized the entire effort as an inappropriate extension of these methods into surgery. Looking at early efforts for controlled testing of radiotherapy, surgery, and chemotherapy for lung cancer, Carsten Timmerman similarly found that surgeons criticized randomization as fully inappropriate for surgery. Trials in other domains of treatment, however, seemed to escape open criticism. Already underway at the time was another large clinical trial in the Veterans Administration (VA) medical system that would eventually enroll 1,357 patients randomized to one of four different surgical procedures to treat peptic ulcer.[37] The VA system seemed to provide a supportive institutional structure for the conduct of such studies, and became home to one of the most widely discussed studies of the period, a clinical trial to test coronary artery bypass surgery against standard medical treatment in a randomized comparison. Here again, however, controversy over the methods and evidence of the RCT rose to public debate, analyzed in its historical context by David Jones.[38]

Although none of these major trials involved—or likely could even have considered—sham surgical controls, the earlier surgical placebo trials remained an important touchstone in the ensuing debate. Resistance to the basic methods of randomization and blinding remained widespread, even within academic surgery. To opponents, placebo or sham surgery exemplified the worst aspects of this new clinical experimentalism.

One of the surgeons' major, persisting criticisms of clinical trials was their static nature. The process of randomizing a sufficient number of subjects in a large trial might take years. During that time the surgical procedure being tested had to be kept unchanged. The procedure used on the last case had to be the same as the first, to allow valid comparison. But critics of the trials, such as the pioneering pediatric surgeon Lawrence Bonchek, were accustomed to look for steady refinement in technique and improvements of a new method in its application. A clinical trial established early in the development of a new procedure might lead to premature rejection of a promising treatment. Clinical testing later, however, seemed potentially unethical, as it might deprive patients randomized to the other treatment of a well-developed, valuable therapy.[39] Timmerman's study of lung cancer documented similar concerns among the surgeons involved with early clinical trials of lung cancer treatment.[40]

Critics of the clinical trials in the 1970s and 1980s, such as Bonchek, conceived of the process of surgical innovation as gradual. Thus the static, episodic nature of prospective clinical trials was disruptive, keeping in use during a long trial an operative procedure that might otherwise have become outmoded through gradual improvement. For Bonchek, the very process of randomization seemed unethical. It assigned a preconceived version of therapy by chance, undermining the ability to vary treatment to suit the needs of the individual patient. In concluding his most critical essay on clinical trials, Bonchek cited the original internal mammary artery experiments as a clear demonstration of experimental hubris, with the use of sham surgery emblematic of the excesses of the experimental approach. The deceptive nature of random assignment and the concealment of what was a nontherapeutic invasion of the patient's body seemed to capture everything that was wrong about the experimental surgical trial.

For enthusiastic advocates of clinical trials such as the physician and medical reformer Thomas Chalmers, medical progress came through winnowing by rigorous testing of all promising innovations. The method of sham controls in surgery held for Chalmers a promise rather than a threat. As the director of the intramural Clinical Center at the NIH in the 1970s, Chalmers was well situated to promote clinical trials and expressed special interest in their application to surgery.[41] Chalmers expressed himself untroubled by the need to halt the development of a new procedure in order to establish a valid clinical trial. Without guidance from well-organized trials, surgeons might continue to change their practices without necessarily improving them. Like his opponents in the debate, Chalmers too cited the sham-surgical trials of the previous decade.[42] They taught a valuable lesson, demonstrating that judgments about therapy based on accumulated experience in a case series might simply be wrong. Surgeons had been convinced of the beneficial effects of internal mammary artery ligation, and no less of a surgical eminence than Owen Wangensteen had considered gastric freezing a major advance. Only the tools of randomization, comparative control groups, blinding, and the use of placebos made possible accurate assessment of a new procedure. As David Jones notes in his examination of trials of coronary artery bypass grafting (CABG), critics of the procedure who were concerned about the overly optimistic embrace of a surgical solution called for randomized controlled trials and "demanded that the burden of proof for CABG be set very high."[43] The need to restrain unfounded surgical enthusiasms required that the surgeon should "randomize the first patient" on every new procedure, as Chalmers famously urged.[44]

The Regulation of Implanted Medical Devices

Despite controversy over the adoption of the RCT, surgeons continued to find uses for even the controversial method of placebo control. Sham surgery was an obvious, if unsettling, way to create a placebo for a surgical trial, but less vivid forms of placebo experimentation were also possible. The gradual interest in implanted medical devices among surgeons created both needs and opportunities for placebo testing. The clinical trials of gastric freezing demonstrated how readily a placebo control for a therapeutic device could be established. It might require nothing more than turning off the device. As surgical innovations increasingly involved the concurrent development of surgical devices, such opportunities—and the opportunity to regulate them—became more common.

The synergy between surgical innovation and the creation of new devices rapidly gained momentum after midcentury, with orthopedic surgery an especially fertile field. The previously mentioned pioneering work of the Swiss AO group on fracture care in the 1960s and 1970s offered a prominent example. The success of John Charnley's prosthetic hip and the development of the Harrington Rods, examined by Beth Linker in this volume, provide parallel examples.[45] Work in cardiology over the same period also produced a host of new "device-assisted" therapies, with the refinement of implanted cardiac pacemakers and prosthetic heart valves leading the way. Whereas implanted devices like aortic valves and spinal stabilizing rods did not lend themselves to ready comparison with placebo or sham controls, related developments in surgically implanted medical devices did provide such opportunities. In 1985, a group organized by neurosurgeons in the Department of Surgery at Dartmouth-Hitchcock Medical Center began enrolling patients in a trial of treatment for Alzheimer's Disease that relied on an implanted pump with an intraventricular catheter. The treatment required surgical implantation of the infusion device, manufactured by Shiley Infusaid, to deliver medication directly into the lateral ventricles of the brain. In a small, exploratory clinical trial, all patients received the implanted device and were assigned randomly to receive infusions of sterile water (placebo) or the active agent, bethanecol chloride, in different sequences over the course of several weeks. No physician in the treatment or the evaluation team, no patients, and no family members were aware of which patients were in which treatment sequence. When the randomization code was unsealed, the results of this placebo-controlled, blinded study were disappointing. The trial was another hybrid that used surgeons in the conduct of a placebo-controlled pharmaceutical trial that involved the invasive placement of a device. Variations on such experimental strategies were soon replicated in a host of new trials for the treatment of chronic, degenerative neurologic conditions.[46]

The acceptance of placebo controls in surgery depended in part on such characteristic niches, emerging with the proliferation of surgically implanted devices that aimed to create subjective therapeutic effects. The degenerative neurological conditions of Alzheimer's and Parkinson's disease remain quite deadly and debilitating, with available treatments weak and imperfect—although improved for Parkinson's disease after the 1960s with L-dopa. Thus the incentive for new therapies has been significant. In addition, both conditions have a fluctuating course, manifested in part through the sufferer's subjective experiences. One of the most widely discussed early sham-surgical experiments to reach the medical literature after a hiatus of over a decade was a pair of placebo-controlled trials of neurosurgical implantation of fetal brain tissue to treat Parkinson's disease.[47] Surgical placement of the fetal tissue required drilling burr holes in the skull. The physicians designing the study were concerned that the placebo effect of this invasive surgical procedure would be significant and would influence the patients' perceptions of treatment efficacy.[48] Although a sham version of the surgery involved drilling the holes in the skull with no therapeutic intent, the investigators' plans for careful, well-informed consent for the experiment and efforts to minimize risks in the placebo arm were deemed to be sufficient ethical precautions. The implantation technique was found, overall, to be only modestly effective in some patients and to cause for others a worsening of symptoms not seen in the placebo group, demonstrating again a potentially valuable role for sham-surgical trials.[49]

Given the obvious difficulties of using placebos in surgery, other forms of therapeutic comparison took precedence in the use of clinical trials in surgery. More commonly, evaluation of surgical treatments in randomized trials involved comparison with other existing surgical procedures or with management through pharmacological or other nonsurgical therapies. Interest in the improvement of methods for such trials spawned many variations. Comparison between a new treatment and established treatments could take the form of an equivalence trial, a noninferiority trial, or a superiority trial, depending on how the trial was organized and analyzed. These methods grew increasingly well-defined and differentiated, in part through the efforts of an emerging cadre of "trialists" with specialized expertise in the design of clinical trials.[50] While certain indications for placebo controls in evaluation, such as treatment of pain or other subjectively evaluated manifestations of disease, have long been evident, and were noted in Henry Beecher's early publications on the sham surgery trials, other new pressures for use of placebo controls have arisen in the nexus of research, discovery, production, marketing, and clinical use within the expanding healthcare sector.

As Shelley McKellar demonstrates in this volume for the case of the cardiac assist pump, the conduct of a modern surgical RCT requires complex agreements among commercial biotechnology firms, federal regulatory agencies, and academic medical centers, with a constantly changing balance of temporary alliances and competitive jostling. Regulatory changes in particular have strongly affected the development of placebo-controlled surgical trials. Already by the 1960s, the FDA established the RCT as the primary tool for regulating pharmaceutical development. The convergence of surgery with biomedical engineering, and the serious risks associated with implanted materials, soon inspired similar attention to invasive medical devices. The FDA had maintained nominal oversight of the introduction of new medical devices since the passage of a 1936 amendment, although no regulatory mechanisms were established until the mid-1970s. By the late-1960s, however, advocates for regulation could point to the quickening pace of medical device development and a series of tragic failures in pacemakers, intrauterine contraceptive devices, and prosthetic cardiac valves. In 1969, Theodore Cooper, then director of the NHLBI, chaired a committee to review the evidence of injuries from failed medical devices. The Cooper Committee, as it was called, estimated that in a ten-year period, there were over 10,000 such injuries, with 731 incidents resulting in death.[51] With the results of the report to support them, reform-minded legislators moved to give the FDA greater regulatory control over devices.

The passage of the Medical Devices Act in 1976 gave the FDA, which had long regulated pharmaceutical approval, parallel authority over medical devices. The law established a process for Pre-Market Approval (PMA) that required manufacturers to submit evidence of the safety and effectiveness of new medical devices before placing them on the market. The FDA divided devices into three categories, assigning the riskiest, typically surgically implanted devices, to the third class requiring clear demonstrations of safety and efficacy for approval. The actual methods for collecting evidence of safety and efficacy were left unspecified and were assumed to vary according to applications and potential risks. At the FDA, the controlled trial was well established as the standard for evaluation of pharmaceuticals, but did not find specific endorsement in the new legislation.[52]

Ambiguity about the standards for evaluation, and the creation of a number of exempt pathways to approval, set the grounds for a slow tug of war between device manufacturers, researchers, and regulators. The first device to win approval by the FDA through the PMA mechanism was an implanted intracaval balloon called the Hunter-Sessions Vena-Cava Occluder. The manufacturer, Concepts Inc., won approval for the device in May 1978 having submitted only a series of case reports on its use. What constituted adequate evidence of effect remained loosely defined. Over the following decade the FDA gradually defaulted into a two-tier system, approving a large number of devices through exempt mechanisms, while gradually tightening standards and promoting evaluation through controlled trials for devices deemed to have a high ration of risk to benefit.[53] Nonetheless, the FDA came under fire intermittently for blocking potentially beneficial innovation through strict regulation. Sham surgery became again a convenient shorthand for the excesses of clinical experimentalism. In seeking to highlight barriers to regulatory approval, the *Wall Street Journal* cited use of sham surgical testing as evidence of the extremes to which device manufacturers were being pushed to prove the effectiveness of their products.[54]

The rigors of placebo testing may at times have constituted a barrier for device development, but it was apparently also treated as an opportunity, as they say in business. The manufacturer of an implanted device to close defects in the septum of the heart initially planned to market the device to prevent embolic strokes caused by embolic clots escaping through such a septal defect. In seeking FDA approval, they submitted a PMA application proposing to establish effectiveness through a randomized trial comparing the device to usual medical care. This clinical trial, however, once completed, suggested that the device did not confer such benefits. But rather than abandon the device as a complete loss, the developers elected to pursue a high-stakes gambit. They reconceived of the closure device as an unorthodox treatment for migraine headaches. Drawing on the novel hypothesis of a collaborating neurologist, they postulated that the device could be used in migraine sufferers to block the hypothetical passage of migraine-inciting substances through defects the cardiac septum (and also secure proof for an original and exciting hypothesis about a possible cause of migraine headaches). The company's prospectus pointed out that among the millions of partially treated migraine patients there would be a sizable market. Evaluation of the treatment would, however, rely heavily on the subjective reports of migraine patients. To gain FDA approval, the manufacturers proposed to conduct a large, multicenter, placebo-controlled, randomized trial comparing implantation of the device against a similar, sham procedure, in blinded fashion. Following a strategy familiar among biotechnology firms pursuing single-drug development, the company streamlined its holdings, so that rights on this one device remained a sole asset. With all the eggs now in this single basket, the placebo-controlled trial became an all-or-nothing gamble on the future of the company. When the multicenter trial subsequently returned unfavorable results, the company dropped from sight.[55]

Not all such high-stakes placebo-controlled tests resulted in failure, keeping open the apparent promise of validation through a single experimental event (with the allure, it has been suggested, of competition against a nonspecific therapy rather than another active treatment). An entirely different surgical procedure for relief of migraines, which was thought to lack an agreed-on basis in physiological effect, nevertheless gained a national podium based largely on ability to exceed the (positive) effects of sham-surgical controls in a randomized clinical trial.[56] The use of such trials has remained, however, an unusual, high-stakes endeavor, given the costs and complexity of large, randomized controlled trials, as well as a prominent record of negative outcomes in controversial trials of internal mammary artery ligation and gastric freezing. A parallel development that drew perhaps more attention to the placebo-surgery trial in the late century was their well-established capacity for debunking established surgical techniques.

Sham Arthroscopy and the Advantages of Bioethical Proceduralism

At the vanguard of efforts to moderate the risks and invasiveness of surgical procedures were advances in what became known as minimally invasive surgery, which used a flexible operative scope and fiber-optic illumination with indirectly manipulated cutting and grasping devices. Surgeons could employ these scopes (depending on the body cavity) for laparoscopy, mediastinoscopy, pleuroscopy, and arthroscopy. The technique inspired several large, randomized trials comparing their use with established, conventional surgical procedures.[57] In the setting of rapidly growing surgical use of endoscopic procedures, the sham-surgical control regained a place in the conventional toolbox of clinical trial methods. In an experiment that reignited many of the lingering controversies surrounding sham surgery, a surgeon in Houston began a trial testing arthoscopic debridement of cartilage in osteoarthritis against a sham-surgical control group.

This sham-arthroscopy experiment came out of the efforts of J. Bruce Moseley, a young surgeon from Baylor University, and Nelda P. Wray, a health services researcher associated with the VA hospital where the trial would take place. The project started with curiosity about a widely used procedure for arthroscopic treatment of the knee cartilage. Using arthroscopy, surgeons would treat arthritic pain and debility by washing out the knee joint and trimming back frayed edges of cartilage, a procedure called lavage and debridement. Patients generally felt better after the procedure, but the results were sometimes transient. Moseley and Wray speculated that the physiological effects of the treatment could not well account for the perceived benefits, since the procedure did not fundamentally affect the underlying disease. Wray was convinced that accurate evaluation of arthroscopic treatment of osteoarthritis would require placebo testing, and began working with Moseley to devise a sham-controlled test. The greatest obstacle to such a trial, they saw, was approval for the ethics of sham controls, before the fetal-tissue implantation studies were widely known. Concerns about the ethical use of sham surgery had grown since the first sham-surgery trials.[58]

In the 1960s, the early mammary artery ligation trials were treated as ethically complex but potentially acceptable. The Boston anesthesiologist Henry Beecher brought the trials to public notice because of the light they shed on placebo effects in surgery. Beecher was also an important early leader in the ethical critique of medical research, but he expressed no ethical objections to the sham surgeries in his discussions. He identified the patient's consent as critical to the internal mammary artery trials. But Beecher recognized that the patients in Seattle were informed only that they were entering an experimental trial, without mention of sham surgery. Elsewhere Beecher suggested that a valid comparison of placebo controls in a study of pain relief might need to be exempted from the requirement of a full disclosure, at least in cases of "no discernible risk."[59] Beecher's ambivalence was consistent with shared medical opinion in the 1960s about the nature of placebo controlled experiments and patient consent. Prominent physicians argued that a subject's knowledge of placebo use would affect their experience and invalidate experimental results. Conscientious physician-scientists believed that they could fairly conduct trials without disclosing the use of placebos, as long as they were truly undecided about the therapeutic value of the real therapy.[60] There were also voices of dissent, but so muddled were prevailing views on the issue that half of American physicians surveyed in the late 1960s found it acceptable not to reveal to a patient that "she had been enrolled in a double blind clinical trial of an experimental anticancer drug and was currently receiving a placebo."[61]

In the wake of gradually more rigorous scrutiny of medical research and public exposure of a series of gross violations in research in the 1970s, medical views on the ethical nature of sham surgical research grew more cautious. Journal articles and surgical textbooks began to identify sham surgical experiments as ethically unacceptable.[62]

Although ethical misgivings inhibited the early acceptance of sham surgical trials, it was, ironically, the growing regulatory oversight of research and especially the institutionalization of bioethics that helped to smooth the path back into use. In the late 1970s and 1980s, bioethics secured a role advising on the conduct and regulation of medical research as the internal dynamics of medical practice opened to greater public scrutiny and critique.[63] Without dispelling certain fundamental ethical concerns about sham surgery, a well-founded bioethical proceduralism helped to make possible cautious use of placebos in surgery. The organization of Moseley and Wray's sham-arthroscopy trial owed much to the involvement of Baruch Brody, one among an early generation of philosophically trained, full-time bioethicists. The preliminary publication of the trial in 1996 stressed the meticulous care taken to document informed consent from participants.[64] The team also took steps to reduce the risk to patients in the placebo arm, and worked out independently a full ethical analysis of the use of surgical placebos to guide their process. Both have continued to pursue scholarship on the general ethical and organizational requirements of surgical clinical trials.[65] The ethical regulation of all clinical trials involving human subjects over the last few decades has taken place within an increasingly elaborate system of oversights and precautions, vividly described for the testing of the cardiac assist pumps by Shelley McKellar in her contribution to this volume.

While the procedures of informed consent and risk analysis made the sham-arthroscopy trial possible, these mechanisms did not fully dispel ethical concerns. In the late 1990s, with the publication of sham surgical trials of knee arthroscopy and neurosurgical treatment of Parkinson's disease, the bioethics community divided sharply over the ethics. Rigorous attention to informed consent in both projects helped to move that issue to a secondary concern, but concerns about imposed risk remained unresolved. Ruth Macklin, another prominent member of a founding cohort of philosophically trained ethicists, sided with surgeons in a traditional approach to the question.[66] Placebos, Macklin suggested, were only permissible in research when their attendant risks were trivial, since by definition they carried deceptive intent and conferred no material benefit. This criterion of harmlessness was satisfied in placebo-controlled drug trials, since a sugar pill was inert and presumptively free of risk. Sham surgeries, however, could not meet this criterion, with their irreducible risks of anesthesia, infection, and surgical incisions. Placebo-controlled surgical trials violated traditional ethical precepts of truthfulness and nonmaleficence.[67]

The ethicists who defended the use of sham surgery promoted a different view of risk. In a parallel editorial, the ethicist Franklin G. Miller faced off against Macklin. Miller argued not that placebo surgery was free of risk, but rather that risk permeated all medical care, including placebo-controlled trials. Miller, like Macklin, was a philosopher, trained at the prestigious ethics program at the University of Virginia. An element of risk was always present in medical experiments, he said, and only need be fully disclosed to meet ethical requirements. The alternative would be the cessation of vital research. Miller agreed that sham surgical trials had a special ethical obligation to minimize risk, up to the limit of what was required for a valid experiment. Even the sugar pill, however, imposed risks, he argued—since if the active treatment proved beneficial, or other potentially beneficial treatments were available, the patient assigned to the sugar pill was necessarily risked being deprived of valuable treatment. And yet the use of sugar pills had been well established. In Miller's view, the twin procedural standards of informed consent and minimized risk permitted the ethical use of sham surgery in trials.[68] The sham-arthroscopy trial organized by Moseley, Wray, and Brody met these standards, passing ethical reviews required by the Department of Veteran's Affairs, which helped to fund the study.[69]

Although the new procedural tools of bioethics made sham surgery ethically defensible, the motivation to conduct these studies arose from other sources. An important allure of the well-designed placebo-controlled study continued to be its effect as an especially rigorous test of surgical effects. Application of placebo-controls in drug testing had repeatedly proven the ability to create surprising and influential new results. This potential was evident already in the 1960s when a nationally organized RCT obtained an unfavorable result for the widely used medication tolbutamide in the University Group Diabetes Control trial, a story expertly told by Jeremy Greene and Harry Marks.[70] The early diabetes trials had a mixed influence on practice. But the results of the CAST trial of antiarrhythmic drugs just a couple of years before planning started for the sham-arthroscopy trial fundamentally reshaped the perceptions of flecainide and encainide when they unexpectedly fell short of placebo in keeping patients alive.[71] The controlled clinical trial obviously had the power to influence practice.

It was this potential to reshape practice, rather than ethical qualms, that moved to the center of the debate with the publication of the placebo-arthroscopy trial. By 2002, concerns about medical utilization, reimbursement, and healthcare costs dominated the discussion of a surgical procedure that had become one of the most expensive lines in a soaring national budget for medical care. The sham-arthroscopy article opened with a statement of the annual cost in the United States of arthroscopy for treatment of osteoarthritis of the knee. The discussion section then closed with the findings that the procedure was very similar to a placebo in its effects and a call to put to better use "the billions of dollars spent on such procedures annually."[72] In response, one of the sharpest criticisms of the study among the many letters received by the editor after publication included the warning that with the release of Moseley's paper, the Veterans Administration had issued a federal directive eliminating the service of knee arthroscopy from covered benefits—a sharp blow to orthopedic surgeons who specialized in the procedure.[73] The nexus of profits, innovation, and clinical trials would move to the center of controversies surrounding the progress of increasingly large and well-organized sham-controlled surgical trials of the following decades.[74]

Conclusion

This brief examination of placebo control in testing surgical procedures and implanted devices helps to trace the slow and partial introduction into surgery of clinical experimental methods that swept into medicine in the second half of the twentieth century. The career of sham surgery reminds us that the randomized controlled trial was not a single experimental method, but a set of techniques that followed differing paths into use. There were specific openings and incentives for sham surgical controls within the changing nature of surgical innovation in the last decades of the twentieth century. Greater attention to the patient's subjective experience and concern about nonspecific therapeutic effects from surgical attention advanced the surgical ambition to treat chronic, disabling conditions and enhanced the value of placebo controls. Institutional change, with the growth of regulatory oversight and the routinization of bioethical practices, also helped in legitimating this alternative experimental method of sham surgery. In addition, the steadily rising cost of medical care and the prominence of expensive and popular surgical procedures inspired renewed interest in the 1990s in a method capable of debunking even widely accepted devices and procedures. Alternately, the existence of a well-recognized high bar for testing created a powerful validating process for the few bold experimentalists willing to try to clear the hurdle. As Shelley McKellar demonstrates in this volume in an examination of the HeartMate technology, the definitive clinical trial could become a "legitimizing moment" that allowed a new procedure or device to move into wider application, opening the way for ongoing modification and redeployment.

A potential trend in the recent use of sham surgical trials bears comment. Several notable recent sham controlled trials aiming to debunk existing surgical and invasive procedures have been conducted outside the United States: an ongoing trial for follow-up on the results of the partial meniscectomy trial in Finland; an ongoing sham-controlled trial of shoulder arthroscopy for impingement at ten sites in the United Kingdom; and a similar placebo-controlled trial of arthroscopic labral tear repair of the hip headquartered in Oslo, Norway.[75] Notably, these countries have some form of universal health care with a closed, centralized budget—giving surgeons smaller economic investments in particular procedures and perhaps a stronger collective sense of stewardship of their budget. The potential advantages of sham-controlled studies have depended strongly on the context in which they were deployed.

The conference that gave rise to this book examined alternatives within surgical innovation and explored the relationships among novel therapeutics, evaluation, and surgical progress. Sham surgery and the associated mechanisms of the RCT provided an alternative means for evaluating surgery, as they entered use alongside the older metrics of individual experience and the organized case series. Randomized controlled trials remain a minor element among methods for evaluating surgical procedures, with surgeons continuing to rely on large case series and case registries. The even rarer and certainly controversial use of sham surgery, however, became a touchstone in a general debate over research methods in surgery. The use of fake surgical procedures as an experimental control seemed to showcase both the best and worst of the new clinical experimentalism—dramatically debunking strongly endorsed procedures, but exposing the lengths to which the enthusiastic experimentalist would go. Observers of sham surgery's rocky course have split in their appraisals, differing in their understanding of therapeutic innovation, whether its progress is inherently episodic or continuous, and whether each surgical novelty is more apt to harbor new therapeutic potential or overrated surgical enthusiasms. Opinion on the ethical nature of sham surgery remains equally unsettled. Enthusiasts who see progressive value in clinical trials point to the power of placebo control to protect individual patients and society from enticing, but ineffective, surgical procedures. By contrast, its critics find the use of sham surgery to be emblematic of a willingness to sacrifice the interests of the individual patient to the quest for exact knowledge about therapeutic effects.

Notes

Volker Hess and J. Andrew Mendelsohn, "Case and Series: Medical Knowledge and Paper Technology, 1600–1900," *History of Science* 48, nos. 3/4 (2010): 287–314; Warwick Anderson, "The Case of the Archives," *Critical Inquiry* 39 (2013): 532–46; Jonathan A. Cook, "The Challenges Faced in the Design, Conduct and Analysis of Surgical Randomised Controlled Trials," *Trials* 10 (2009): 1–9.

2. A. F. Jarman, N. P. Wray, D. M. Wenner et al., "Trials and Tribulations: The Professional Development of Surgical Trialists," *American Journal of Surgery* 204, no. 3 (2012): 339–46; Patrick Vavken, "Rationale for and Methods of Superiority, Noninferiority, or Equivalence Designs in Orthopaedic, Controlled Trials," *Clinical Orthopaedics and Related Research* 469, no. 9 (2011): 2645–53.

3. In the seminar that produced this paper, we began with insights from David Edgerton, *The Shock of the Old: Technology and Global History since 1900* (London: Profile Books, 2006); also see Shelley McKellar, "Disruptive Potential: The 'Landmark' REMATCH Trial, Left Ventricular Assist Device (LVAD) Technology, and the Surgical Treatment of Heart Failure in the United States," chapter 6 of this volume.

4. The term "placebo effect" can be used for a variety of related phenomena. Here I will try to stay close to what seems the intended uses of the individual authors. For a look at the diversity of meanings historically, see Arthur K. Shapiro and Elaine Shapiro, *The Powerful Placebo: From Ancient Priest to Modern Physician* (Baltimore: Johns Hopkins University Press, 1997). For a lively examination of the roots of the placebo-controlled trial, see T. J. Kaptchuk, "Intentional Ignorance: A History of Blind Assessment and Placebo Controls in Medicine," *Bulletin of the History of Medicine* 72, no. 3 (1998): 389–433.

5. An early and emphatic statement of the view appears in Archie L. Cochrane, *Effectiveness and Efficiency: Random Reflections on Health Services* (London: Nuffield Provincial Hospitals Trust, 1972), see, for example, the section on reducing the use of tonsillectomy through the RCT, 60–61.

6. For a rare example, see the report and commentary: David Dodick, Bahman Guyuron, and Hans Christoph Diener, "Debate Session 1: Surgery Deactivation of the Trigger Sites for Migraine Prevention," Session AHS1313, International Headache Congress, Boston, June 27–30, 2013, http://www.dcprovidersonline.com/ahs; B. Guyuron, D. Reed, J. S. Kriegler et al., "A Placebo-Controlled Surgical Trial of the Treatment of Migraine Headaches," *Plastic and Reconstructive Surgery* 124, no. 2 (2009): 461–68.

7. E. Grey Dimond, C. Frederick Kittle, and James E. Crockett, "Evaluation of Internal Mammary Artery Ligation and Sham Procedure in Angina Pectoris: Abstract," *Circulation* 18, no. 4 (1958): 712–13; Editorial, "Ligation of the Internal Mammary Arteries," *New England Journal of Medicine* 257, no. 8 (1957): 385.

8. For analysis of the sham-surgery trials, see Scott H. Podolsky, "Quintessential Beecher—Surgery as Placebo: A Quantitative Study of Bias," *International Anesthesia Clinics* 45 (Fall 2007): 47–63; also Ernest Barsamian, "The Rise And Fall of Internal Mammary Artery Ligation in the Treatment of Angina Pectoris and the Lessons Learned," in *Costs, Risks, and Benefits of Surgery*, ed. J. P. Bunker, B. A. Barnes, and F. Mosteller (New York: Oxford University Press, 1977), 212–20.

9. Ronald A. Fisher, *The Design of Experiments* (Edinburgh: Oliver and Boyd, 1935); Austin Bradford Hill, *Principles of Medical Statistics* (London: Lancet Limited,

1937). But see Joseph M. Gabriel, "The Testing of Sanocrysin: Science, Profit, and Innovation in Clinical Trial Design, 1926–1931," *Journal of the History of Medicine and Allied Sciences* 69, no. 4 (2014): 604–32.

10. Peter Keating and Alberto Cambrosio, *Cancer on Trial: Oncology as a New Style of Practice* (Chicago: University of Chicago Press, 2014), 9, 14.

11. Leonard A. Cobb, George I. Thomas, Robert A. Bruce et al., "Preliminary Report of a Double Blind Evaluation of Ligation of the Internal Mammary Arteries: Abstract," *Circulation* 18, no. 4 (1958): 704.

12. Allan M. Brandt and Martha Gardner, "The Golden Age of Medicine?," in *Medicine in the Twentieth Century*, ed. Roger Cooter and John Pickstone (Amsterdam: Harwood, 2000), 27. Even in this period of rapid growth, the US gross domestic product grew "only" 47 percent during the same period of five years. For GDP statistics, see www.research.stlouisfed.gov.

13. Jeremy Greene, *Prescribing by Numbers* (Baltimore: Johns Hopkins University Press, 2007), 117–19; Keating and Cambrosio, "Cancer Clinical Trials," in Cantor, *Cancer in the Twentieth Century*, 197–223, 199–200.

14. See Harry M. Marks, *The Progress of Experiment: Science and Therapeutic Reform in the United States, 1900–1990* (Cambridge: University of Cambridge Press, 1997). For an overview of the relationship to the FDA, see Scott H. Podolsky, *The Antibiotic Era: Reform, Resistance, and the Pursuit of a Rational Therapeutics* (Baltimore: Johns Hopkins University Press, 2015), 73–111.

15. E. Grey Dimond, "Reflections," in *The Kansas School of Medicine: Eyewitness Reflections on Its Formative Years*, ed. Stanley R. Friesen and Robert P. Hudson (Kansas City, KS: Stanley R. Friesen, 1996), 150–54; G. I. Thomas, "K. Alvin Merendino: His Contribution to Surgery," *American Journal of Surgery* 149, no. 5 (1985): 574–79.

16. H. K. Beecher, "Surgery as Placebo: A Quantitative Study of Bias," *Journal of the American Medical Association* 176 (1961): 1102–7; William M. Carley, "Research & Ethics," *Wall Street Journal*, June 10, 1965, 1.

17. Stanley Milgram, "Behavioral Study of Obedience," *Journal of Abnormal and Social Psychology* 67(1963): 371–78.

18. Hess and Mendelsohn, "Case and Series"; Anderson, "Case of the Archives."

19. A discussion of the didactic use of case reports is found in Christopher Crenner, *Private Practice: In the Early Twentieth-Century Medical Office of Dr. Richard Cabot* (Baltimore: Johns Hopkins University Press, 2005), 76–81.

20. Thomas Schlich, *Surgery, Science, and Industry: A Revolution in Fracture Care, 1950s–1990s* (New York: Palgrave MacMillan, 2002), 130. On cancer registries as an alternative mechanism to clinical trials, see Keating and Cambrosio, *Cancer on Trial*, 378–79.

21. See also Thomas Schlich, "Risk and Medical Innovation: A Historical Perspective," in *The Risks of Medical Innovation: Risk Perception and Assessment in Historical Context*, ed. Thomas Schlich and Ulrich Tröhler (London: Routledge, 2006), 1–19.

22. David S. Jones, "Surgical Practice and the Reconstruction of the Therapeutic Niche: The Case of Myocardial Revascularization," chapter 8 of this volume.

23. John D. Birkmeyer and Samuel R. G. Finlayson, "Critical Assessment of Surgical Outcomes," in *Sabiston Textbook of Surgery: The Biological Basis of Modern Surgical Practice*, ed. David C. Sabiston, Jr. and H. Kim Lyerly (Philadelphia: W. B. Saunders, 2004), 209–20.

24. See recently P. McCulloch, D. G. Altman, W. B. Campbell et al., "No Surgical Innovation without Evaluation: The IDEAL Recommendations," *Lancet* 374 (2009): 1105–12.

25. Harvey V. Fineberg, "Gastric Freezing—A Study of Diffusion of a Medical Innovation," in *Medical Technology and the Health Care System*, ed. Committee on Technology and Health Care (Washington, DC: National Academy of Sciences, 1979), 173–200; Barsamian, "Rise And Fall of Mammary Artery Ligation."

26. O. H. Wangensteen, E. T. Peter, D. M. Nicoloff et al., "Achieving 'Physiological Gastrectomy' by Gastric Freezing: A Preliminary Report of an Experimental and Clinical Study," *Journal of the American Medical Association* 180, no. 6 (1962): 439–44; Owen Wangensteen, Harlan Root, Conrad B. Jenson et al., "Depression of Gastric Secretion and Digestion by Gastric Hypothermia: Its Clinical Use in Massive Hematemesis," *Surgery* 44, no. 2 (1958): 265–74. See the suggestion of this hypothesis in the letter of O. H. Wangensteen to Ward O. Griffen, MD, February 17, 1960, box 14, folder 424, Department of Surgery, University of Minnesota Archives, Minneapolis, MN (hereafter MN Archives).

27. Owen Wangensteen to Alfred Stoffer, May 22, 1963, box 4, folder 89 "AMA 1961–1963," MN Archives.

28. Wangensteen et al., "Achieving 'Physiological Gastrectomy,'" 439.

29. Fineberg, "Gastric Freezing," 174.

30. Wangensteen et al., "Achieving 'Physiological Gastrectomy,'" 443. Wangensteen modified this procedure constantly over several years, backing away from the idea of "freezing," changing balloons, the coolant, and the attendant treatments. This description applies to the procedure as widely disseminated in its heyday.

31. Owen H. Wangensteen, "Benefactions of Surgery to Man," *Sigma Xi Quarterly* 24, no. 4 (1936): 177; also Dale C. Smith, "Appendicitis, Appendectomy, and the Surgeon," *Bulletin of the History of Medicine* 30 (1996): 414–41. The notion of "elective surgery" is apparent in these developments also, as when the surgeon was encouraged to put the choice of appendectomy in the hands of the patient in uncertain cases; Dale C. Smith, "Appendicitis, Appendectomy, and the Surgeon," *Bulletin of the History of Medicine* 30 (1996): 437.

32. P. H. Lee and A. A. Gawande, "The Number of Surgical Procedures in an American Lifetime in 3 States," *Journal of the American College of Surgery* 207, no. 1 (2008): S75.

33. Bashir A. Zikria, Ramon S. De Jesus, William R. Cunnick et al., "Gastric "Freezing"—A Clinical Double-Blind Study," *American Journal of Gastroenterology* 47 (1967): 208–14, 213, 209; Fineberg, "Gastric Freezing."

34. J. M. Ruffin, J. E. Grizzle, N. C. Hightower et al., "Co-Operative Double-Blind Evaluation of Gastric "Freezing" in the Treatment of Duodenal Ulcer," *New England Journal of Medicine* 281, no. 1 (1969): 16–19.

35. Allen B Weiss, "Conversations in Medicine: Owen H. Wangensteen," *Hospital Practice* 23, no. 3 (1988): 111–31. See M. I. Grossman to Editor, *Journal of the American Medical Association*, December 9, 1966, box 14, folder 408; and letter of O. H. Wangensteen to M. I. Grossman, April 14, 1967, box 13, folder 405; additional letters are also in box 13, folder 405, MN Archives.

36. W. P. Longmire, Jr., J. W. Kuzma, and W. J. Dixon, "The Use of Triethylenethiophosphoramide as an Adjuvant to the Surgical Treatment of Gastric Carcinoma," *Annals of Surgery* 167, no. 3 (1968): 293–312.

37. W. D. Johnson, J. E. Grizzle, and R. W. Postlethwait, "Veterans Administration Cooperative Study of Surgery for Duodenal Ulcer: I. Description and Evaluation of Method of Randomization," *Archives of Surgery* 101, no. 3 (1970): 391–95; R. W. Postlethwait, "Five Year Follow-Up Results of Operations for Duodenal Ulcer," *Surgery, Gynecology & Obstetrics* 137, no. 3 (1973): 387–92.

38. Barron H. Lerner, *The Breast Cancer Wars: Hope, Fear and the Pursuit of Care in Twentieth-Century America* (New York: Oxford University Press, 2001), 115–40; Carsten Timmerman, *A History of Lung Cancer: The Recalcitrant Disease* (New York: Palgrave Macmillan, 2014), 104–8; David S. Jones, "Visions of a Cure: Visualization, Clinical Trials, and Controversies in Cardiac Therapeutics, 1968–1998," *Isis* 91, no. 3 (2000): 520–22. For a compelling study of the development of coronary artery bypass, see David S. Jones, *Broken Hearts: The Tangled History of Cardiac Care* (Baltimore: Johns Hopkins University Press, 2012), as well as chapter 8 in this volume, Jones, "Surgical Practice and the Reconstruction of the Therapeutic Niche."

39. L. I. Bonchek, "The Role of the Randomized Clinical Trial in the Evaluation of New Operations," *Surgical Clinics of North America* 62, no. 4 (1982): 761–69; L. I. Bonchek, "Sounding Board: Are Randomized Trials Appropriate for Evaluating New Operations?," *New England Journal of Medicine* 301, no. 1 (1979): 44–45; Textbooks on clinical research outlined such difficulties in the organization of trials in surgery: Lawrence M. Friedman, Curt D. Furberg, and David L. DeMets, *Fundamentals of Clinical Trials* (Boston: John Wright, 1985), 3–5, 21–23. Restatement of this paradox remains a tenet of the surgical position on clinical trials: see Birkmeyer, "Critical Assessment of Surgical Outcomes," 209.

40. Timmerman, *History of Lung Cancer*, 104–8.

41. Esther B. Fein, "Dr. Thomas C. Chalmers, a President of Mt. Sinai, Dies at 78," *New York Times*, December 29, 1995, http://www.nytimes.com/1995/12/29/nyregion/dr-thomas-c-chalmers-a-president-of-mt-sinai-dies-at-78.html. For Chalmers on the "natural history" of clinical trials, see Keating and Cambrosio, *Cancer on Trial*, 238.

42. Thomas C. Chalmers, "Randomization and Coronary Artery Surgery," *Annals of Thoracic Surgery* 14, no. 3 (1972): 323–27.

43. Jones, "Visions of a Cure," 505.

44. Thomas C. Chalmers, "Randomization of the First Patient," *Medical Clinics of North America* 59 (1975): 1035–38.

45. Julie Anderson, Francis Neary, and John V. Pickstone, *Surgeons, Manufacturers and Patients: A Transatlantic History of Total Hip Replacement* (New York: Palgrave Macmillan, 2007). Beth Linker, "Spines of Steel: A Case of Surgical Enthusiasm in Cold War America," *Bulletin of the History of Medicine* 90, no. 2 (2016): 222–49.

46. R. E. Harbaugh, T. M. Reeder, H. J. Senter et al., "Intracerebroventricular Bethanechol Chloride Infusion in Alzheimer's Disease: Results of a Collaborative Double-Blind Study," *Journal of Neurosurgery* 71, no. 4 (1989): 481–86. More recently, developments in gene therapy have precipitated a similar trial design. See, for example, W. J. Marks Jr., R. T. Bartus, J. Siffert et al., "Gene Delivery of AAV2-Neurturin for Parkinson's Disease: A Double-Blind, Randomised, Controlled Trial," *Lancet Neurol.* 12, no. 9 (2010): 1164–72, doi:10.1016/S1474–4422(10)70254–4.

47. C. R. Freed, P. E. Greene, R. E. Breeze et al., "Transplantation of Embryonic Dopamine Neurons for Severe Parkinson's Disease," *New England Journal of Medicine* 344, no. 10 (2001): 710–19.

48. T. B. Freeman, D. E. Vawter, P. E. Leaverton et al., "Use of Placebo Surgery in Controlled Trials of a Cellular-Based Therapy for Parkinson's Disease," *New England Journal of Medicine* 341, no. 13 (1999): 988–92. Subsequent evaluation of the placebo effects measured in various therapeutic trials for Parkinson's disease did show that surgical placebos had the greatest likelihood of inducing a significant short-term improvement in disease ratings: C. G. Goetz, J. Wuu, M. P. McDermott et al., "Placebo Response in Parkinson's Disease: Comparisons among 11 Trials Covering Medical and Surgical Interventions," *Mov Disord* 23, no. 5 (2008): 690–99.

49. Freed et al., "Transplantation of Embryonic Dopamine Neurons," 710; A. Bjorklund, S. B. Dunnett, P. Brundin et al., "Neural Transplantation for the Treatment of Parkinson's Disease," *Lancet Neurol* 2, no. 7 (2003): 437–45.

50. The evidence is easy to trace in the development of textbooks such as, Friedman, Furberg, and DeMets, *Fundamentals of Clinical Trials.* See also Jarman et al., "Professional Development of Surgical Trialists."

51. Office of Technology Assessment, *Federal Policies and the Medical Devices Industry* (Washington, DC: US Congress, Office of Technology Assessment, 1984), 165, 338–39; Daniel Schultz, "Regulating Medical Devices," in *Perspectives on Risk and Regulation: The FDA at 100,* ed. Arthur Daemmrich and Joanna Radin (Philadelphia: Chemical Heritage Foundation, 2007), 52–64.

52. Office of Technology Assessment, *Medical Devices Industry,* 112–14.

53. Rodney R. Munsey, "Trends and Events in FDA Regulation of Medical Devices over the Last Fifty Years," *Food and Drug Law Journal* 50 (1995): 163–77.

54. Scott Gottlieb, "The FDA Wants You for Sham Surgery; There Are Better Ways to Test Medical Devices Than by Having Patients Be Placebos Who Get Fake Operations," *Wall Street Journal (online),* February 18, 2014, http://online.wsj.com/public/page/archive.html.

55. John D. Carroll, "Migraine Intervention with STARFlex Technology Trial: A Controversial Trial of Migraine and Patent Foramen Ovale Closure," *Circulation* 117 (2008): 1358–60; Andrew Dowson, Michael J. Mullen, Richard Peatfield et al., "Migraine Intervention with STARFlex Technology (MIST) Trial: A Prospective, Multicenter, Double-Blind, Sham-Controlled Trial to Evaluate the Effectiveness of Patent Foramen Ovale Closure with STARFlex Septal Repair Implant to Resolve Refractory Migraine Headache," *Circulation* 117, no. 11 (2008): 1397–1404; Welton M. Gersony and Deborah R. Gersony, "Migraine Headache and the Patent Foramen Ovale," *Circulation* 121 (2012): 1377–78; S. Claiborne Johnston, "Patent Foramen Ovale Closure—Closing the Door Except for Trials," *New England Journal of Medicine* 366, no. 11 (2012): 1048–50. See a succession of financial reports by NMT Medical, Inc., "Form 10-K," US Securities and Exchange Commission (Boston, 2002, 2004, 2010), available publically in the SEC database: http://www.sec.gov/edgar/searchedgar/.

56. Dodick, Guyuron, and Diener, "Debate Session 1"; Guyuron et al., "Placebo-Controlled Surgical Trial"; J. E. Janis, "Discussion: A Placebo-Controlled Surgical Trial of the Treatment of Migraine Headaches," *Plastic and Reconstructive Surgery* 124, no. 2 (2009): 469–70. In promoting the technique, advocates said that sham surgical testing "represents the definitive proof," whereas opponents expressed concerns about the technical conduct of the trials, saying that the sham control "was not a sham." Guyuron, and Diener, "Debate Session 1."

57. See, for example, D. J. Raab, D. A. Fischer, J. P. Smith et al., "Comparison of Arthroscopic and Open Reconstruction of the Anterior Cruciate Ligament: Early Results," *American Journal of Sports Medicine* 21, no. 5 (1993): 680–83; discussion 683–84.

58. J. Bruce Moseley Jr., Nelda P. Wray, David Kuykendall et al., "Arthroscopic Treatment of Osteoarthritis of the Knee: A Prospective, Randomized, Placebo-Controlled Trial Results of a Pilot Study, "*American Journal of Sports Medicine* 24, no. 1 (1996): 28–34; J. B. Moseley Jr., K. O'Malley, N. J. Petersen et al., "A Controlled Trial of Arthroscopic Surgery for Osteoarthritis of the Knee," *New England Journal of Medicine* 347, no. 2 (2002): 81–88. A detailed account, based on Wray's experience, can be found in Carol M. Ashton and Nelda P. Wray, *Comparative Effectiveness Research: Evidence, Medicine, and Policy* (New York: Oxford University Press, 2013), 4–10.

59. Carley, "Research & Ethics," *Wall Street Journal*, June 10, 1965; H. K. Beecher, "Ethics and Clinical Research," *New England Journal of Medicine* 274, no. 24 (1966): 1354–60; H. K. Beecher, "The Placebo Effect and Sound Planning in Surgery," *Surgery, Gynecology & Obstetrics* 114 (1962): 507–9. On exemptions to consent, see Beecher, "Consent in Clinical Experimentation: Myth and Reality," *Journal of the American Medical Association* 195, no. 1 (1966): quote on 34. Beecher suggested in his discussion of the mammary artery trials that permission must be granted by patients for such experiments, but the patients in Kansas City seem to have been given even less information about the experiment than in Seattle (Beecher, "Surgery as Placebo," 92).

60. Jay Katz, *Experimentation with Human Beings: The Authority of the Investigator, Subject, Professions, and State in the Human Experimentation Process* (New York: Russell Sage Foundation, 1972), 686–90.

61. Ruth Faden and Tom L. Beauchamp, with the assistance of Nancy M. P. King, *A History and Theory of Informed Consent* (New York: Oxford University Press, 1986), 89.

62. Jens Thomsen, Poul Bretlau, Mirko Tos et al., "Placebo Effect in Surgery for Ménière's Disease: A Double-Blind, Placebo-Controlled Study on Endolymphatic Sac Shunt Surgery," *Archives of Otolaryngology* 107 (May 1981): 271–77; Frederick Mosteller, John P. Gilbert, and Buchnam McPeek, "Controversies in Design and Analysis of Clinical Trials," in *Clinical Trials: Issues and Approaches*, ed. Stanley H. Shapiro and Thomas A. Louis (New York: Marcel Dekker, 1983), 13–64. Podolsky makes this point as well in "Quintessential Beecher." Recent surgical textbooks continue to report that sham surgical trials are "difficult ethically to perform": Robin S. McLeod, "Evidence-Based Surgery," in *Surgery: Basic Science and Clinical Features*, ed. Jeffrey A. Norman et al. (New York: Springer, 2001), 59.

63. There is a large literature offering varying accounts of the growth of bioethics. For recent insight to the development of the fundamental mechanism of the institutional review board, see Laura Stark, *Behind Closed Doors: IRBs and the Making of Ethical Research* (Chicago: University of Chicago Press, 2012), 81–111, 159–66.

64. Moseley et al., "Arthroscopic Treatment"; Ashton and Wray, *Comparative Effectiveness Research*, 8.

65. Baruch A. Brody, Kimberly Wristers, Nancy J. Petersen et al., "Criteria for Legitimate Placebo-Controlled Surgery Trials," typescript manuscript, n.p., n.d., included with e-mail communication to the author from Nelda Wray, August 27, 2013.

66. Renee C. Fox, "The Evolution of American Bioethics: A Sociological Perspective," in *Social Science Perspecitive on Medical Ethics*, ed. George Weisz

(Philadelphia: University of Pennsylvania, 1990), 201–17, 41–42; R. Macklin, "The Ethical Problems with Sham Surgery in Clinical Research," *New England Journal of Medicine* 341, no. 13 (1999): 992–96.

67. Macklin, "Ethical Problems."

68. Sam Horng and Franklin G. Miller, "Is Placebo Surgery Unethical?," *New England Journal of Medicine* 347, no. 2 (2002): 137–39. Note that this debate appeared in the same issue that published the sham-arthroscopy trial, seeming to tip the editors' hand with regard to the ethical status of sham surgery.

69. The proposal was reviewed by university and hospital IRB committees: Moseley et al., "Controlled Trial of Arthroscopic Surgery."

70. Marks, *Progress of Experiment*, 204–28; Greene, *Prescribing by Numbers*, 115–23.

71. The Cardiac Arrhythmia Suppression Trial Investigators, "Preliminary Report: Effect of Encainide and Flecainide on Mortality in a Randomized Trial of Arrhythmia Suppression after Myocardial Infarction," *New England Journal of Medicine* 321, no. 6 (1989): 406–12.

72. Moseley et al., "Controlled Trial of Arthroscopic Surgery," 81.

73. Correspondence regarding "A Controlled Trial of Arthroscopic Surgery for Osteoarthritis of the Knee," *New England Journal of Medicine* 347, no. 21 (2002): 1717–19. Also see Robert W. Jackson, "Debate on the Use of Arthroscopic Surgery for Osteoarthritis of the Knee," *Proceedings of Baylor University Medical Center* 61, no. 1 (2003): 27–29.

74. A well-planned series of sham-controlled studies have steadily narrowed the indications for the procedure while emphasizing the enormous costs of their widespread use: J. D. Bradley, D. K. Heilman, B. P. Katz et al., "Tidal Irrigation as Treatment for Knee Osteoarthritis: A Sham-Controlled, Randomized, Double-Blinded Evaluation," *Arthritis Rheum* 46, no. 1 (2002): 100–108; A. Kirkley, T. B. Birmingham, R. B. Litchfield et al., "A Randomized Trial of Arthroscopic Surgery for Osteoarthritis of the Knee," *New England Journal of Medicine* 359, no. 11 (2008): 1097–1107; and Raine Sihvonen, Mika Paavola, Antti Malmivaara et al., "Arthroscopic Partial Meniscectomy versus Sham Surgery for a Degenerative Meniscal Tear," *New England Journal of Medicine* 369, no. 26 (2013): 2515–24.

75. Development of Knee Osteoarthritis after Arthroscopic Partial Resection of Degenerative Meniscus Tear, Teppo Jarvinen, Helsinki University Central Hospital, NIH trials ID: NCT01052233; D. J. Beard, Rees, I. Rombach et al., "The CSAW Study (Can Shoulder Arthroscopy Work?)—A Placebo-Controlled Surgical Intervention Trial Assessing the Clinical and Cost Effectiveness of Arthroscopic Subacromial Decompression for Shoulder Pain: Study Protocol for a Randomised Controlled Trial," *Trials* 16 (2015): 210; Arthroscopic Surgical Procedures vs. Sham Surgery for Patients with Femoroacetabular Impingement and/or Labral Tears, May Arna Risberg, Oslo University Hospital, NIH Trials ID: NCT02692807. But see also the controlled trial with a sham arm: D. F. Kallmes, B. A. Comstock, P. J. Heagerty et al., "A Randomized Trial of Vertebroplasty for Osteoporotic Spinal Fractures," *New England Journal of Medicine* 361 (2009): 569–79, which was organized at the Mayo Clinic with sites in the United States, United Kingdom, and Australia. Ongoing trials listed at www.clinicaltrials.gov.

Chapter Eight

Surgical Practice and the Reconstruction of the Therapeutic Niche

The Case of Myocardial Revascularization

David S. Jones

Speaking at a conference in Houston in 1985, the surgeon René Favaloro described 1968 as "the year of revolution."[1] He was not referring to the assassinations of Martin Luther King Jr. or Robert Kennedy or the protests against the Vietnam War. Instead, his revolution was the development of coronary artery bypass grafting (CABG) to treat coronary artery disease (CAD). For that operation, 1968 was indeed transformative. In April Favaloro published the results from his first fifty-five patients. By the summer of 1970 he and his colleagues at the Cleveland Clinic had performed CABG on over one thousand patients.[2] Their success was matched by surgical teams in Milwaukee and New York City.[3] Surgeons throughout the country took note. By 1977, surgeons in the United States completed over one hundred thousand CABG operations each year.[4]

The CABG "revolution" provides an important case study of surgical innovation. Over a single decade the procedure emerged from obscurity to become one of the most common major surgical procedures. Many aspects of the innovation are interesting. First, its rise was not the result of a new discovery: Alexis Carrel had first attempted to place a bypass graft between the aorta and a coronary artery in 1910.[5] Second, it was not the

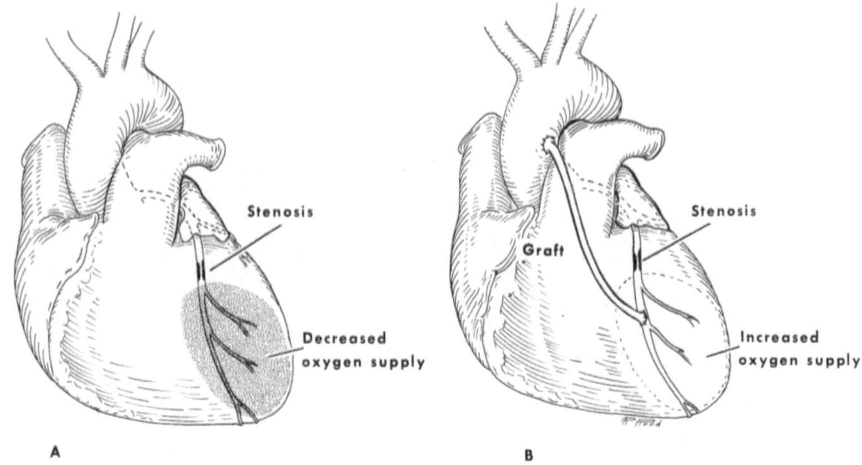

Figure 8.1. Coronary artery bypass graft surgery. The before (A) and after (B) drawings show how the graft can increase oxygen supply to the heart. Illustration by Robert Reed, 1973. Reproduced by permission from the Cleveland Clinic Center for Medical Art & Photography.

result of a lone genius, or the group at the Cleveland Clinic. Instead, researchers worldwide had tried to make Carrel's technique a success for decades, conducting extensive animal research and occasional human trials in the 1950s and 1960s. They had also developed dozens of other surgical techniques to treat CAD. Third, it was not the result of a landmark clinical trial, of the sort described by Shelley McKellar in this volume.[6] In fact, Favaloro later downplayed the magnitude of the innovation, describing it in 1998 as a simple progression through a series of related procedures: "The evolution took place in just a few months from patch graft to interposition graft to bypass graft."[7]

Favaloro's concise account obscures a far more interesting dynamic, one that changed in a fundamental way how physicians thought about CAD. The advent of CABG for treatment of CAD was not simply an innovation in surgical technique: CABG transformed CAD itself. It did not change the phenomenology of the disease, as insulin changed diabetes and protease inhibitors changed AIDS. Instead, CABG transformed the concept of CAD. Before 1968 most surgeons, including Favaloro and his colleagues in Cleveland, saw CAD primarily as a diffuse process, one not amenable to direct surgical repair of the sort promised by CABG. They enthusiastically deployed other operations that brought new blood to the heart through indirect paths. After 1968, their perception of the disease changed. They saw CAD as a focal process, one that CABG could fix (fig. 8.1). This demonstrates an important aspect of surgical innovation: the dynamic exchange between theory and practice. The disease model that became most popular was the one that helped to make the most popular therapy make sense.[8]

This paper traces the linked history of disease theory and surgical practice for CAD, from the initial proposal to use CABG to treat syphilitic heart disease, through the development of an astonishing diversity of techniques to treat coronary atherosclerosis, to the 1968 reemergence of CABG. Over this sixty-year period, the mission of surgery changed repeatedly. Efforts to reduce the heart's demand for blood gave way to efforts to increase the heart's supply of blood. Indirect techniques, which predominated until 1968, gave way to a direct technique, CABG. By tracing the prehistory and eventual advent of CABG, it is possible to understand how and why surgeons developed different understandings of CAD, how these understandings defined a shifting therapeutic niche, and how CABG transformed the niche itself. The history of coronary revascularization from 1910 to 1970 is not one driven by the kinds of clinical trials described by Christopher Crenner and Shelley McKellar.[9] Instead, it is one in which outcomes data, largely from case reports and case series, interacted with changing models of disease, new surgical techniques, and surgical intuition to fuel innovation in surgery.

The Therapeutic Niche

In the simplest models of medical innovation, physicians identify a problem and work to develop a solution. This is easy to understand in many areas of surgical practice. If a tumor is found, then surgeons want to remove it. If a bone has been fractured, then surgeons will try to mend it. The model applies to pharmaceuticals as well. Paul Ehrlich famously sought a magic bullet for syphilis, a specific drug that would kill the bacteria while leaving the patient intact. Proponents of rational drug design now seek new molecular targets for pharmaceutical intervention. In each of these cases, the model of innovation assumes that the problem exists prior to the solution: it is a fixed target that the innovation aims to strike.

Actual innovation is never so straightforward. Thomas Schlich has shown how even the most mechanistic of surgical procedures, the operative repair of fractures, required careful coordination of theory and practice and of clinic and industry.[10] Jack Pressman, who sought to explain why lobotomy worked in the 1940s but no longer does, documented the subtle interplay between scientific rationale, social need, and surgical practice. He argued that the efficacy of a treatment could only be understood in the context of the particular problem the treatment hoped to solve: "the extent to which a treatment flourishes is directly dependent upon the specific features of the day's clinical landscape. In the long haul, viability is a matter of ecology, not virtue." In the 1930s, asylums overflowed with patients, hopelessness, and horror. Psychiatrists desperately sought new treatments. Lobotomy, which could calm some patients (at the cost of damaging their personality), offered "human salvage." It appealed to patients, their families, and psychiatrists. The metaphor was explicit: "from an ecological perspective, the treatment rapidly penetrated into a niche of almost limitless size that as yet had no competitors."[11]

The niche model has intuitive appeal, invoking familiar imagery of evolution and adaptation. One aspect, however, requires fuller development. The niche, as envisioned by historians of medicine, is not an intrinsic property of the medical landscape. Instead, the existence of any particular niche is the result of the convergence of many forces. Pressman described how the appalling conditions in psychiatric hospitals created a demand for better solutions. Ian Hacking, who used a niche model to account for the rise and fall of psychiatric diagnoses was explicit: "one fruitful idea for understanding transient mental illness is the ecological niche, not just social, not just medical, not just coming from the patient, not just from the doctors, but from the concatenation of an extraordinarily large number of diverse types of elements which for a moment provide a stable home for certain manifestations of illness."[12] A niche, whether diagnostic or therapeutic, is not a given, but a result.

Evolutionary biologists have recognized this as well. In the 1970s Richard Lewontin popularized the idea of "niche construction."[13] As subsequent theorists have explained, "Organisms, through their metabolism, their activities, and their choices, define, partly create, and partly destroy their own niches."[14] Recognition that organisms construct their niches, rather than simply adapting to them, requires a new formulation of the meaning of natural selection. Evolution becomes a coupled process in which organisms are functions of their environment and environments are functions of their organisms.[15]

This mode of analysis lends itself easily to histories of therapeutics.[16] Historians' analyses of pharmaceuticals demonstrate this well. One frequent claim is that pharmaceutical companies have worked to create a market—a niche—in order to sell their products. They popularized previously neglected diseases and created new ones where none had existed before. Jeremy Greene and David Healy have described two important examples. When diuretics and tricyclic antidepressants appeared in the 1950s, Merck and other companies distributed educational materials to popularize the diseases—hypertension and depression—that the drugs could treat.[17] This set a precedent for marketing many diseases, and their drugs, from social anxiety disorder to restless leg syndrome or erectile dysfunction.[18]

Coronary revascularization demonstrates the value of niche construction for understanding surgical innovation. Its history is not one in which a disease category was created in order to sell an intervention. CAD rose to prominence in the early to mid-twentieth century for many reasons, independent of surgeons' efforts. Instead, niche construction here is a subtler phenomena, about the parameters of the therapeutic niche provided by CAD. Specifically, was CAD the sort of disease that could be managed surgically? And, if so, what sort of interventions made sense? Physicians sought treatments that could prevent heart attacks and prolong survival. They needed to determine whether coronary atherosclerosis provided appropriate targets for surgical intervention. The basic question, about whether disease is focal or diffuse, is a familiar one for historians of medicine, having played out most famously with breast cancer.[19]

The focal or diffuse nature of CAD should be a simple matter of anatomic fact. But facts about bodies and diseases are never simple. Over the course of the twentieth century, physicians examined the anatomy of CAD with ever increasing technological sophistication, from inspection and palpation to catheter-based ultrasound scanners and near-infrared spectroscopy. Despite this increasing diagnostic capability, answers to the question of whether CAD was focal or diffuse depended less on what was revealed by diagnostic technology than on what could be done by surgical or pharmaceutical intervention. The history of coronary revascularization between 1950 and 1970 reveals a dynamic interaction between disease concept and therapeutic fashion. As different therapeutic interventions have come and gone, disease models have changed. Understanding this dynamic is essential for understanding the efficacy of surgical interventions.

The Diversity of Surgeries

After William Heberden described the now-familiar syndrome of angina pectoris in 1768, Edward Jenner suggested a link between angina and CAD. By 1799 Caleb Parry had concluded that CAD was its most common cause.[20] Consensus, however, was not easily achieved. Reviewing the problem in 1880, Frederick Winsor noted that there was no lesion of the heart "with which angina has any constant or necessary condition."[21] German pathologists debated whether the coronary arteries were end arteries, vulnerable to occlusion, or linked by collateral vessels into resilient networks. In his famous 1912 account of the clinical features of coronary obstruction, James

Herrick argued that collateral vessels allowed patients to survive what would otherwise have been lethal infarctions.[22]

Heart disease received increasing attention after 1910, when it reached the top of the mortality charts in the United States.[23] By 1930s concerned officials named it the "American Disease."[24] By the time of President Dwight D. Eisenhower's heart attack in 1955, few doubted the severity of the problem.[25] Throughout this time, medical thinking focused on coronary occlusion. M. H. Nathanson, for instance, described in 1925 how the gradual progression of coronary atherosclerosis culminated abruptly with an occlusive thrombus.[26] *Reader's Digest* described this fate in 1966: "Coronary arteries that nourish the heart were choked with disease. Soon, if the disease ran its normal course, they would close entirely. Then the starved heart would die. This is the script that sends upwards of half a million North Americans to their graves each year."[27]

Physicians had long recognized the value of prevention. Winsor, in 1880, urged "the importance of a most temperate, guarded, and unexciting mode of life."[28] At a 1936 address before the Massachusetts Medical Society, John Sproull described how he warned his patients to avoid emotional arousal, whether from gambling, detective stories, or sexual intercourse. Laurence Chapin added his own admonitions: "If your daughter is out on a blind date, take a grain and a half of phenobarbital. When a member of an opposing political party is on the air, turn off the radio. When your tax bill comes in, be nonchalant—light a cigarette."[29] However, physicians were very aware that patients did not always heed their advice. The Cleveland surgeon Claude Beck hoped that the disease would be preventable, but concluded that "there is little evidence that this will be accomplished in the near future."[30] Meyer Friedman doubted whether Americans could prevent CAD through perfect adherence to advice about diet, smoking, exercise, and stress: "we are confronted with a constantly increasing incidence of a disease which is almost totally preventable but at a cost few of us are willing to pay."[31] The Houston surgeon Denton Cooley, narrating a 1984 Orson Welles film about heart disease, concluded that until prevention mastered CAD, "treatment is the responsibility of the medical profession."[32]

But how could CAD be treated? Perceiving CAD to be a disease of supply and demand, surgeons recognized two basic strategies. As two New York physicians wrote in 1942, "The rationale of surgery in the treatment of coronary arterial disease is to decrease the myocardial demand or increase the coronary supply."[33] This basic framework guided the surgical assault on CAD throughout the twentieth century.

The earliest attempt came in 1910 when Alexis Carrel, a French surgeon on staff at the Rockefeller Institute, suggested that coronary occlusions could be bypassed by using a piece of saphenous vein, taken from the leg, to make a bridge between the aorta and coronary artery. He was interested in angina pectoris caused by syphilis in the aorta, with its focal lesions confined to placed where the right and left coronary arteries branched off of the aorta. A successful bypass would reach a healthy distal artery. Carrel had prodigious skill with needle and thread: he had learned to embroider silk as a child to support his family after his father's death.[34] The *New York Times* named him "a wizard of the medical world."[35] Yet he could not make the technique work. As he described at a symposium of the New York Academy of Medicine, "It was, for many reasons, a difficult operation."[36] The constant motion of the heart made it difficult to dissect and suture the coronary artery. He had to stop flow through the coronary artery to perform the anastomosis, but the dog's heart went into ventricular fibrillation. The dog died despite cardiac massage. Carrel concluded that the procedure had to be completed in under three minutes, something he had not achieved: "The technique of these operations is far from being completely developed. They must not be used on human beings under their present form."[37]

When surgeons began to focus in the 1920s and the 1930s on coronary artery disease caused by atherosclerosis, they believed that Carrel's direct approach was not possible. Instead, they developed many other approaches to coronary disease. Their work demonstrates extraordinary imagination and a willingness to reengineer the body's tissues to suit their purposes.

Knowing that the sympathetic nervous system stimulated the heart to beat more forcefully and more quickly, surgeons attacked these nerves to reduce cardiac work. Surgical techniques—severing the nerves—came first. Proposed in 1899 and first performed in 1916, sympathectomy persisted for decades. Other approaches soon appeared, including the use of alcohol injections or radiation to kill the nerves. Many groups reported excellent outcomes.[38] Reviewing the experience at Massachusetts General Hospital in 1933, James White observed that "In each case where we have been sure of a successful interruption of the above mentioned structures, angina pectoris has disappeared."[39] Critics, meanwhile, deemed these procedures "disastrous from the therapeutic point of view."[40] Angina pectoris provided a crucial warning to patients that their heart was in danger; removing that warning was foolhardy. White, defending the procedures in 1948, offered dubious consolation: "If fatal coronary infarction takes place [in patients who have had these procedures], it is usually painless."[41]

Other surgeons targeted the thyroid gland. Motivated by an incidental 1902 finding of angina relief after surgical removal of the thyroid, and by observations of patients whose angina became worse in the setting of hyperthyroidism, surgeons in the 1920s began to remove thyroid glands to reduce the body's metabolic activity, reduce demand on the heart, and treat angina. As a team at Boston's Beth Israel Hospital reported in 1933, "In terms of the law of supply and demand, we may say that the supply of the blood has not been increased, but the demands have been reduced to such an extent that the reduced supply is now adequate to the ordinary needs of daily life under these new circumstances."[42] Their colleagues at the Peter Bent Brigham Hospital described the procedure's "immediate and strikingly beneficial results."[43] This enthusiasm was not widely shared, not even in Boston. Surgeons at Massachusetts General Hospital tried thyroidectomy in twenty-one patients and obtained "relatively poor results," with improvement in only one quarter.[44] When radioactive iodine became available after World War II, physicians realized that they could achieve the same result—hypothyroidism—without surgery. The Beth Israel team found that in eleven of seventeen patients, "the therapeutic result has been decidedly worth while"; four patients, previously incapacitated, had returned to work.[45]

Surgeons also worked the other side of supply and demand. As Claude Beck wrote in 1958, "The starting point for effective treatment of coronary heart disease concerns blood supply to ischemic muscle. Any medicament or any surgical operation that increases the amount of blood in ischemic muscle (distal to stenosis or occlusion in an artery) is obviously beneficial. This statement may be considered as an axiom or as a self-evident truth concerning treatment of this disease."[46] What could be done? There were few limits on the surgical imagination. One approach used irritants to provoke vascular scars between the heart and pericardium. Surgeons tried powdered bone, iron filings, iodine, oils, resins, sand, cotton, talc, clay, formaldehyde, horse serum, and even dried, sterilized human skin. Asbestos "produced the most favorable reaction."[47] They sutured other tissues onto the surface of the heart, hoping that blood would flow to the heart's ischemic tissues. Candidates included pericardium, pericardial fat, mediastinal tissues, pleura, diaphragm, and substernal muscles.[48] Omentum, believed to lend its aid to damaged abdominal organs, became the most popular cardiac graft.[49] Surgeons also wrapped sponges around the heart, in hopes that the trabecular structure would provide a scaffolding across which blood vessels would grow into the heart.[50] Beck pioneered a series of combination techniques. He stripped the epicardium off the heart, applied asbestos to promote adhesions, sutured the omentum onto its surface, and performed a partial ligation of the coronary sinus to slow venous drainage. He achieved relief of angina in over 80 percent of his patients, and nearly as many returned to work.[51] Even an "implausible operation"—ligation of the internal mammary artery—flourished between 1939 and 1960. Christopher Crenner, in this volume, describes how skeptical surgeons used sham operations to discredit this procedure.[52]

Enthusiasm for revascularization intensified in the 1950s as surgeons debated the relative merits of two new surgical techniques: coronary endarterectomy and implantation of the internal mammary artery into the myocardium. The Montreal surgeon Arthur Vineberg, who had gained extensive experience with omentum grafts and sponge procedures, developed the implant procedure. Careful analysis of autopsy specimens had convinced him that the myocardium had a unique system of porous arteries and capillaries, a "veritable sponge-work of vessels." He believed that if he inserted the bleeding end of another artery into the myocardium, these venous sinusoids would absorb the blood and perfuse the heart. He began experiments on dogs in 1945 and performed his first human procedure in April 1950.[53] Enthusiastic coverage in *Reader's Digest* and the *Wall Street Journal* explained the logic of the procedure: "Within a few months, if all goes well, the end of the artery implanted to the heart muscle has established itself and is providing the muscle with a new supply of blood."[54] But skeptics wanted to know more. "What *proof* could he offer of any benefits derived?"[55] Vineberg, relying on the traditional method of case series, described invalids who returned to work after the procedure—farmers, machinists, and others. He reported one patient who experienced a coronary occlusion after the operation, but survived: "it would appear that his mammary artery implant protected most probably against death, and most definitely against infarction."[56]

Many surgeons feared that the bleeding implant would simply produce a large pool of blood—a bruise—in the heart wall. Skepticism dissipated in January 1962 when the Cleveland Clinic cardiologist Mason Sones performed coronary angiography on one of Vineberg's patients. Sones saw the implant "giving off small radicals into the myocardium." This provided "clear-cut and uncompromising evidence of [e]ffective myocardial perfusion."[57] Donald Effler, a cardiac surgeon at Cleveland who had been skeptical of implants, became a convert. Within four years he had done over three hundred implant procedures.[58] Surgeons in Boston, Houston, Milwaukee, New Orleans, Uppsala, and London began implanting vessels into hearts—arteries and veins, alone or in combination. Surgeons at the Peter Bent Brigham were especially pleased that their patients reported relief only on a timeframe that made sense (that is, only after the time required for new vascular connections to form): "Angina continued unabated for three to six months after surgery before marked and progressive relief began to evolve." Implants also cut the heart attack rate in half. They published a glowing review in the *New England Journal of Medicine*.[59]

Coronary endarterectomy emerged in parallel. Endarterectomy, in which an atherosclerotic plaque is scraped out of the artery, had been used by vascular surgeons for peripheral vascular disease and renal artery stenosis in the 1940s and 1950s. Surgeons in the mid-1950s explored whether the technique could be applied to the much smaller coronary arteries. They tested the procedure in animals and human cadavers. The procedure was difficult, but possible.[60] Beck, who had the most extensive experience with coronary revascularization, was skeptical: "The widespread involvement of the coronary tree by the disease, often including secondary branches of coronary arteries in a large percentage of cases, the possibility of changing stenosis into occlusion by the surgical manipulation, and the possibility of creating an imbalance and electrocuting currents are considerations that will determine success of failure of this manipulation."[61] Other surgeons, however, were willing to try.

Charles Bailey, in Philadelphia, reported the first successful human coronary endarterectomy 1956. He removed the plaque, a 7-mm tubular cast of the vessel, and watched "restoration of vigorous pulsatile flow."[62] His first patient remained alive three months after the procedure. His second patient was "'markedly improved' in his words and in those of his cardiologist." William Longmire began performing the procedure in Los Angeles in 1957. He was convinced that "the most effective means of increasing myocardial blood flow would be to remove the obstructing atheromatous plaques from the coronary arteries themselves."[63] Some of his patients became asymptomatic, with normal stress tests, and returned to work. Outcomes, however, were mixed. Effler began endarterectomies in 1962. Although three of his first ten patients died, six showed "very significant improvement."[64] The Los Angeles team lost eleven of its first twenty-seven patients (40.7 percent); with careful work, and the use of cardiopulmonary bypass, they reduced operative mortality to 23 percent.[65] When they presented their work at the American Association of Thoracic Surgery in New Orleans in 1965, Effler praised their tenacity: "This is 'heart-rending' work, and the fact they have had the courage to continue, even with a rather forbidding initial mortality, is much to their credit."[66]

Effler came to prefer a promising new variant, the patch graft technique. The procedure began with endarterectomy: the surgeon opened the vessel and removed the plaque. But instead of just closing the incision in the vessel directly, the surgeon used a piece of another tissue (e.g., saphenous vein, from the leg, or pericardium, the sac that surrounds and protects the heart) as a patch to repair the site of the endarterectomy. This left an enlarged vessel that resembled the "Vista Dome" of tourist railroad cars.[67] Effler learned about the technique from a vascular surgeon at the Cleveland Clinic and began laboratory experiments "to develop worktable techniques" for coronary arteries.[68] Effler first tried a patch graft on a patient in January 1962. The procedure was not a simple one: "the graft reconstruction was best characterized as an acrobatic feat rather than a surgical procedure." He was pleased by his early results. Postoperative angiography revealed "obvious improvement." However, as had happened with endarterectomy, procedures on the left coronary arteries met with a "formidable mortality rate": eleven of fourteen patients died.[69] But successful operations were "rewarded by dramatic rehabilitation of the patient and relief of all symptoms."[70] Effler concluded that "direct, surgical attack upon segmental arterial obstruction offers 'instant revascularization.'"[71]

Surgeons' Assessments of Surgical Effectiveness

A simple taxonomy helps to make sense of these procedures. The first distinction is between supply and demand. Whereas some techniques sought to reduce demand on the heart by cutting nerves that make it beat more powerfully, or by reducing the body's overall metabolic activity, others sought to increase the supply of blood to the heart through adhesions, tissue grafts, or replumbing. The second distinction is within supply-side therapeutics, between direct and indirect techniques. Direct techniques, like Carrel's aortocoronary bypass or Effler's patch graft, targeted the coronary arteries and their lesions in order to restore flow through the native vessels. Indirect approaches ignored the damaged coronary arteries and sought to bring the blood to the myocardium by other—indirect—means, for instance by implanting the internal mammary artery into the ventricular muscle. Surgeons' decisions among these options depended on three questions. First, what could the surgical techniques accomplish? Second, what benefits could surgeons demonstrate in their patients? Third, did the treatment make sense, given surgeons' understanding of the pathology of CAD? This depended on whether they saw CAD as focal or diffuse.

The surgical innovators had big plans for what they hoped these procedures could accomplish. All of the procedures demonstrated a particular attitude toward the body, a conception of the body as a malleable toolkit. Its parts could be moved around and recombined in order to restore a lost function or create a new one. As an editorial in the *New England Journal of Medicine* described in 1957, "The implantation of tissues bearing vasculature, the plunging of a pulsating and bleeding artery into myocardial tissue, the creation of pericardial adhesions and attempts to augment, by irritating epicardial substances, intercoronary anastomoses have placed the myocardium in a class by itself as an object of surgical assault."[72] This surgical reengineering was far more ambitious than usual surgical tasks of draining infections, removing tumors, or setting bones.[73]

Human tissues, however, constrained surgeons' design ambitions. The heart is a concrete, material thing with limited tolerances as a living organ. Surgeons had intimate experience with this. If they pushed too hard, the heart let them know. Effler's operative notes demonstrate this well. He often used a Beck rasp to abrade the epicardium. In a 1959 procedure he did this "as vigorously as possible within the limits of toleration," until the surface of the heart "showed frank bleeding . . . the patient was given frequent rest periods to allow the heart to return to a stable rhythm. It was necessary to give the patient some vasopressors to maintain normal blood pressure."[74] In a 1962 operation, "The heart was quite irritable and frequent rest periods were necessary as the blood pressure fluctuated a good deal during this portion of the procedure."[75] Different operations presented different hazards.

As a surgeon implanted the internal mammary artery into the myocardium, the severed side branches "bleed so furiously that literally the entire surgical team gets bathed with these tiny jets of blood."[76]

Surgeons were also surprised by the complications of seemingly successful procedures. In 1963 Sones performed an angiography on a patient who had had a Vineberg implant by a surgeon in New York. Instead of remaining within the wall of the heart, the implant extended into the chamber of the ventricle itself. As Effler wryly told Vineberg, "You'll have to see this to believe it!": "In systole, the contracting myocardium shuts off the internal mammary artery; in diastole, the dye makes a beautiful ventriculogram. This is a very interesting variation of the Vineberg procedure and one that I would not have thought possible."[77] Nonetheless, skillful surgeons learned how to accomplish what they set out to do. Sympathetic nerves could be cut, thyroid glands removed, sponges wrapped around abraded hearts, and arteries implanted into the myocardium. Tragedies and misadventures notwithstanding, surgeons concluded that they could reengineer the heart.

But did the procedures work? Surgeons knew that their surgical imagination would have to answer to the clinical outcomes. Assessment of outcomes, however, was often elusive. As Charles Rosenberg, Harry Marks, Jack Pressman, and other historians of medicine have shown, evaluation of therapeutic outcomes is a complex social and scientific process.[78] In the decades after World War II, randomized clinical trials rose to prominence as the most rigorous way to determine the efficacy of medical interventions. As Crenner describes in this volume, however, clinical trials have had a vexed relationship with surgery, with far less impact on surgery than randomized trials have had on internal medicine.[79] Sometimes a clinical trial has proven decisive for a new surgical procedure. McKellar, in this volume, describes how the REMATCH study legitimized the use of left ventricular assist devices for long-term therapy.[80] However, all of the surgical procedures for CAD, described here, rose to prominence not because of a successful clinical trial but because of case reports and case series. And in these reports, surgeons evaluated their procedures with many different measures.

Surgeons cared greatly about operative mortality, but they took a stoic approach and saw the often appalling mortality as the inevitable cost of innovation. It was rare for cardiac surgeons to abandon a procedure simply because of high mortality in their first attempts.[81] At the same time, they knew that survival was not a good enough outcome. As Effler noted in 1967, surgeons often believed "that the mere fact that the patient is alive and warm, he must be better." For CAD patients, the standard had to be higher: "Survival is all-important and it is a very welcome thing, we certainly agree with that, but the patient must have both subjective and objective demonstration that he is better."[82]

Surgeons deployed all sorts of objective and subjective claims to demonstrate that their patients were better. Many patients, including "intractable cardiac cripples," had returned to their former occupations.[83] Some reduced their need for medications. One of Vineberg's first sponge patients, for instance, decreased his use of nitroglycerin from more than thirty tablets each day to only ten each week.[84] When another patient died in a fight after spending a night with a prostitute, Vineberg claimed success: the patient "had improved sufficiently after the operation, to return to work and do those things that lead to his death."[85] Effler returned the humor: "if you emphasized the effect of your operation on the libido, it might provoke more enthusiasm among our medical colleagues."[86] Jokes aside, cardiac surgeons faced a serious problem. As their experience accumulated, they realized that anything they did—physiologically sound or not—relieved angina in patients and allowed them to resume their former activities. Some reported immediate relief even when surgeons knew that physiologic benefit should not materialize for months. Surgeons concluded that patients could not be trusted to provide reliable assessments of therapeutic success.

Two influential studies, analyzed by Crenner, drove this home.[87] As the popularity and notoriety of internal mammary artery ligation increased in the 1950s, surgeons in Seattle used a sham procedure in 1959 to test its efficacy in seventeen unsuspecting patients: eight were ligated, while nine received the sham.[88] Patients in each group reported dramatic relief of angina, reduced need for nitroglycerin, and improved exercise tolerance. One patient in the sham group even had better results on an exercise electrocardiogram. A Kansas City group published similar results from their own sham controlled trial the next year.[89] These studies provided compelling evidence of the placebo effects of surgery. The Seattle team concluded that "The value of the usual clinical evaluation of any form of surgical therapy designed to relieve the symptoms of angina pectoris is considered highly speculative."[90] The Kansas City team warned surgeons to find ways to distinguish true physiological benefit from the "psychotherapy of surgery."[91] The lesson was heard loud and clear. David Sabiston, the chairman of surgery at Duke University, warned in 1966 that "the bias of suggestion is, in itself, often sufficient to produce dramatic symptomatic improvement."[92] The next year Favaloro described his similar misgivings: "Relief of angina pectoris by an operative procedure is not a certain index of surgical success."[93]

Coronary angiography provided a partial solution to the question of outcome. After his accidental 1959 discovery that a patient could survive an injection of radio-opaque contrast material into the coronary arteries, Mason Sones worked closely with engineers from the North American Philips Corporation to design customized x-ray sources, image amplifiers, and movie cameras. He soon had a working system of coronary cine-angiography.[94] Sones's technique achieved what Lorraine Daston and Peter

Galison call "mechanical objectivity."[95] It produced images and movies of the contrast agent flowing through coronary arteries in living patients. Filling defects indicated the presence of atherosclerotic plaques. As high-quality angiography spread from Cleveland in the 1960s, it changed how surgeons selected patients for coronary surgery and assessed their outcomes. It led to the demise of many older techniques. Although sponge procedures, abrasions, irritants, and the others had all relieved angina, none of them met the standard of angiography. Effler completed 120 cases of abrasion and omental graft without finding a single one in which postoperative angiography demonstrated that the operation provided additional blood flow to heart. He abandoned the technique.[96] As he explained at a conference in New York in 1967, "Perhaps we are in error on this; but we are holding to the thesis that we will believe only what we see—and right now all we see is what the arteriographers can show us."[97]

Angiography, in effect, triggered a mass extinction. Vineberg implants, endarterectomy, and patch grafts survived, but all other surgical treatments for CAD disappeared. Consolidation of practice around these three procedures reflected a major change in treatment design. In the 1930s surgeons had set out to increase supply or reduce demand. As angiography increasingly captured their attention in the 1960s, they focused on what angiography could reveal: whether or not the operation had increased blood flow to the heart. The therapeutic niche had changed, and it would soon change again.

Focal or Diffuse? A Malleable Niche

As the therapeutic niche narrowed, leaving space only for procedures that increased the supply of blood to the heart, it focused attention on the third question: Did the different treatments make sense, given physicians' understanding of the pathophysiology of CAD? The most vigorous debates focused on whether coronary atherosclerosis was predominantly focal or diffuse. If the disease was focal, then endarterectomy and patch grafts could provide a direct and useful solution. But if the disease was diffuse, then surgeons needed an indirect technique, such as Vineberg implants, that brought blood to the heart without relying on the major coronary arteries. Whether atherosclerosis was focal or diffuse ought to have been a simple anatomic matter of fact, a descriptive claim about the distribution of atherosclerotic lesions in the coronary tree. The fact, however, proved to be ambiguous.

Clinical histories and physical exams could diagnose coronary artery disease, but not localize its pathology. Electrocardiograms could identify which coronary artery was affected, but not reveal the distribution of the lesions. As glossed by *Reader's Digest*, "Doctors could listen with a stethoscope for strange sounds and guess the extent of a damage by the patient's chest pains. They learned what they could from the tracings on electrocardiograms. But it was, says Dr. Donald B. Effler, the Cleveland Clinic's famed heart surgeon, 'like trying to navigate without a map.'"[98]

Effler, unlike most other physicians, had direct access to coronary arteries during surgery. In his early years of coronary work he routinely inspected and palpated the arteries during surgery. His descriptions are concrete and evocative. In a 1962 operation, he described how "by direct inspection and by palpation the coronary vessels are characterized by deposits of atheromatous material giving the vessels a typical beaded appearance."[99] The coronary arteries of another patient "had the typical rosary effect produced by multiple atheromatous deposits."[100] The implications of his physical findings were often self-evident: "by palpation, the coronary arteries, both right and left, feel like uncooked noodles. There is obvious extensive atherosclerosis in all of the vessels."[101]

Effler, however, came to distrust his senses. He explained to an audience at the 1966 meeting of the American Association of Thoracic Surgery in Vancouver: "Any attempt to identify a segmental coronary artery occlusion by indirect means (for example, direct palpation or visualization in the operating room) is not only unreliable but foolhardy."[102] He instead emphasized the importance of coronary angiography, which promised to reveal the extent and location of coronary lesions: angiography "has made it possible to select patients intelligently and to tailor the operative procedure to the needs of the individual patient and his specific disease."[103] It was "the *sine qua non* of revascularization surgery."[104] But even this was imperfect. As Effler admitted in 1969, "Frequently, the localized segmental obstruction, visualized at operation, is more extensive than suggested by the preoperative coronary arteriograms."[105] Plans for direct procedures had to be reassessed when surgeons found how extensive the disease actually was.

What did pathologists think? Ever since the development of anatomic pathology in the nineteenth century, pathologists had promised to provide definitive answers to clinical questions. Pathologists at Boston's Beth Israel Hospital thought that they had answered the question of whether CAD was focal or diffuse in 1941. They developed a fastidious method: they injected a colored lead agar mass into the coronary vessels, x-rayed the heart, and then dissected its arteries. Performed properly, the "technic discloses all narrowings, occlusions and anastomoses of the coronary arteries in every heart examined."[106] They studied 400 hearts and found 198 occlusions. Two-thirds were focal, less than 5 millimeters long, and half were proximal, within the first 4 centimeters of the major arteries. When they did this work initially, they were not interested in its therapeutic implications: they simply wanted to guide pathologists' search for possible coronary lesions. However, when the advent of endarterectomy in 1956 renewed interest in the distribution of

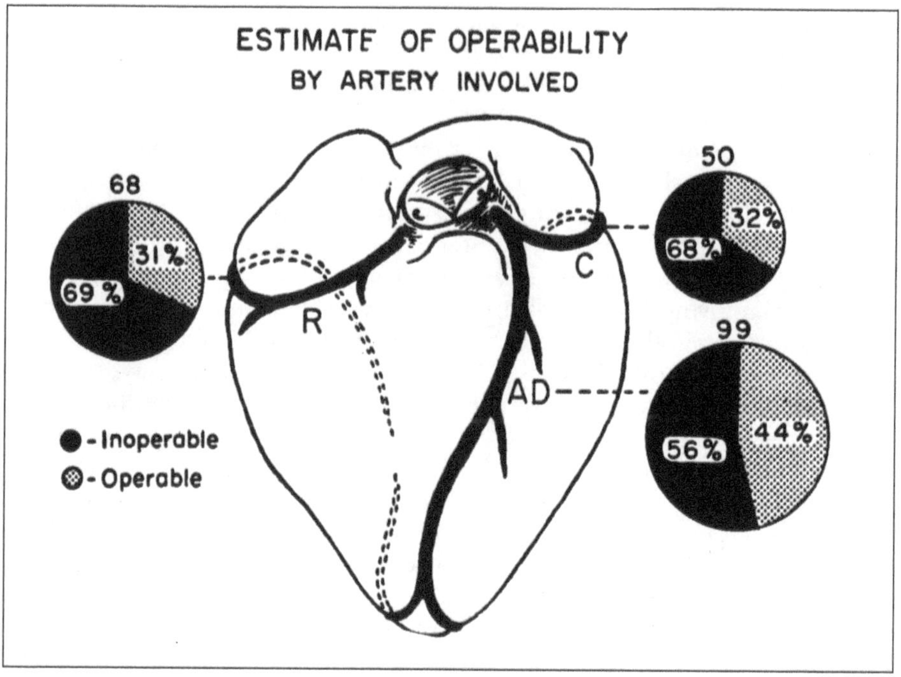

Figure 8.2. The relative incidence of operable and inoperable occlusive lesions in the main coronary artery branches. Note that these authors deemed most lesions to be inoperable. D. Szialagyi et al., "The Applicability of Angioplastic Procedures in Coronary Atherosclerosis: An Estimate through Postmortem Injection Studies," *Annals of Surgery* 148, no. 3 (1958): 457, fig. 14. Reproduced by permission from Wolters Kluwer Health, Inc.

coronary plaques, the team reviewed their old data in 1959 and concluded that "lesions are mostly localized and segmental and consequently make surgical correction feasible." This left the Boston pathologists guardedly optimistic about the prospects of endarterectomy: "one may anticipate gratifying results if suitable patients can be accurately selected by radiography without undue hazard and if the technical difficulties of the appropriate surgical procedures can be surmounted."[107]

Other pathologists disagreed. Surgeons at the University of Minnesota, eager to pursue new surgical approaches, acknowledged their pathologists' pessimistic findings: "it is true that the majority of patients dying with severe coronary artery disease have fairly diffuse involvement." Only five of thirty patients were suitable for a direct surgical approach.[108] A Detroit team deemed 44 percent of the patients they examined inoperable, 35 percent might experience some benefit, but only 21 percent were potentially curable (fig. 8.2). The problem was the nature of the disease: "the atheromatous segments are set close together, tend to coalesce and often render surgical interference difficult or impossible."[109]

Patients, surgeons, cardiologists, and pathologists each had a different way of knowing the disease. This echoes what Anne-Marie Mol encountered in her ethnography of peripheral vascular disease in a Dutch hospital.[110] The varied enactments convinced Mol that multiple different atheroscleroses coexisted simultaneously. Surgeons, however, were more interested in surgery than epistemology. They struggled to integrate different ways of knowing to answer the question: was CAD focal or diffuse? Amid imperfect methods and inconsistent results, CAD existed in multiple conditions of possibility.

Charles Bailey, who performed the first coronary endarterectomy, cited the Beth Israel team and described the disease as "segmental in localization, affecting only one or more narrow zones."[111] Longmire's team, which also favored endarterectomy, reported that "in every instance the obliterative disease was typically segmental."[112] Other surgeons came to the opposite conclusion. Vineberg, who promoted implants—an indirect approach—found that only "13 to 18 per cent of cases have segmental disease. . . . These studies have been made at autopsy."[113] He was astonished by the number of people who had disease in all of the major coronary arteries, even citing the Beth Israel studies as evidence that this should have been expected. The therapeutic consequence was clear: "the disease effects a stranglehold upon the coronary artery inflow tract which is so diffuse that direct surgical relief of coronary artery obstruction is impracticable."[114] Effler agreed. Speaking at the AATS in Houston in 1963, he described how only four of over fifteen hundred patients studied by Sones had segmental disease. Endarterectomy could have only an "extremely limited place in the treatment of occlusive coronary artery disease. This limitation is imposed by the nature of the disease itself. The overwhelming majority of patients studied with selective coronary arteriography demonstrate a diffuse pattern of coronary atherosclerosis."[115] This explained the unpopularity of direct procedures: speaking in Philadelphia in 1965, Effler estimated that in the cumulative experience of cardiac surgery, "only about *200 patients have survived such procedures.*"[116]

Effler and his protege René Favaloro gradually moved toward a more nuanced position. As they gained confidence with patch graft reconstructions, they wrote: "Our original belief that the direct approach should be limited to the few patients whose disease was confined to a single proximal occlusion is both restrictive and unimaginative. It is now evident that there not only is a place for the direct surgical approach but that it is applicable to a rather wide group of coronary artery problems."[117] By 1966 they had done 76 direct procedures on the over 6,000 patients studied by Sones.[118] But this shift in attitude was subtle. They still diagnosed the overwhelming majority of their patients with diffuse disease and treated them with

Vineberg implants, often performing a double procedure that tunneled both of the internal mammary arteries into the myocardium. Between January 1962 and March 1967 they performed 1,088 revascularization operations, including 839 implant procedures (717 single, 122 double) but only 134 patch grafts.[119]

Sometimes, and perhaps most intriguingly, a middle ground appeared. Favaloro found a particular pattern of atherosclerosis in some patients: diffuse in the left coronary artery and focal in the right. He began doing combination procedures: an implant into the left ventricle and a patch graft on the right coronary artery.[120] This was a convenient way of seeing and treating coronary artery disease. Only the left ventricle was thick enough to receive an implant. Only on the right coronary could a patch safely be done. Favaloro's interpretation of CAD justified the operations that he could actually perform.

The distribution of atherosclerotic lesions, in the end, was no simple matter of fact. Instead, it was an opportunity. Autopsies, angiography, and direct palpation produced ambivalent data that granted surgeons considerable discretion. Despite the seeming material reality of the heart, it remained open to reinterpretation according to surgical fashion. Proponents of direct surgical approaches described focal disease. Proponents of indirect techniques described diffuse disease. Poised on the edge of this malleable therapeutic niche, surgeons saw a world of promise. As Effler wrote in 1966, "A new era of surgery for coronary arterial disease has opened."[121]

CABG and the Rise of Focal CAD

Within five years, however, everything had changed: the interpretation of CAD, the choice of surgical procedures, and the scale of cardiac surgery. All were transformed by a single technique, coronary artery bypass grafting (CABG). The idea itself was not new—it was exactly the technique that Alexis Carrel had tried in a dog in 1910. Carrel concluded that the procedure could not be done quickly enough to make it feasible. However, over the decades that followed, as surgeons developed the range of techniques described above, they continued to dabble in CABG.

Most of the research took place in surgical laboratories. Toronto's Gordon Murray, for instance, conducted extensive studies of coronary artery surgery in the 1940s and 1950s, including excision of atherosclerotic segments, interposition grafts, and bypass grafts from the carotid, axillary, or internal mammary arteries.[122] Surgeons encountered many problems in their animal studies, especially ventricular fibrillation and postoperative thromboses.[123] In 1964 Michael DeBakey surveyed the field and found twelve surgical laboratories at work on direct surgical approaches to CAD, but with a success rate (e.g., patent grafts) of only 50 percent at six months. He concluded that the procedures were not yet ready for human use.[124]

Robert Goetz was the first to try CABG in a patient. After practicing a technique of sutureless anastomosis—one that Carrel had proposed in 1910—in twelve dogs, he performed an internal mammary artery to coronary artery bypass at Van Etten Hospital in the Bronx in May 1960. However, he only mentioned this patient as an addendum to an article about his animal work, and he was never able to attempt another.[125] David Sabiston, Michael DeBakey, and Donald Kahn each attempted a saphenous vein CABG (in 1962, 1964, and 1966, respectively); unsatisfied with the results, they did not publish until years later (1974, 1973, and 1971).[126] William Longmire reported two cases in a French journal in 1966: one patient died during the surgery, and the graft failed in the second. He concluded that Vineberg implants were "the most promising method."[127] Parallel efforts took place in Leningrad. Vasilli Kolessov performed a bypass procedure in 1964 and published an article on it in Russian in 1965.[128] When he published his experiences with twelve patients to the *Journal of Thoracic and Cardiovascular Surgery* in 1966, the journal's editor added a disclaimer that the Russian work was "at variance with the concepts of many surgeons in the United States."[129] The editor solicited a commentary from Effler, who critiqued the Kolessov for performing coronary artery surgery without preoperative angiography.[130]

Amidst all of these efforts, it was Favaloro who successfully established CABG as the preferred approach.[131] Favaloro, an Argentinian surgeon, flew to Cleveland in February 1962 with only a letter of introduction, hoping to gain research and surgical experience with Effler. He arrived at an opportune moment, just one month after Effler's first patch graft and Sones's first angiographic demonstration of flow through a Vineberg implant. He worked with Effler on the full range of indirect and direct techniques in the mid-1960s. Frustrated by the difficulty and failure rate of patch grafts, and inspired by vascular surgeons at the Cleveland Clinic who used saphenous vein grafts to repair renal artery stenosis, he began to wonder in 1966 whether vein grafts could be used on coronary arteries.[132] He performed his first saphenous vein interposition graft in May 1967. He described the operation's immediate success: when the team removed the clamps, they "could see the branches of the right coronary fill with blood."[133] Postoperative angiography showed "excellent function of the graft."[134] Favaloro had not practiced this technique on laboratory animals. He later defended his decision, saying that he had accumulated substantial experience performing other operations on hundreds of patients, and he knew that animal work by Murray and others had demonstrated proof of principle.[135]

After performing an interposition graft in 14 patients, Favaloro began doing saphenous vein CABG (fig. 8.1).[136] The Cleveland team went slowly at first because they were not aware of any of the prior human cases and because they were not sure that the grafts would hold up.[137] Favaloro published the results on his first 15 patients in April 1968, with another 40 mentioned in an addendum.[138] By the end of 1968 he had performed 171 CABG operations.[139] At first he often combined CABG with a Vineberg implant, as he had done with patches (e.g., CABG to RCA, Vineberg implant to left ventricle): of his first 100 CABG patients, 41 also received an implant.[140] By May 1969 the Cleveland team had bypassed 303 patients and become increasingly fond of the direct approach. They described how CABG "has the distinct advantage of its immediate effect both in better myocardial perfusion and in symptomatic improvement."[141] By 1970, Favaloro and Effler had done over 1,000 CABG operations.

As news of the Cleveland work spread in 1968, it was buttressed by reports from two other surgeons: Dudley Johnson in Milwaukee and George Green at New York University.[142] Surgeons everywhere quickly abandoned endarterectomies and implants and adopted CABG. By 1977 surgeons in the United States performed over one hundred thousand each year.[143] CABG had obvious appeal. Unlike many of the earlier procedures, it was simple and elegant: no vigorous abrasion, no oozing ventricles, no tiny jets of blood. Like arterial implants, it brought a new source of blood to the heart, but it did so immediately. Like patch grafts, it directly restored flow through coronary arteries, but it did so with less trauma. Its success could be seen with postoperative angiography. As the Cleveland team wrote, the direct approach of CABG "has the distinct advantage of its immediate effect both in better myocardial perfusion and in symptomatic improvement."[144] Providing instant gratification, CABG "increases the indications for revascularization procedures."[145]

Economics also played a role. Surgeons marketed the procedure to an eager public and were inundated with patients. By 1973, Donald Effler billed over $1 million each year. Since he had a salary of under $100,000, money poured into the Cleveland Clinic's coffers.[146] Denton Cooley, the charismatic founder of the Texas Heart Institute, earned $9,865,000 from his medical practice in 1987, much of it from CABG.[147] Surgeons' lavish lifestyles (and homes) were celebrated in popular periodicals, from *Life* to *Architectural Digest.*[148]

Before CABG, most surgeons had seen coronary atherosclerosis as a diffuse process. From 1962 until 1968 Effler and Favaloro had done sixteen times as many implants as patches (2,675 vs. 163).[149] Yet by 1970, surgeons—especially Effler and Favaloro—used CABG as "practically the sole means" of treating coronary artery disease.[150] Patients presented with the same chief complaints and clinical histories, and cardiologists used the same angiography machines, but surgeons rationalized a different procedure. Coming at the end of a decade of debate about whether CAD was focal or diffuse, in which diffuse had the upper hand, CABG transformed surgeons' understanding of the disease—it was now focal—such that only CABG made sense as a treatment. The operation re-created the therapeutic niche in its own image.

Cardiologists were quick to follow this lead. Building on prior work by the Oregon radiologist Charles Dotter, the German angiologist Andreas Grüntzig developed coronary transluminal angioplasty.[151] He used a balloon-tipped catheter to compress atherosclerotic plaques. Angioplasty shared much of the intuitive appeal of CABG. It offered a direct and immediate solution to the problem of large (and focal) coronary plaques. Angioplasty also had distinct advantages: it was "comparatively simple and has the advantage of providing instantaneous revascularization without the need for open-heart surgery." His early hopes were modest. In 1979 he estimated that angioplasty might be an option for "10 to 15 per cent of candidates for bypass surgery."[152] His ambitions grew quickly. After moving to Atlanta and establishing angioplasty in the United States, Grüntzig and his new colleagues expanded their vision of when angioplasty should be done. Their experience supported its use not just in patients with severe lesions, but also "its preventive application for mild stenosis at an earlier stage of coronary artery disease." As they explained, "timely early intervention by PTCA [angioplasty] before double- and triple-vessel disease develops and irreversible myocardial damage occurs might appear logical and justified, even though symptoms are mild."[153] With the advent of coronary artery stents, use of angioplasty increased dramatically. By 1996 it had surpassed the number of CABG procedures in the United States (666,000 vs. 598,000).[154] Since 1999 over 1 million angioplasty procedures have been performed annually.[155] Coronary revascularization (i.e., angiography, CABG, and angioplasty) now provided one-third of the revenue of many medical centers.[156]

Epilogue: The Ongoing Debate

Given that American medicine now has a $100 billion annual commitment to the direct techniques of coronary revascularization—CABG and angioplasty—and their model of disease—focal atherosclerosis—you might think that the controversy would have been resolved. But it has not. Debate persists in part because the choice "focal or diffuse" is too simplistic. The pattern of disease can vary within an individual and between individuals. And the debate persists in part because of ongoing therapeutic competition, not between CABG and angioplasty (which certainly exists), but between revascularization procedures and pharmaceutical treatments of coronary disease. Even as angioplasty rose to prominence in the 1970s and 1980s, researchers developed statins and other agents that lowered serum cholesterol and stabilized coronary plaques.[157] Cardiologists recognized that aspirin and other platelet inhibitors could mitigate the consequences of plaque rupture and prevent coronary thrombosis.[158] Those drugs, like the procedures, have become a multibillion dollar industry.

Competition between the procedures and medications renewed interest in the old question of whether CAD was focal or diffuse. CABG and angioplasty, especially when used prophylactically to prevent future heart attacks, rely on the assumption that CAD is focal and predictable. Proponents of medications argue that coronary atherosclerosis is a diffuse process and that risk is scattered across large and small lesions throughout the coronary tree. They argue that doctors must treat "the entire coronary tree" by lowering cholesterol and stabilizing plaques or platelets.[159] A *New York Times* reporter captured the critique well in 2006. Since angioplasty and stenting targeted only a few of the countless at-risk plaques, interventional cardiologists faced "a losing game of medical whack-a-mole."[160]

Now, as in the 1960s, coronary artery disease exists in multiple conditions of possibility. The therapeutic niche, redefined in 1968 by CABG, has been destabilized and broadened by statins, aspirin, and other medications. Is CAD focal, diffuse, or both? The distribution of lesions in a patient can be characterized by coronary angiography, but the distribution of risk remains a topic of debate. It is not a matter of fact, but an opportunity. Despite the rising tide of evidence-based medicine, physicians still exercise discretion. Many patients and doctors hedge their bets by pursuing both revascularization and a lifelong regimen of pharmaceutical prophylaxis. They benefit, as do hospitals and the device and pharmaceutical industries, from the coexistence of different therapeutic approaches and the ways in which therapeutic practice continues to refashion the therapeutic niche.

Notes

1. René G. Favoloro, quoted in *THI Today* (December 1985): 2, in Institutional Collection #43 (Texas Heart Institute), box 2, folder "THI Today, 1985," John P. McGovern Historical Collections and Research Center (Houston Academy of Medicine), Texas.

2. René G. Favaloro, "Saphenous Vein Autograft Replacement of Severe Segmental Coronary Artery Occlusion," *Annals of Thoracic Surgery* 5 (1968): 334–39; René G. Favaloro, Donald B. Effler, Laurence K. Groves, William C. Sheldon, Earl K. Shirey, and F. Mason Sones, "Severe Segmental Obstruction of the Left Main Coronary Artery and Its Divisions," *Journal of Thoracic and Cardiovascular Surgery* 60 (197): 469–82.

3. W. Dudley Johnson, Robert J. Flemma, Derward Lepley, and Edwin H. Ellison, "Extended Treatment of Severe Coronary Artery Disease: A Total Surgical Approach," *Annals of Surgery* 170 (1969): 460–69; George E. Greene, Simon H. Stertzer, and Edmund H. Reppert, "Coronary Arterial Bypass Grafts," *Annals of Thoracic Surgery* 5 (1968): 443–50.

4. Henry D. McIntosh and Jorge A. Garcia, "The First Decade of Aortocoronary Bypass Grafting, 1967–1977: A Review," *Circulation* 57 (1978): 405–31.

5. Alexis Carrel, "On the Experimental Surgery of the Thoracic Aorta and the Heart," *Annals of Surgery* 52 (1910): 83–95.

6. Shelley McKellar, "Disruptive Potential: The 'Landmark' REMATCH Trial, Left Ventricular Assist Device (LVAD) Technology, and the Surgical Treatment of Heart Failure in the United States," chapter 6 of this volume.

7. René G. Favaloro, "Oral History" (March 3, 1997), in *Pioneers of Cardiac Surgery*, ed. William S. Stoney (Nashville: Vanderbilt University Press, 2008), 364.

8. Elsewhere I have argued a parallel case: that the advent of statins and platelet inhibitors in the late 1980s and early 1990s made an old hypothesis about the cause of heart attacks—the plaque-rupture hypothesis—newly relevant. David S. Jones, *Broken Hearts: The Tangled History of Cardiac Care* (Baltimore: Johns Hopkins University Press, 2013).

9. Christopher Crenner, "Placebos and the Progress of Surgery," chapter 7 of this volume; McKellar, "Disruptive Potential."

10. Thomas Schlich, *Surgery, Science, and Industry: A Revolution in Fracture Care, 1950s–1990s* (New York: Palgrave Macmillan, 2002).

11. Jack Pressman, *Last Resort: Psychosurgery and the Limits of Medicine* (Cambridge: Cambridge University Press, 1998), quotations on 14, 10, 190.

12. Ian Hacking, *Mad Travelers: Reflections on the Reality of Transient Mental Illness* (Charlottesville: University of Virginia Press, 1998), 13.

13. Richard Lewontin, "Adaptation," *Scientific American* 239 (September 1978): 215.

14. F. John Odling-Smee, Kevin N. Laland, and Marcus W. Feldman, "Niche Construction," *American Naturalist* 147 (1996): 641.

15. Richard Lewontin, "Gene, Organism, Environment," in *Evolution from Molecules to Men*, ed. D. S. Bendall (Cambridge: Cambridge University Press, 1983), 282.

16. For a fuller discussion, see David S. Jones, "Therapeutic Evolution or Revolution? Metaphors and Their Consequences," in *Therapeutic Revolutions: Pharmaceuticals and Social Change in the Twentieth Century*, ed. Jeremy A. Greene, Flurin Condrau, and Elizabeth Siegel Watkins (Chicago: University of Chicago Press, 2016), 269–301.

17. David Healy, *The Antidepressant Era* (Cambridge: Harvard University Press, 1997); Jeremy A. Greene, *Prescribing by Numbers: Drugs and the Definition of Disease* (Baltimore: Johns Hopkins University Press, 2007).

18. Ray Moynihan and David Healy, "The Fight against Disease Mongering: Generating Knowledge for Action," *PLoS Medicine* 3 (2006): e191.

19. Barron H. Lerner, *The Breast Cancer Wars: Hope, Fear, and the Pursuit of a Cure in Twentieth-Century America* (New York: Oxford University Press, 2001).

20. Leon Michaels, *The Eighteenth-Century Origin of Angina Pectoris: Predisposing Causes, Recognition, and Aftermath* (London: The Wellcome Trust, 2002).

21. [Frederick] Winsor, "Angina Pectoris with Rupture of the Heart," as reported in George E. Putney, "Extracts from the Records of the Middlesex East District Medical Society," *Boston Medical and Surgical Journal* 103 (October 21, 1880): 398.

22. James Herrick, "Clinical Features of Sudden Obstruction of the Coronary Arteries," *Journal of the American Medical Association* 59 (December 7, 1912): 2015–20.

23. Centers for Disease Control and Prevention, "Leading Causes of Death, 1900–1998," last updated November 12, 2009, http://www.cdc.gov/nchs/nvss/mortality_historical_data.htm.

24. Timothy Leary, "Mallory Institute Dedication," December 13, 1933, in Timothy Leary Papers, B MS c 40, box 4, Countway Library, Boston, Massachusetts.

25. W. Bruce Fye, *American Cardiology: The History of a Specialty and Its College* (Baltimore: John Hopkins University Press, 1996); W. Bruce Fye, *Caring for the Heart: Mayo Clinic and the Rise of Specialization* (New York: Oxford University Press, 2015).

26. M. H. Nathanson, "Diseases of the Coronary Arteries," *American Journal of Medical Sciences* 170 (1925): 240–55.

27. J. D. Ratcliff, "New Life for Failing Hearts," *Reader's Digest*, February 1966, 181.

28. Winsor, "Angina Pectoris," 398.

29. John Sproull, "A General Practitioner's View on the Treatment of Angina Pectoris," *New England Journal of Medicine* 215 (1936): 443–52; and Laurence Chapin, "Discussion [of Sproull]," 452.

30. Claude S. Beck, "Operations for Coronary Artery Disease," *Journal of the International College of Surgeons* 21 (1954): 314.

31. Meyer Friedman, *Pathogenesis of Coronary Artery Disease* (New York: McGraw-Hill, 1969), 223.

32. Denton Cooley, Introduction to Orson Welles, "A Matter of Life" [film] (1984), WG 300 VC #160, 1984, Texas Heart Institute Library & Learning Resource Center.

33. Samuel Alcott Thompson and Milton J. Raisbeck, "Cardio-Pericardiopexy: The Surgical Treatment of Coronary Arterial Disease by the Establishment of Adhesive Pericarditis," *Annals of Internal Medicine* 16 (1942): 495.

34. R. M. Langer and B. D. Kahan, "Alexis Carrel's Legacy: Visionary of Vascular Surgery and Organ Transplantation," *Transplantation Proceedings* 34 (2002): 1061–65.

35. "Heart Surgery Is Science's Latest Marvel: Dr. Alexis Carrel of the Rockefeller Institute Successfully Performs Operations That May Revolutionize Surgery," *New York Times*, March 27, 1910, SM4.

36. Carrel, "On the Experimental Surgery," 93.

37. Ibid., 95.

38. See, for examples: Elliott C. Cutler and Jacob Fine, "Sympathectomy in Angina Pectoris," *Journal of the American Medical Association* 86 (1926): 1972–79; Marcy L. Sussman, "The Treatment of Angina Pectoris by Para-Vertebral Short Wave Radiation," *American Journal of Roentgenology* 24 (1930): 163–68. For an extremely useful chronicle of the history of this and the subsequent techniques, see Richard L. Mueller, Todd K. Rosengart, and O. Wayne Isom, "The History of Surgery for Ischemic Heart Disease," *Annals of Thoracic Surgery* 63 (1997): 869–78.

39. James C. White, "Experimental and Clinical Studies in the Surgical Treatment of Angina Pectoris," *Annals of Internal Medicine* 7 (1933): 238.

40. D. Daniélopolu, "The Pathology and Surgical Treatment of Angina Pectoris," *British Medical Journal* 2 (1924): 556.

41. James C. White and Edward F. Bland, "The Surgical Relief of Severe Angina Pectoris," *Medicine* 27 (1948): 39.

42. Herrman L. Blumgart, Joseph E. F. Riseman, David Davis, and David D. Berlin, "Therapeutic Effect of Total Ablation of Normal Thyroid on Congestive Heart Failure and Angina Pectoris," *Annals of Internal Medicine* 52 (1933): 876.

43. Elliott C. Cutler and Max T. Schnitker, "Total Thyroidectomy for Angina Pectoris," *Annals of Surgery* 100 (1934): 578.

44. Richard J. Clark, James H. Means, and Howard B. Sprague, "Total Thyroidectomy for Heart Disease," *New England Journal of Medicine* 214 (1936): 294.

45. Herrman L. Blumgart, A. Stone Freedberg, and George S. Kurland, "Treatment of Incapacitated Euthyroid Cardiac Patients by Producing Hypothyroidism with Radioactive Iodine," *New England Journal of Medicine* 245 (1951): 83.

46. Claude S. Beck, David S. Leighninger, Bernard L. Brofman, and Jess F. Bond, "Some New Concepts of Coronary Heart Disease," *Journal of the American Medical Association* 168 (1958): 2110.

47. Paul Schildt, Eugene Stanton, and Claude S. Beck, "Communications between the Coronary Arteries Produced by the Application of Inflammatory Agents to the Surface of the Heart," *Annals of Surgery* 118 (1943): 44.

48. Claude S. Beck and V. L. Tichy, "The Production of Collateral Circulation of the Heart," *American Heart Journal* 10 (1935): 849–73.

49. Arthur Vineberg, Rosendo Criollos, Claude Mercier, Roque Pifarre, and Samir Ragheb, "Apparent Reversion to Trophism of a Free Omental Graft: A Preliminary Report," *Canadian Medical Association Journal* 87 (1962): 1074–76. See also Ratcliff, "New Life for Failing Hearts": 188.

50. Arthur Vineberg, T. Deliyannis, and Gil Pablo, "Myocardial Nutrition after the Ivalon Sponge Operation: The Return of a 400 Million Year Old System," *Canadian Medical Association Journal* 80 (1959): 948–58.

51. Beck et al., "Some New Concepts," 2110–17.

52. For an enthusiastic American report, see Robert P. Glover, Julio C. Davilla, Robert H. Kyle, John C. Beard, Robert G. Trout, and J. Roderick Kitchell, "Ligation of the Internal Mammary Arteries as a Means of Increasing Blood Supply to the Myocardium," *Journal of Thoracic Surgery* 34 (1957): 661–78. A prominent editorial deemed it "implausible": "Ligation of the Internal Mammary Arteries," *New England Journal of Medicine* 257 (1957): 385. For discussions of this case, see: Ernest M. Barsamian, "The Rise and Fall of Internal Mammary Artery Ligation in the Treatment of Angina Pectoris and the Lessons Learned," in *Costs, Risks, and Benefits of Surgery*, ed. John P. Bunker, Benjamin A. Barnes, and Frederick Mosteller (New York: Oxford University Press, 1977), 213–20; Scott H. Podolsky, "Quintessential Beecher—Surgery as Placebo: A Quantitative Study of Bias," *International Anesthesia Clinics* 45 (Fall 2007): 47–63; Crenner, "Placebos and the Progress of Surgery."

53. Arthur Vineberg and Douglas Miller, "Functional Evaluation of an Internal Mammary Coronary Artery Anastomosis," *American Heart Journal* 45 (1953): 875.

54. Jerry E. Bishop, "Healing the Heart," *Wall Street Journal*, May 17, 1966, 1.

55. Ratcliff, "New Life for Failing Hearts," 186. Emphasis in the original.

56. Arthur Vineberg, "Internal Mammary Artery Implant in the Treatment of Angina Pectoris: A Three Year Follow Up," *Canadian Medical Association Journal* 70 (1954): 378. For a discussion of the role of case series in surgical, research, see Crenner, "Placebos and the Progress of Surgery."

57. Mason Sones, "Angiography Report," January 12, 1962, "P126/C8, 250 Sones," Vineberg Fronds, Osler Library of the History of Medicine, McGill University. The report says "defective," not "effective," but the intended meaning is clear from the context.

58. Donald B. Effler, Laurence K. Groves, and Mason Sones, "Myocardial Revascularization by Internal Mammary Artery Implantation," *Vascular Disease* 3 (1966): 42–48.

59. Richard Gorlin and Warren J. Taylor, "Selective Revascularization of the Myocardium by Internal-Mammary-Artery Implant," *New England Journal of Medicine* 275 (1966): 283–90.

60. Angelo M. May, "Coronary Endarterectomy: Curettement of Coronary Arteries in Dogs," *American Journal of Surgery* 93 (1957): 969–73.

61. Claude S. Beck, "Coronary Heart Disease after Twenty-five Years," *Journal of Thoracic Surgery* 36 (1958): 350.

62. Charles P. Bailey and Angelo M. May, "Survival after Coronary Endarterectomy in Man," *Journal of the American Medical Association* 164 (1957): 641, 643.

63. William P. Longmire, Jack A. Cannon, and Albert A. Kattus, "Direct-Vision Coronary Endarterectomy for Angina Pectoris," *New England Journal of Medicine* 259 (1958): 993.

64. Sones to E. P. Roy, December 12, 1963, "Cardiology Annual Reports, 1975–1985" (#1554), A08–27/1, Cleveland Clinic Foundation Archives, Cleveland, Ohio.

65. Ralph B. Dilley, Jack A. Cannon, Albert A. Kattus, Rex N. MacAlpin, and William P. Longmire, "The Treatment of Coronary Occlusive-disease by Endarterectomy," *Journal of Thoracic and Cardiovascular Surgery* 50 (1965): 511–26.

66. Effler, discussion of Dilley et al., "The Treatment," 523.

67. Donald B. Effler, Laurence K. Groves, Renesto L. Suarez, and René G. Favaloro, "Direct Coronary Artery Surgery with Endarterectomy and Patch-Graft Reconstruction," *Journal of Thoracic and Cardiovascular Surgery* 53 (1967): 93–101.

68. Donald B. Effler, Mason Sones, René G. Favaloro, and Groves, "Coronary Endarterotomy with Patch-Graft Reconstruction," *Annals of Surgery* 162 (1965): 591. See also "Doctor Tells Clinic of Artery Patching," *Cleveland News*, January 8, 1959.

69. Effler et al., "Coronary Endarterotomy," 591 (acrobatic), 595 (obvious), 597 (formidable). For the mortality rate, see W. Dudley Johnson, "Oral History" (June 5, 2003), in *Pioneers of Cardiac Surgery*, ed. William S. Stoney (Nashville, TN: Vanderbilt University Press, 2008), 384.

70. Effler et al., "Direct Coronary Artery Surgery": 100.

71. Donald B. Effler, "Surgical Treatment of Myocardial Ischemia," *Clinical Symposia* 21 (1969): 6.

72. Editorial, "Ligation of the Internal Mammary Arteries," 385.

73. The ambitions of cardiac surgeons were rivaled by those of reconstructive surgeons and transplant surgeons. For example, see Thomas Schlich, *The Origins of Organ Transplantation: Surgery and Laboratory Science, 1880–1930* (Rochester, NY: University of Rochester Press, 2010).

74. Effler, "Operative Report," July 8, 1959, "P126/C8,54 Cleveland Clinic," Vineberg Fronds.

75. Effler, "Operative Report," November 23, 1962, "P126/C8,54 Cleveland Clinic," Vineberg Fronds.

76. Leonard Gordon, "Surgical Approaches to Coronary Artery Disease," *Medical Tribute*, February 13–14, 1965, 17.

77. Effler to Vineberg, April 12, 1963, "P126/C8,78 Effler," Vineberg Fronds. Effler to Vineberg, July 11, 1963, "P126/C8,54 Cleveland Clinic," Vineberg Fronds.

78. Charles Rosenberg, "The Therapeutic Revolution: Medicine, Meaning, and Social Change in Nineteenth-century America," *Perspectives in Biology and Medicine* 20 (1977): 485–506; Harry Marks, *The Progress of Experiment: Science and Therapeutic Reform in the United States, 1900–1990* (Cambridge: Cambridge University Press, 1997); Pressman, *Last Resort*.

79. Crenner, "Placebos and the Progress of Surgery."

80. McKellar, "Disruptive Potential."

81. Jones, *Broken Hearts*, 117, 121–22.

82. Effler, in Arthur Vineberg, Donald B. Effler, Goffredo G. Gensini, John Shanks, and William C. Sheldon, "Revascularization of the Myocardium," *Industrial Medicine and Surgery* 36 (1967): 527.

83. Blumgart, Freedberg, and Kurland, "Treatment of Incapacitated Euthyroid Cardiac Patients," 4.

84. Arthur Vineberg and T. Deliyannis, "The Sponge Operation for Myocardial Revascularization: An Experimental Study," *Canadian Medical Association Journal* 78 (1958): 612.

85. Vineberg to Sones, April 12, 1960, "P126/C8,78 Effler," Vineberg Fronds.

86. Effler to Vineberg, April 25, 1960, "P126/C8,78 Effler," Vineberg Fronds,

87. Crenner, "Placebos and the Progress of Surgery."

88. Leonard A. Cobb, George I. Thomas, David D. Dillard, K. Alvin Merendino, and Robert A. Bruce, "An Evaluation of Internal-Mammary-Artery Ligation by a Double-Blind Technic," *New England Journal of Medicine* 260 (1959): 1115–18.

89. E. Grey Dimond, C. Frederick Kittle, James E. Crockett, "Comparison of Internal Mammary Artery Ligation and Sham Operation for Angina Pectoris," *American Journal of Cardiology* 5 (1960): 483–86.

90. Cobb et al., "An Evaluation," 1118.

91. Dimond et al., "Comparison," 486.

92. David C. Sabiston, "Role of Surgery in the Management of Myocardial Ischemia," *Modern Concepts of Cardiovascular Disease* 35 (1966): 126.

93. René G. Favaloro, Donald B. Effler, Laurence K. Groves, Mason Sones, and David J. G. Ferguson, "Myocardial Revascularization by Internal Mammary Artery Implant Procedures: Clinical Experience," *Journal of Thoracic and Cardiovascular Surgery* 54 (1967): 367.

94. Sones and Shirey, "Cine Coronary Angiography," *Modern Concepts of Cardiovascular Disease* 31 (July 1962): 735–38; Sones to Roy. For the best account of the development of angiography, see Fye, *Caring for the Heart*, 315–39.

95. Lorraine Daston and Peter Galison, *Objectivity* (Cambridge: Zone Books, 2007).

96. Donald B. Effler, "A New Era of Surgery for Ischemic Heart Disease," *Chest* 54 (1968): 399–400.

97. Effler, in discussion of Favaloro et al., "Myocardial Revascularization," 370.

98. Ratcliff, "New Life for Failing Hearts," 182.

99. Effler, "Operative Report," June 13, 1962, "P126/C8,54 Cleveland Clinic," Vineberg Fronds.

100. Effler, "Operative Report," January 22, 1962, "P126/C8,78 Effler," Vineberg Fronds.

101. Effler, "Operative Report," October 19, 1962, "P126/C8,78 Effler," Vineberg Fronds.

102. Effler et al., "Direct Coronary Artery Surgery," 93.

103. Effler, "Surgical Treatment," 3.

104. Donald B. Effler, René G. Favaloro, and Laurence K. Groves, "Myocardial Revascularization: Cleveland Clinic Experience," *Journal of Cardiovascular Surgery* 12 (1971): 2.

105. Effler, "Surgical Treatment," 8.

106. Monroe J. Schlesinger and Paul M. Zoll, "Incidence and Localization of Coronary Artery Occlusions," *Archives of Pathology* 32 (1941): 178.

107. Blumgart, Zoll, and Kurland, "Direct Relief of Coronary Occlusion," *Archives of Internal Medicine* 104 (1959): 862, 868.

108. Alan Thal, John F. Perry, Fletcher A. Miller, and Owen H. Wangensteen, "Direct Suture Anastomosis of the Coronary Arteries in the Dog," *Surgery* 40 (1956): 1029.

109. D. Emerick Szilagyi, Richard T. McDonald, and Lloyd C. France, "The Applicability of Angioplastic Procedures in Coronary Atherosclerosis: An Estimate through Postmortem Injection Studies," *Annals of Surgery* 148, no. 3 (1958): 451, 457.

110. Anne-Marie Mol, *The Body Multiple: Ontology in Medical Practice* (Durham, NC: Duke University Press, 2002).

111. Bailey and May, "Survival," 641.

112. Cannon, Longmire, and Kattus, "Considerations of the Rationale and Technique of Coronary Endarterectomy for Angina Pectoris," *Surgery* 46 (1959): 207.

113. Arthur Vineberg, "Surgery of Coronary Artery Disease," *Progress in Cardiovascular Disease* 4 (1962): 397.

114. Arthur Vineberg, John Shanks, Roque Pifarré, Rosendo Criollos, Yutaka Kato, and K. S. Baichwal, "Myocardial Revascularization by Omental Graft without Pedicle: Experimental Background and Report on 25 Cases Followed 6 to 16 Months," *Journal of Thoracic and Cardiovascular Surgery* 49 (1965): 103.

115. Effler, Groves, Sones, and Shirey, "Endarterectomy in the Treatment of Coronary Artery Disease," *Journal of Thoracic and Cardiovascular Surgery* 47 (1964): 104.

116. Effler et al., "Coronary Endarterotomy," 590.

117. Ibid., 591.

118. Effler et al., "Direct Coronary Artery Surgery," 93.

119. Favaloro et al., "Myocardial Revascularization," 360.

120. René G. Favaloro, Donald B. Effler, Laurence K. Groves, Medhi Razavi, and Yair Lieberman, "Combined Simultaneous Procedures in the Surgical Treatment of Coronary Artery Disease," *Annals of Thoracic Surgery* 8 (1969): table 1, p. 21.

121. Donald B. Effler, "A New Era of Coronary Artery Surgery," *Surgery, Gynecology & Obstetrics* 123 (1966): 1311.

122. Gordon Murray, J. Hilario, R. Porcheron, and W. Roschlau, "Surgery of Coronary Heart Disease," *Angiology* 4 (1953): 526–31. This part of Murray's work is described briefly in Shelley McKellar, *Surgical Limits: The Life of Gordon Murray* (Toronto: University of Toronto Press, 2003).

123. Lester R. Sauvage, Stephen J. Wood, Kenneth M. Eyer, and Alexander H. Bill, "Experimental Coronary Artery Surgery: Preliminary Observations of Bypass Venous Grafts, Longitudinal Arteriotomies, and End-to-End Anastomoses," *Journal of Thoracic and Cardiovascular Surgery* 46 (1963): 826–35. See also: Blumgart et al., "Direct Relief";

and David C. Sabiston and Alfred Blalock, "Physiologic and Anatomic Determinants of Coronary Blood Flow and Their Relationship to Myocardial Revascularization," *Surgery* 44 (1958): 417.

124. M. E. DeBakey, "Oral History" (1998), in Stoney, *Pioneers of Cardiac Surgery*, 156.

125. Robert H. Goetz, Michael Rohman, Jordan D. Haller, Ronald Dee, and Stephan S. Rosenak, "Internal Mammary-Coronary Artery Anastomosis: A Nonsuture Method Employing Tantalum Rings," *Journal of Thoracic and Cardiovascular Surgery* 41 (1961): 378–86; Igor E. Konstantinov, "Robert H. Goetz: The Surgeon Who Performed the First Successful Clinical Coronary Artery Bypass Operation," *Annals of Thoracic Surgery* 69 (2000): 1966–72.

126. David C. Sabiston, "The Coronary Circulation," *Johns Hopkins Medical Journal* 134 (1974): 320–21; H. Edward Garrett, Edward W. Dennis, and DeBakey, "Aortocoronary Bypass with Saphenous Vein Graft: Seven-Year Follow-Up," *Journal of the American Medical Association* 223 (1973): 792–94; Donald Kahn, in discussion of Donald B. Effler, René G. Favaloro, Laurence K. Groves, and Floyd D. Loop, "The Simple Approach to Direct Coronary Artery Surgery: Cleveland Clinic Experience," *Journal of Thoracic and Cardiovascular Surgery* 62 (1971): 509.

127. Longmire, Dilley, and Kattus, "Various Direct Surgical Techniques Utilized in the Treatment of Obstructive Coronary Artery Diseases," *Bulletin de la Société Internationale de Chirurgie* 25 (1966): 523.

128. Igor Konstantinov, "The First Coronary Artery Bypass Operation and Forgotten Pioneers," *Annals of Thoracic Surgery* 64 (1997): 1522–23.

129. V. I. Kolessov, "Mammary Artery-Coronary Artery Anastomosis as a Method of Treatment for Angina Pectoris," *Journal of Thoracic and Cardiovascular Surgery* 54 (1967): 535–44; Brian Blades, "Foreword," 535.

130. Donald B. Effler, "Comment," in Kolessov, "Mammary Artery-Coronary Artery Anastomosis," 543.

131. A full discussion of this claim cannot be provided here. But for an example of the consensus about this point, see Mueller, Rosengart, and Isom, "History of Surgery," 876. See also Fye, *Caring for the Heart*, 340–62.

132. René G. Favaloro, "Direct Myocardial Revascularization: A Ten Year Journey," *American Journal of Cardiology* 43 (1979): 110; René G. Favaloro, "The Present Era of Myocardial Revascularization—Some Historical Landmarks," *International Journal of Cardiology* 4 (1983): 331–44; Favaloro "Oral History," 364.

133. René G. Favaloro, *The Challenging Dream of Heart Surgery: From the Pampas to Cleveland* (New York: Little, Brown, 1994), 96.

134. Favaloro, "Saphenous Vein Autograft," 337.

135. Favaloro, *Challenging Dream,* 98; Favaloro, "Direct Myocardial Revascularization," *Surgical Clinics of North America* 51 (1971): 1035.

136. Favaloro, "Saphenous Vein Autograft," 337.

137. Favaloro, "Present Era," 335.

138. Favaloro, "Saphenous Vein Autograft."

139. René G. Favaloro, "Saphenous Vein Graft in the Surgical Treatment of Coronary Artery Disease: Operative Technique," *Journal of Thoracic and Cardiovascular Surgery* 58 (1969): 178.

140. René G. Favaloro, Donald B. Effler, Laurence K. Groves, William C. Sheldon, and Mohammed Riahi, "Direct Myocardial Revascularization with Saphenous Vein Autograft: Clinical Experience in 100 Cases," *Diseases of the Chest* 56 (1969): 279.

141. William C. Sheldon, René G. Favaloro, Mason Sones, and Donald B. Effler, "Reconstructive Coronary Artery Surgery: Venous Autograft Technique," *Journal of the American Medical Association* 213 (1970): 78.

142. Johnson et al., "Extended Treatment"; Greene et al., "Coronary Arterial Bypass Grafts."

143. McIntosh and Garcia, "First Decade."

144. Sheldon et al., "Reconstructive Coronary," 78.

145. René G. Favaloro, Donald B. Effler, Laurence K. Groves, William C. Sheldon, and Mason Sones, "Direct Myocardial Revascularization by Saphenous Vein Graft," *Annals of Thoracic Surgery* 10 (1970): 109.

146. John G. Mearns, "Effler and Sones and the Boys at Cleveland Clinic Have Taken the You-Bet-Your-Life Out of Heart Surgery," *Cleveland Magazine*, November 1973, 10.

147. "In re: Denton A. Cooley . . ." Case No. 88–00154-H5–11 (chapter 11), United States Bankruptcy Court for the Southern District of Texas, Houston Division, "First Amended Disclosure Statement," March 28, 1988, in Denton A. Cooley Papers (Manuscript Collection #43), box "Chapter 11 Court Records," John P. McGovern Historical Collections and Research Center, Houston, Texas.

148. Rich Gore, "The Ace of Hearts They Call 'Ted Terrific,'" *Life*, October 13, 1972, 82–89; Richard Conniff, "Profile: Denton Cooley," *Architectural Digest*, May 1987, 194–201, 246.

149. This is an estimate based on a cumulative count of procedures in their periodicals; it is not always possible to sort out overlapping case series that appear across multiple publications, and it is possible that not all of their cases were included in their publications.

150. Angelo M. May, William E. Neville, William R. Rumel, "Report of the Subcommittee on Surgery for Coronary Disease American College of Chest Physicians," *Chest* 61 (1972): 477.

151. Ramona Braun, "Voyaging in the Vein: Medical Experimentation with Heart Catheters in the Twentieth Century," *Nuncius* 26 (2011): 132–58.

152. Andreas R. Grüntzig, Åke Senning, and Walter E. Siegenthaler, "Nonoperative Dilatation of Coronary-Artery Stenosis," *New England Journal of Medicine* 301 (1979): 65, 61.

153. Thomas Ischinger, Andreas R. Gruentzig, Jay Hollman, Spencer King III, John Douglas, Bernhard Meier, James Bradford, and Rose Tankersley, "Should Coronary Arteries with Less Than 60% Diameter Stenosis Be Treated by Angioplasty?," *Circulation* 68 (July 1983): 148, 152.

154. E. J. Graves and M. F. Owings, "1996 Summary: National Hospital Discharge Survey: Advance Data from Vital and Health Statistics; no. 301" (Hyattsville, MD: National Center for Health Statistics, 1998).

155. J. R. Popovic and M. J. Hall, "1999 National Hospital Discharge Survey: Advance Data from Vital and Health Statistics; no. 319" (Hyattsville, MD: National Center for Health Statistics, 2001).

156. "Doctor-Owned Specialty Hospitals Spur Investor Interest, Capital Hill Worries," *BNA's Health Care Policy Report* 11 (2003): 532–33; Stephanie Desmon and Robert Little, "St. Joe's, Cardiology Group Probed: Hospital, Midatlantic Involved in Business, Legal Disputes," *Baltimore Sun*, March 24, 2009.

157. Daniel Steinberg, "An Interpretive History of the Cholesterol Controversy, Part V: The Discovery of the Statins and the End of the Controversy," *Journal of Lipid Research* 47 (2006): 1339–51; Jeremy A. Greene, "The Abnormal and the Pathological: Cholesterol, Statins, and the Threshold of Disease," in *Medicating Modern America: Pharmaceutical Drugs in History*, ed. Andrea Tone and Elizabeth Watkins (New York: New York University Press, 2007), 183–228.

158. Jones, *Broken Hearts*, 80–83.

159. William C. Little, Martin Constantinescu, Robert J. Applegate, Michael A. Kutcher, Mark T. Burrows, Frederic R. Kahl, and William P. Santamore, "Can Coronary Angiography Predict the Site of a Subsequent Myocardial Infarction in Patients with Mild-to-Moderate Coronary Artery Disease," *Circulation* 78 (November 1988): 1157.

160. Barnaby J. Feder, "In Quest to Improve Heart Therapies, Plaque Gets a Fresh Look," *New York Times*, November 27, 2006.

Bibliography of Secondary Sources

Anderson, Warwick. "The Case of the Archives." *Critical Inquiry* 39 (2013): 532–46.

Angelos, Peter. "The Art of Medicine: The Ethical Challenges of Surgical Innovation for Patient Care." *Lancet* 376 (2010): 1046.

Aronowitz, Robert. *Unnatural History: Breast Cancer and American Society.* Cambridge: Cambridge University Press, 2007.

Asher, Marc A. *Dogged Persistence: Harrington, Post-Polio Scoliosis, and the Origin of Spinal Instrumentation.* Traverse City, MI: Chandler Lake Books, 2015.

Asher, Marc A., and Douglas C. Burton. "Reflection: Paul Randall Harrington (1911–1980)." *Journal of Bone & Joint Surgery* 93, no. 24 (2011): 151–52.

Baehr, Peter. "The 'Iron Cage' and the 'Shell as Hard as Steel': Parsons, Weber, and the Stahlhartes Gehäuse Metaphor in the Protestant Ethic and the Spirit of Capitalism." *History and Theory* 40, no. 2 (2001): 153–69.

Barkun, Jeffrey S., et al. "Evaluation and Stages of Surgical Innovations." *Lancet* 374 (2009): 1089–96.

Barsamian, Ernest. "The Rise And Fall of Internal Mammary Artery Ligation in the Treatment of Angina Pectoris and the Lessons Learned." In *Costs, Risks, and Benefits of Surgery,* edited by J. P. Bunker, B. A. Barnes, and F. Mosteller, 212–20. New York: Oxford University Press, 1977.

Basalla, G. *The Evolution of Technology.* Cambridge: Cambridge University Press, 1988.

Belofsky, Nathan. *Strange Medicine: A Shocking History of Real Medical Practices through the Ages.* New York: Penguin, 2013.

Berrios, German E. "The Origins of Psychosurgery: Shaw, Burckhardt and Moniz." *History of Psychiatry* 8, no. 29 (1997): pt. 1, 61–81.

Bijker, Wiebe E., Thomas P. Hughes, and Trevor Pinch. "General Introduction." In *The Social Construction of Technological Systems: New Directions in the Sociology and History of Technology,* edited by Wiebe E. Bijker, Thomas P. Hughes, and Trevor Pinch, 1–15. Boston: MIT Press, 1987.

Blackbourn, David. *History of Germany, 1780–1918: The Long Nineteenth Century.* Malden, MA: Blackwell, 2002.

Bliss, Michael. *Harvey Cushing: A Life in Surgery.* New York: Oxford University Press, 2005.

Blume, Stuart. *The Artificial Ear: Cochlear Implants and the Culture of Deafness.* New Brunswick, NJ: Rutgers University Press, 2010.

Bodenhamer, David J., Robert G. Barrows, and David Gordon Vanderstel. *The Encyclopedia of Indianapolis.* Bloomington: Indiana University Press, 1994.

Bonow, Robert O., MD, Douglas L. Mann, MD, FACC, Douglas P. Zipes, MD, and Peter Libby, eds. *Braunwald's Heart Disease.* 9th ed. Philadelphia, PA: Elsevier/Saunders, 2012.

Bonner, Thomas Neville. *Becoming a Physician: Medical Education in Great Britain, France, Germany, and the United States, 1750–1945.* New York: Oxford University Press, 1995.

Bosk, Charles. *Forgive and Remember: Managing Medical Failure.* Chicago: University of Chicago Press, 1979.

Brandt, Allan M., and Martha Gardner. "The Golden Age of Medicine?" In *Medicine in the Twentieth Century,* edited by Roger Cooter and John Pickstone, 21–37. Amsterdam: Harwood, 2000.

Braun, Ramona. "Voyaging in the Vein: Medical Experimentation with Heart Catheters in the Twentieth Century." *Nuncius* 26 (2011): 132–58.

Breidbach, Olaf. "Karl Friedrich Burdach." *In Naturphilosophie nach Schelling,* edited by Thomas Bach and Olaf Breidbach, 73–106. Stuttgart: Frommann-Holzboog, 2005.

Broman, Thomas. *The Transformation of German Academic Medicine, 1750–1820.* New York: Cambridge University Press, 2002.

———. "University Reform in Medical Thought at the End of the Eighteenth Century." *Osiris,* 2nd ser., 5 (January 1, 1989): 36–53.

Brüdermann, Stefan. *Göttinger Studenten und akademische Gerichtsbarkeit im 18. Jahrhundert.* Göttingen: Vandenhoeck & Ruprecht, 1990.

Casey, Brian P. "The Surgical Elimination of Violence? Conflicting Attitudes towards Technology and Science during the Psychosurgery Controversy of the 1970s." *Science in Context* 28, no. 1 (2015): 99–129.

Cavallo, Sandra. *Artisans of the Body in Early Modern Italy: Identities, Families and Masculinities: Gender in History.* Manchester, England: Manchester University Press, 2010.

Christensen, Clayton M. *The Innovator's Dilemma: The Revolutionary Book That Will Change the Way You Do Business.* New York: Harper Business, 1997; repr. 2011.

———. *The Innovator's Dilemma: When New Technologies Cause Great Firms to Fail.* Boston, MA: Harvard Business School Press, 1997.

Clapp, Elizabeth J. *Mothers of All Children: Women Reformers and the Rise of Juvenile Courts in Progressive Era America.* University Park: Pennsylvania State University Press, 1998.

Comfort, Nathaniel C. *The Science of Human Perfection: How Genes Became the Heart of American Medicine.* New Haven, CT: Yale University Press, 2012.

Crenner, Christopher. *Private Practice: In the Early Twentieth-Century Medical Office of Dr. Richard Cabot.* Baltimore: Johns Hopkins University Press, 2005.

Cunningham, Andrew. *The Anatomist Anatomis'd: An Experimental Discipline in Enlightenment Europe.* England: Ashgate Publishing, 2010.

———. "The Pen and the Sword: Recovering the Disciplinary Identity of Physiology and Anatomy before 1800—II: Old Anatomy—the Sword." *Studies in History and Philosophy of Science* 34, no. 1 (2003): 51–76.

———. "The Pen and the Sword: Recovering the Disciplinary Identity of Physiology and Anatomy before 1800—I: Old Physiology—the Pen," *Studies in History and Philosophy of Science* 33, no. 4 (2002): 631–65.

Dally, Ann. *Women under the Knife: A History of Surgery*. London: Hutchinson Radius, 1991.

Daston, Lorraine, and Peter Galison. *Objectivity*. Cambridge: Zone Books, 2007.

Davis, Kathy. *Dubious Equalities and Embodied Differences: Cultural Studies on Cosmetic Surgery*. Oxford: Rowman & Littlefield, 2003.

Dowbiggin, Ian Robert. *Keeping America Sane: Psychiatry and Eugenics in the United States and Canada, 1880–1940*. Cornell Studies in the History of Psychiatry. Ithaca, NY: Cornell University Press, 1997.

Duden, Barbara. *The Woman Beneath the Skin: A Doctor's Patients in Eighteenth-Century Germany*. Cambridge, MA: Harvard University Press, 1998.

Dunn, Jacob Piatt. *Greater Indianapolis: The History, the Industries, the Institutions, and the People of a City of Homes*. Vol. 2. Chicago: The Lewis Publishing Company, 1910.

Edgerton, David. "From Innovation to Use: Ten Eclectic Theses on the Historiography of Technology." *History and Technology* 16 (1999): 111–36.

———. "Innovation, Technology, or History: What Is the Historiography of Technology About?" *Technology and Culture* 51 (2010): 680–97.

———. *The Shock of the Old: Technology and Global History since 1900*. London: Profile Books, 2006.

Ellis, Harold. *A History of Surgery*. Cambridge: Cambridge University Press, 2001.

English, Peter C. *Shock, Physiological Surgery, and George Washington Crile: Medical Innovation in the Progressive Era*. Westport. CT: Greenwood Press, 1980.

Ergina, Patrick L., et al. "Challenges in Evaluating Surgical Innovation." *Lancet* 374 (2009): 1097–1104.

Faden, Ruth, and Tom L. Beauchamp, with the assistance of Nancy M. P. King. *A History and Theory of Informed Consent*. New York: Oxford University Press, 1986.

Farrokhyar, Forough, et al. "Randomized Clinical Trials of Surgical Interventions." *Annals of Surgery* 251, no. 3 (2010): 409–16.

Faulkner, Alex. "Casing the Joint: The Material Development of Artificial Hips." In *Artificial Parts, Practical Lives: Modern History of Prosthetics*, edited by Katherine Ott, David Serlin, and Stephen Mihm, 199–226. New York: New York University Press, 2002.

Favaloro, René G. *The Challenging Dream of Heart Surgery: From the Pampas to Cleveland*. New York: Little, Brown, 1994.

Fineberg, Harvey V. "Gastric Freezing—A Study of Diffusion of a Medical Innovation." In *Medical Technology and the Health Care System*, edited by the Committee on Technology and Health Care, 173–2000. Washington, DC: National Academy of Sciences, 1979.

Flamm, Eugene S. "From Signs to Symptoms: The Neurosurgical Management of Head Trauma from 1517 to 1867." In Greenblatt, Dagi, and Epstein, *History of Neurosurgery in Its Scientific and Professional Contexts*, 65–82.

Fox, Renee C. "The Evolution of American Bioethics: A Sociological Perspective." In *Social Science Perspecitive on Medical Ethics*, edited by George Weisz, 201–20. Philadelphia: University of Pennsylvania, 1990.

Fox, Renee C., and Judith P. Swazey. *The Courage to Fail: A Social View of Organ Transplants and Dialysis*. Chicago: University of Chicago Press, 1978.

———. *Spare Parts: Organ Replacement in American Society*. New York: Oxford University Press, 1992.

Fram, Joel, and Sandra Salmans. *Weird Cures: The Most Hilarious, Disgusting and Downright Dangerous Medical Treatments Ever.* Philadelphia: Running Press, 2006.

Frampton, Sally. "The Debris of Life: Diseased Ovaries in Eighteenth-Century Medicine." In *The Secrets of Generation: Reproduction in the Long Eighteenth Century,* edited by Raymond Stephanson and Darren N. Wagner, 344–63. Toronto: University of Toronto Press, 2015.

———. "'The Most Startling Innovation': Ovarian Surgery in Britain, c. 1740–1939." PhD diss., University College London, 2013.

———. "Patents, Priority Disputes and the Value of Credit: Towards a History (and Pre-History) of Intellectual Property in Medicine." *Medical History* 55 (2011): 322.

Friedman, Lawrence M., Curt D. Furberg, and David L. DeMets. *Fundamentals of Clinical Trials.* Boston: John Wright, 1985.

Fye, W. Bruce. *American Cardiology: The History of a Specialty and Its College.* Baltimore: John Hopkins University Press, 1996.

———. *Caring for the Heart: Mayo Clinic and the Rise of Specialization.* New York: Oxford University Press, 2015.

Gabriel, Joseph M. "The Testing of Sanocrysin: Science, Profit, and Innovation in Clinical Trial Design, 1926–1931." *Journal of the History of Medicine and Allied Sciences* 69, no. 4 (2014): 604–32.

Gavrus, Delia. "Men of Dreams and Men of Action: Neurologists, Neurosurgeons, and the Performance of Professional Identity, 1920–1950." *Bulletin of the History of Medicine* 85, no. 1 (2011): 57–92.

———. "Men of Strong Opinions: Identity, Self-Representation, and the Performance of Neurosurgery, 1919–1950." PhD diss., University of Toronto, 2011.

———. "Skill, Judgement and Conduct for the First Generation of Neurosurgeons, 1900–1930." *Medical History* 59, no. 3 (2015): 361–78.

Genschorek, Wolfgang. *Wegbereiter der Chirurgie: Johann Friedrich Dieffenbach, Theodor Billroth.* Leipzig: S. Hirzel, 1983.

Getis, Victoria. *The Juvenile Court and the Progressives.* Urbana: University of Illinois Press, 2000.

Gillick, Muriel R. "The Technological Imperative and the Battle for Hearts in America." *Perspectives in Biology and Medicine* 50, no. 2 (2007): 283.

Gilman, Sander. *Creating Beauty to Cure the Soul: Race and Psychology in the Shaping of Aesthetic Surgery.* Durham, NC: Duke University Press, 1998.

———. *Making the Body Beautiful: A Cultural History of Aesthetic Surgery.* Princeton, NJ: Princeton University Press, 2001.

Godin, Benoît. "Social Innovation : Utopias of Innovation from c. 1830 to the Present." Project on the Intellectual History of Innovation, Working Paper no. 11, INRS, Montreal, 2012, 8. http://www.csiic.ca/PDF/SocialInnovation_2012.pdf.

Greenblatt, Samuel H., T. Forcht Dagi, and Mel H. Epstein, eds. *A History of Neurosurgery in Its Scientific and Professional Contexts.* Park Ridge, IL: American Association of Neurological Surgeons, 1997.

Greene, Jeremy A. "The Abnormal and the Pathological: Cholesterol, Statins, and the Threshold of Disease." In *Medicating Modern America: Pharmaceutical Drugs in History,* edited by Andrea Tone and Elizabeth Watkins, 183–228. New York: New York University Press, 2007.

———. *Prescribing by Numbers: Drugs and the Definition of Disease.* Baltimore: Johns Hopkins University Press, 2007.

Guenther, Katja. *Localization and Its Discontents: A Genealogy of Psychoanalysis and the Neuro Disciplines.* Chicago: University of Chicago Press, 2015.

Hacking, Ian. "Degeneracy, Criminal Behavior, and Looping." In *Genetics and Criminal Behavior*, edited by David Wasserman and Robert Wachbroit, 141–67. Cambridge: Cambridge University Press, 2001.

———. *Mad Travelers: Reflections on the Reality of Transient Mental Illness.* Charlottesville: University of Virginia Press, 1998.

———. "Making Up People." In *Reconstructing Individualism: Autonomy, Individuality, and the Self in Western Thought*, edited by Thomas C. Heller, David E. Wellbery, and Morton Sosna, 222–36. Stanford, CA: Stanford University Press, 1986.

———. *The Taming of Chance.* Cambridge: Cambridge University Press, 1990.

Haegler, Carl S. *Händereinigung, Händedesinfektion und Händeschutz.* Basel: Schwabe, 1900.

Haiken, Elizabeth. *Venus Envy: A History of Cosmetic Surgery.* Baltimore: Johns Hopkins University Press, 1997.

Hamilton, David. *A History of Organ Transplantation: Ancient Legends to Modern Practice.* Pittsburgh, PA: University of Pittsburgh Press, 2013.

Haraway, Donna J. *Simians, Cyborgs, and Women: The Reinvention of Nature.* New York: Routledge, 2013.

Harrington, Anne, *Medicine, Mind, and the Double Brain: A Study in Nineteenth-Century Thought.* Princeton, NJ: Princeton University Press, 1987.

Hawes, Joseph M. *Children in Urban Society: Juvenile Delinquency in Nineteenth-Century America.* New York: Oxford University Press, 1971.

Healy, David. *The Antidepressant Era.* Cambridge: Harvard University Press, 1997.

Hellerström, Patricia. "Johann Friedrich Dieffenbach: Leben und Wirken und sein Einfluß auf die moderne Medizin." Diss., Freie Universität Berlin, 1997.

Hess, Volker, and J. Andrew Mendelsohn, "Case and Series: Medical Knowledge and Paper Technology, 1600–1900." *History of Science* 48, nos. 3/4 (2010): 287–314.

Horwitz, Morton J. *The Transformation of American Law, 1870–1960: The Crisis of Legal Orthodoxy.* New York: Oxford University Press, 1992.

Howell, Joel D. *Technology in the Hospital: Transforming Patient Care in the Early Twentieth Century.* Baltimore: Johns Hopkins University Press, 1995.

Jones, David S. *Broken Hearts: The Tangled History of Cardiac Care.* Baltimore: Johns Hopkins University Press, 2012.

———. "Therapeutic Evolution or Revolution? Metaphors and Their Consequences." In *Therapeutic Revolutions: Pharmaceuticals and Social Change in the Twentieth Century*, edited by Jeremy A. Greene, Flurin Condrau, and Elizabeth Siegel Watkins, 269–301. Chicago: University of Chicago Press, 2016.

———. "Visions of a Cure: Visualization, Clinical Trials, and Controversies in Cardiac Therapeutics, 1968–1998." *Isis* 91, no. 3 (2000): 504–41.

Jones, David S., and Jeremy A. Greene. "The Decline and Rise of Coronary Heart Disease." *American Journal of Public Health* 103, no. 7 (2013): 1207–18.

Jones, Stuart. "Review of *The Invention of Altruism*, by Thomas Dixon." *Reviews in History*, April 2009. http://www.history.ac.uk/reviews/review/757.

Jütte, Robert. *Ärzte, Heiler und Patienten: Medizinischer Alltag in der frühen Neuzeit.* Munich: Artemis & Winkler, 1991.

Kaptchuk, T. J. "Intentional Ignorance: A History of Blind Assessment and Placebo Controls in Medicine." *Bulletin of the History of Medicine* 72, no. 3 (1998): 389–433.

Katz, Jay. *Experimentation with Human Beings: The Authority of the Investigator, Subject, Professions, and State in the Human Experimentation Process.* New York: Russell Sage Foundation, 1972.

Keating, Peter, and Alberto Cambrosio. "Cancer Clinical Trials." In *Cancer in the Twentieth Century*, edited by David Cantor, 197–227. Baltimore: Johns Hopkins University Press, 2008.

———. *Cancer on Trial: Oncology as a New Style of Practice.* Chicago: University of Chicago Press, 2014.

Kernahan, Peter J. "Causation and Cleanliness: George Callender, Wounds, and the Debates over Listerism." *Journal of the History of Medicine and Allied Sciences* 64 (2008): 1–36.

Kevles, Daniel J. *In the Name of Eugenics: Genetics and the Uses of Human Heredity.* New York: Knopf, 1985.

Kline, Ronald. "Where are the Cyborgs in Cybernetics?" *Social Studies of Science* 39, no. 3 (2009): 331–62.

Lamb, S. D. *Pathologist of the Mind: Adolf Meyer and the Origins of American Psychiatry.* Baltimore: Johns Hopkins University Press, 2014.

Landecker, Hannah. *Culturing Life: How Cells Became Technologies.* Cambridge, MA: Harvard University Press, 2009.

———. "Living Differnetly in Time: Plasticity, Temporality and Cellular Biotechnologies." In *Technologized Images, Technologized Bodies*, edited by Jeanette Edwards, Penelope Harvey, and Peter Wade, 211–36. New York: Berghahn Books, 2010.

Langer, R. M., and B. D. Kahan. "Alexis Carrel's Legacy: Visionary of Vascular Surgery and Organ Transplantation." *Transplantation Proceedings* 34 (2002): 1061–65.

Laqueur, Thomas. *Making Sex: Body and Gender from the Greeks to Freud.* Cambridge, MA: Harvard University Press, 1990.

Largent, Mark A. *Breeding Contempt: The History of Coerced Sterilization in the United States.* New Brunswick, NJ: Rutgers University Press, 2008.

Latour, Bruno. *Reassembling the Social: An Introduction to Actor-Network-Theory.* Oxford: Oxford University Press, 2005.

Law, John. "Technology and Heterogeneous Engineering: The Case of Portuguese Expansion." In Bijker, Hughes, and Pinch, *Social Construction of Technological Systems*, 111–34.

Lawrence, Christopher. "Democratic, Divine and Heroic: The History and Historiography of Surgery." In Lawrence, *Medical Theory, Surgical Practice*, 1–47.

———. *Medical Theory, Surgical Practice: Studies in the History of Surgery.* New York: Routledge, 1992.

Lederer, Susan E. *Flesh and Blood: Organ Transplantation and Blood Transfusion in Twentieth-Century America.* Oxford: Oxford University Press, 2008.

———. *Subjected to Science: Human Experimentation in America before the Second World War.* Baltimore: Johns Hopkins University Press, 1995.

Lenoir, Timothy. "Teleology without Regrets: The Transformation of Physiology in Germany, 1790–1847." *Studies in History and Philosophy of Science*, Part A, 12, no. 4 (1981): 293–354.

Lepore, Jill. "The Disruption Machine: What the Gospel of Innovation Gets Wrong." *New Yorker*, June 16, 2014. http://www.newyorker.com/magazine/2014/06/23/the-disruption-machine.

Lerner, Barron H. *The Breast Cancer Wars: Hope, Fear, and the Pursuit of Care in Twentieth-Century America.* New York: Oxford University Press, 2001.

Linker, Beth. "A Dangerous Curve: The Role of History in America's Scoliosis Screening Programs." *American Journal of Public Health* 102, no. 4 (2012): 606–16.

———. "Spines of Steel: A Case of Surgical Enthusiasm in Cold War America." *Bulletin of the History of Medicine* 90, no. 2 (2016): 222–49.

———. *War's Waste: Rehabilitation in World War I America.* Chicago: University of Chicago Press, 2011.

Longo, Lawrence D. "The Rise and Fall of Battey's Operation: A Fashion in Surgery." *Bulletin of the History of Medicine* 53 (1979): 244–67.

Löwy, Ilana. "Medicine and Change." In *Medicine and Change: Historical and Sociological Studies of Medical Innovation*, edited by Ilana Löwy et al., 1–4. Paris: INSERM.

MacCallum, W. G. *William Stuart Halsted, Surgeon.* Baltimore: Johns Hopkins University Press, 1930.

MacLeod, Christine. *Heroes of Invention: Technology, Liberalism and British Identity: 1750–1914.* Cambridge: Cambridge University Press, 2007.

Macmillan, Malcolm. *An Odd Kind of Fame: Stories of Phineas Gage.* Cambridge, MA: MIT Press, 2000.

Manring, M. M., and Jason Calhoun. "Joseph C. Risser Sr., 1892–1982." *Clinical Orthopaedics and Related Research* 468, no. 3 (2010): 643–45.

Marks, Harry M. *The Progress of Experiment: Science and Therapeutic Reform in the United States, 1900–1990.* Cambridge: Cambridge University Press, 1997.

Mau, A., and Edgar Biemer. "Johann-Friedrich Dieffenbach: The Pioneer of Plastic Surgery," *Annals of Plastic Surgery* 33, no. 1 (1994): 112–15.

McKinlay, J. B., "From 'Promising Report' to 'Standard Procedure': Seven Stages in the Career of a Medical Innovation." *The Milbank Memorial Fund Quarterly* 59, no. 3 (1981): 374–411.

McKellar, Shelley. "Artificial Hearts: A Technological Fix More Monstrous Than Miraculous?" In *The Technological Fix: How People Use Technology to Create and Solve Problems*, edited by Lisa Rosner, 11–26. New York: Routledge University Press, 2004.

———. "Negotiating Risk: The Failed Development of Atomic Hearts in America, 1967–77." *Technology and Culture* 54, no. 1 (2013): 1–39.

———. *Surgical Limits: The Life of Gordon Murray.* Toronto: University of Toronto Press, 2003.

McLeod, R. S. "Evidence-Based Surgery." In *Surgery: Basic Science and Clinical Features*, edited by Jeffrey A. Norman et al., 21–35. New York: Springer, 2001.

Meldrum, Marcia. "Departures from the Design: The Randomized Clinical Trial in Historical Context, 1946–1970." PhD diss., State University of New York at Stony Brook, 1994.

Mennel, Robert M. *Thorns & Thistles: Juvenile Delinquents in the United States, 1825–1940.* Hanover, NH: The University Press of New England, 1973.

Merton, Robert K. *The Sociology of Science.* Chicago: University of Chicago Press, 1973.

Michaels, Leon. *The Eighteenth-Century Origin of Angina Pectoris: Predisposing Causes, Recognition, and Aftermath.* London: The Wellcome Trust, 2002.

Moen, Kathleen Y., and Alf L. Nachemson. "Treatment of Scoliosis: An Historical Perspective." *Spine* 24, no. 24 (1999): 2570–75.

Mol, Anne-Marie. *The Body Multiple: Ontology in Medical Practice.* Durham, NC: Duke University Press, 2002.

Morantz-Sanchez, Regina. *Conduct Unbecoming a Woman: Medicine on Trial in Turn-of-the-Century Brooklyn.* Oxford: Oxford University Press, 1999.

Moscucci, Ornella. *The Science of Woman: Gynaecology and Gender in England, 1800–1929.* Cambridge: Cambridge University Press, 1990.

Mros, Bodo. *Der Arzt Johann Friedrich Dieffenbach (1792–1847) in seiner Zeit.* Berlin: Humboldt Universität, 1965.

Mueller, Richard L., Todd K. Rosengart, and O. Wayne Isom. "The History of Surgery for Ischemic Heart Disease." *Annals of Thoracic Surgery* 63 (1997): 869–78.

Muhammad, Khalil Gibran. *The Condemnation of Blackness: Race, Crime, and the Making of Modern Urban America.* Cambridge, MA: Harvard University Press, 2010.

Myers, Tamara. "Embodying Delinquency: Boys' Bodies, Sexuality, and Juvenile Justice History in Early Twentieth-Century Quebec." *Journal of the History of Sexuality* 14, no. 4 (2006): 383–414.

Neary, Francis, and John V. Pickston. *Surgeons, Manufacturers and Patients: A Transatlantic History of Total Hip Replacement.* New York: Palgrave Macmillan, 2007.

Nyhart, Lynn. *Biology Takes Form: Animal Morphology and the German Universities, 1800–1900.* Chicago: University of Chicago Press, 1995.

Odem, Mary E. *Delinquent Daughters: Protecting and Policing Adolescent Female Sexuality in the United States, 1885–1920.* Chapel Hill: University of North Carolina Press, 1995.

Odling-Smee, F. John, Kevin N. Laland, and Marcus W. Feldman. "Niche Construction." *American Naturalist* 147 (1996): 641.

Ojanuga, Durrenda. "The Medical Ethics of the 'Father of Gynaecology,' Dr. J. Marion Sims." *Journal of Medical Ethics* 19 (1993): 28–31.

Pernick, Martin S. *The Black Stork: Eugenics and the Death of "Defective" Babies in American Medicine and Motion Pictures since 1915.* New York: Oxford University Press, 1996.

Peters, Günter. *Der zerrissene Engel: Genieästhetik und literarische Selbstdarstellung im achtzehnten Jahrhundert.* Stuttgart: Metzler, 1982.

Pickstone, John V. "Introduction." In *Medical Innovations in Historical Perspective,* edited by John V. Pickstone, 1–16. Basingstoke, England: MacMillan Press, 1992.

Pinch, Trevor J., and Wiebe E. Bijker. "The Social Construction of Facts and Artifacts: Or How the Sociology of Science and the Sociology of Technology Might Benefit Each Other." In Bijker, Hughes, and Pinch, *Social Construction of Technological Systems,* 17–50.

Podolsky, Scott H. *The Antibiotic Era: Reform, Resistance, and the Pursuit of a Rational Therapeutics.* Baltimore: Johns Hopkins University Press, 2015.

———. "Antibiotics and the Social History of the Controlled Clinical Trial, 1950–1970." *Journal of the History of Medicine and Allied Sciences* 65, no. 3 (2010): 327–67.

———. "Quintessential Beecher—Surgery as Placebo: A Quantitative Study of Bias." *International Anesthesia Clinics* 45 (Fall 2007): 47–63.

Pols, Hans. "Beyond Clinical Frontiers: The American Mental Hygiene Movement, 1910–1945." In *International Relations in Psychiatry: Britain, Germany, and the United States to World War II*, edited by Volker Roelcke, Paul Weindling, and Louise Westwood, 111–33. Rochester, NY: University of Rochester Press, 2010.

Porter, Roy. *The Greatest Benefit to Mankind: A Medical History of Humanity.* New York: W. W. Norton, 1999.

Prentice, Rachel. *Bodies in Formation: An Ethnography of Anatomy and Surgery Education.* Durham, NC: Duke University Press, 2013.

Pressman, Jack D. *Last Resort: Psychosurgery and the Limits of Medicine.* Cambridge: Cambridge University Press, 2002.

———. *The Origins of Organ Transplantation: Surgery and Laboratory Science, 1880–1930.* Rochester, NY: University of Rochester Press, 2010.

Rafter, Nicole Hahn. *Creating Born Criminals.* Urbana: University of Illinois Press, 1997.

Reiser, Stanley Joel. *Technological Medicine: The Changing World of Doctors and Patients.* New York: Cambridge University Press, 2009.

Richards, Robert. *The Romantic Conception of Life: Science and Philosophy in the Age of Goethe.* Chicago: University of Chicago Press, 2002.

Rogers, Naomi. *Dirt and Disease: Polio before FDR.* New Brunswick, NJ: Rutgers University Press, 1992.

———. *Polio Wars: Sister Elizabeth Kenny and the Golden Age of American Medicine.* New York: Oxford University Press, 2014.

Rosenberg, Charles E. "Introduction, Framing Disease: Illness, Society, and History." In *Framing Disease: Studies in Cultural History*, edited by Charles E. Rosenberg and Janet Lynne Golden, xiii–xxvi. New Brunswick, NJ: Rutgers University Press, 1992.

———. "The Therapeutic Revolution: Medicine, Meaning, and Social Change in Nineteenth-century America." *Perspectives in Biology and Medicine* 20 (1977): 485–506.

Rothman, David J. *Conscience and Convenience: The Asylum and Its Alternatives in Progressive America.* rev. ed. New York: Aldine de Gruyter, 2002.

Royal College of Surgeons. *From Innovation to Adoption: Successfully Spreading Surgical Innovation.* London: Royal College of Surgeons, 2014.

Rüegg, Walter. *A History of the University in Europe*, vol. 3, *Universities in the Nineteenth and Early Twentieth Centuries (1800–1945).* Cambridge: Cambridge University Press, 2004.

Santoni-Rugiu, Paolo, and Philip Sykes. *A History of Plastic Surgery.* New York: Springer, 2007.

Sass, Edmund J. *Polio's Legacy: An Oral History.* Lanham, MD: University Press of America, 1996.

Schatzberg, Eric. *Wings of Wood, Wings of Metal: Culture and Technical Choice in American Airplane Materials, 1914–1945.* Princeton, NJ: Princeton University Press, 1999.

Schlich, Thomas. "Asepsis and Bacteriology: A Realignment of Surgery and Laboratory Science." *Medical History* 56 (2012): 308–43.

———. "The Art and Science of Surgery: Innovation and Concepts of Medical Practice in Operative Fracture Care, 1960s–1970s." *Science, Technology & Human Values* 32, no. 1 (2007): 65–87.

———. "'The Days of Brilliancy Are Past': Skill, Styles and the Changing Rules of Surgical Performance, ca. 1820–1920." Unpublished manuscript, 2014.

———. "Ein Netzwerk von Kontrolltechnologien: Eine neue Perspektive auf die Entstehung der modernen Chirurgie." *NTM Journal of the History of Science, Technology and Medicine* 16 (2008): 333–61.

———. "How Gods and Saints Became Transplant Surgeons: The Scientific Article as a Model for the Writing of History." *History of Science* 33 (1995): 311–31.

———. "Negotiating Technologies in Surgery: The Controversy about Surgical Gloves in 1890s." *Bulletin of the History of Medicine* 87 (2013): 170–97.

———. "'One and the Same the World Over'—The International Culture of Surgical Exchange in an Age of Globalization, 1870–1914." *Journal of the History of Medicine and Allied Sciences* (online February 16, 2016), doi:10.1093/jhmas/jrw003.

———. *The Origins of Organ Transplantation: Surgery and Laboratory Science, 1880s–1930s.* Rochester, NY: University of Rochester Press, 2010.

———. "'Physiological Surgery': Laboratory Science as the Epistemic Basis of Modern Surgery (and Neurosurgery)." Unpublished manuscript, 2014.

———. "Risk and Medical Innovation: A Historical Perspective." In *The Risks of Medical Innovation: Risk Perception and Assessment in Historical Context,* edited by Thomas Schlich and Ulrich Tröhler, 1–19. London: Routledge, 2006.

———. *Surgery, Science, and Industry: A Revolution in Fracture Care, 1950s–1990s.* New York: Palgrave MacMillan, 2002.

———. "Why Were Surgical Gloves Not Used Earlier? History of Medicine and Alternative Paths of Innovation." *Lancet* 386, no. 10,000 (2015): 1234–35.

Schmidt, Jochen. *Die Geschichte des Genie-Gedankens in der deutschen Literatur, Philosophie und Politik, 1750–1945: Von der Aufklärung bis zum Idealismus.* 2 vols. 3rd ed. Heidelberg: Winter, 2004.

———. *Die Geschichte des Genie-Gedankens in der deutschen Literatur, Philosophie und Politik, 1750–1945: Von der Romantik bis zum Ende des Dritten Reichs.* 2 vols. Heidelberg: Winter, 2004.

Schultheiss, Dirk, et al. "Johann Friedrich Dieffenbach (1792–1847) als Begründer der Plastischen Chirurgie." *Mund-, Kiefer- Und Gesichtschirurgie* 2, no. 6 (1998): 309–15.

Schultz, Daniel. "Regulating Medical Devices." In *Perspectives on Risk and Regulation: The FDA at 100,* edited by Arthur Daemmrich and Joanna Radin, 52–64. Philadelphia: Chemical Heritage Foundation, 2007.

Scull, Andrew. *Madhouse: A Tragic Tale of Megalomania and Modern Medicine.* New Haven, CT: Yale University Press, 2004.

———. *Madness in Civilization: A Cultural History of Insanity, from the Bible to Freud, from the Madhouse to Modern Medicine.* Princeton, NJ: Princeton University Press, 2015.

Serlin, David. *Replaceable You: Engineering the Body in Postwar America.* Chicago: University of Chicago Press, 2004.

Shapiro, Arthur K., and Elaine Shapiro. *The Powerful Placebo: From Ancient Priest to Modern Physician.* Baltimore: Johns Hopkins University Press, 1997.

Sharp, Lesley A. *The Transplant Imaginary: Mechanical Hearts, Animal Parts and Moral Thinking in Highly Experimental Science.* Berkeley: University of California Press, 2014.

Smith, Dale C. "Appendicitis, Appendectomy, and the Surgeon." *Bulletin of the History of Medicine* 30 (1996): 414–41.

Stanley, Peter. *For Fear of Pain: British Surgery, 1790–1850.* New York: Penguin, 2003.

Stanton, Jennifer. "Introduction." In *Innovations in Health and Medicine: Diffusion and Resistance in the Twentieth Century,* edited by Jennifer Stanton, 1–15. London: Routledge, 2002.

———. "Making Sense of Technologies in Medicine." *Social History of Medicine* 12 (1999): 437–48.

Stark, Laura. *Behind Closed Doors: IRBs and the Making of Ethical Research.* Chicago: University of Chicago Press, 2012.

Steinberg, Daniel. "An Interpretive History of the Cholesterol Controversy, Part V: The Discovery of the Statins and the End of the Controversy." *Journal of Lipid Research* 47 (2006): 1339–51.

Stern, Alexandra Minna. "Sterilized in the Name of Public Health: Race, Immigration, and Reproductive Control in Modern California." *American Journal of Public Health* 95, no. 7 (2005): 1128–38.

Stevens, Rosemary. *In Sickness and in Wealth: American Hospitals in the Twentieth Century.* New York: Basic Books, 1989.

Sullivan, Deborah. *Cosmetic Surgery: The Cutting Edge of Commercial Medicine in America.* New Brunswick, NJ: Rutgers University Press, 2001.

Terrall, Mary. *Catching Nature in the Act: Réaumur and the Practice of Natural History in the Eighteenth Century.* Chicago: University of Chicago Press, 2014.

Timmerman, Carsten. *A History of Lung Cancer: The Recalcitrant Disease.* New York: Palgrave Macmillan, 2014.

Tobbell, Dominique. "Charitable Innovations: The Political Economy of Thalassemia Research and Drug Development in the United States, 1960–2000." In *Perspectives on Twentieth Century Pharmaceuticals,* edited by Judy Slinn and Vivianne Quirke, 303–38. Bern: Peter Lang, 2009.

Tomes, Nancy. "Merchants of Health: Medicine and Consumer Culture in the United States, 1900–1940." *Journal of American History* (2001): 519–47.

Tone, Andrea. *The Age of Anxiety: A History of America's Turbulent Affair with Tranquilizers.* New York: Basic Books, 2008.

Tröhler, Ulrich. *Auf dem Weg zur physiologischen Chirurgie: Der Nobelpreisträger Theodor Kocher 1841–1917.* Basel: Birkhäuser, 1984.

Trost, Jennifer. *Gateway to Justice: The Juvenile Court and Progressive Child Welfare in a Southern City.* Athens: University of Georgia Press, 2005.

Tuchman, Arleen. *Science, Medicine, and the State in Germany: The Case of Baden, 1815–1871.* New York: Oxford University Press, 1993.

Ulrich, U., and C. Lauritzen. "Johann Friedrich Dieffenbach (1792–1847): 'Vater der Plastischen Chirurgie' in Deutschland." *Deutsche Medizinische Wochenschrift* 117, no. 30 (1992): 1165–67.

Valenstein, Elliot S. *Great and Desperate Cures: The Rise and Decline of Psychosurgery and Other Radical Treatments for Mental Illness.* New York: Basic Books, 1986.

Wall, L. Lewis. "The Medical Ethics of Dr. J. Marion Sims: A Fresh Look at the Historical Record." *Journal of Medical Ethics* 32 (2006): 346–50.

Watkins, Elizabeth Siegel. *On the Pill: A Social History of Oral Contraceptives, 1950–1970.* Baltimore: Johns Hopkins University Press, 2011.

Weiss, Allen B. "Conversations in Medicine: Owen H. Wangensteen." *Hospital Practice* 23, no. 3 (1988): 111–31.

Wilde, Sally. *History of Surgery: Trust, Patient Autonomy, Medical Dominance and Australian Surgery, 1890–1940.* Byron Bay, Australia: Finesse Press, 2010.

Williamson, Bess. "Electric Moms and Quad Drivers: People with Disabilities Buying, Making, and Using Technology in Postwar America." *American Studies* 52, no. 1 (2012): 5–29.

Willrich, Michael. *City of Courts: Socializing Justice in Progressive Era Chicago.* Cambridge: Cambridge University Press, 2003.

———. *Pox: An American History.* London: Penguin Books, 2011.

———. "The Two Percent Solution: Eugenic Jurisprudence and the Socialization of American Law, 1900–1930." *Law and History Review* 16, no. 1 (1998): 63–111.

Wilson, Daniel J. "And They Shall Walk: Ideal versus Reality in Polio Rehabilitation in the United States." *Asclepio* 61, no. 1 (2009): 175–92.

———. *Living with Polio: The Epidemic and Its Survivors.* Chicago: University of Chicago Press, 2005.

Wooten, Heather Green. *The Polio Years in Texas: Battling a Terrifying Unknown.* College Station: Texas A&M University Press, 2009.

Worboys, Michael. *Spreading Germs: Disease Theories and Medical Practice in Britain, 1865–1900.* Cambridge: Cambridge University Press, 2000.

Young, Robert Maxwell. *Mind, Brain and Adaptation in the Nineteenth Century: Cerebral Localization and Its Biological Context from Gall to Ferrier.* Oxford: Carendon Press, 1970.

Zetka, James R. *Surgeons and the Scope.* Ithaca, NY: Cornell University Press, 2003.

Zimmerman, Leo, and Ilza Veith. *Great Ideas in the History of Surgery.* San Francisco: Norman Publishing, 1993.

Zloczower, Awraham. *Career Opportunities and the Growth of Scientific Discovery in Nineteenth-Century Germany.* New York: Arno Press, 1981.

Contributors

CHRISTOPHER CRENNER, MD, PhD, is the Ralph Major and Robert Hudson Professor and Chair of the Department of History and Philosophy of Medicine at the University of Kansas Medical Center, where he is also faculty in the Department of Internal Medicine. He is presently the editor of the *Journal of the History of Medicine and Allied* Sciences. His research looks at the history of American medicine in the nineteenth and twentieth centuries and especially the interface of science and medical practice. His book *Private Practice* (Johns Hopkins University Press, 2005) examines the history of doctor-patient interactions and the influence of medical technology on practice. He also works regularly as a volunteer physician at the free Jaydoc Health Clinic.

SALLY FRAMPTON, PhD, is a postdoctoral researcher at the Faculty of English at the University of Oxford. Her current research looks at the development of the medical press in the nineteenth century and at public participation in medicine through movements such as first aid and antivaccination campaigns. She has published on the history of ovarian disease, intellectual property in surgery, and on the introduction of minimally invasive therapies into surgery in the twentieth century.

DELIA GAVRUS is assistant professor of the history of science at the University of Winnipeg in Canada. She has published on the history of neuroscience and the history of surgery, and is currently working on a book about the development of neurosurgery in Canada and the United States (under advanced contract with McGill-Queen's University Press) and on an edited collection about technique in the history of the mind and brain sciences.

LISA HAUSHOFER, MD, is a PhD candidate at the Department of the History of Science at Harvard University. Her research examines the emergence of a new category of medicinal consumables located at the unstable conceptual and regulatory boundary of medicine and food in late nineteenth- and early twentieth-century Britain and the United States. She also coedits the history of medicine blog Remedia.

DAVID S. JONES, MD, PhD, is the inaugural A. Bernard Ackerman Professor of the Culture of Medicine at Harvard University. His initial research focused on epidemics among American Indians (*Rationalizing Epidemics: Meanings and Uses of American Indian Mortality since 1600*, Harvard University Press, 2004). Next he examined the history of decision making in cardiac therapeutics (*Broken Hearts: The Tangled History of Cardiac Care*, Johns Hopkins University Press, 2013). He is currently at work on two books. *On the Origins of Therapies* will trace the evolution of coronary-artery surgery. The other book examines the history of heart disease and cardiac therapeutics in India.

BETH LINKER is associate professor at the University of Pennsylvania in the Department of the History and Sociology of Science. She is the author of *War's Waste: Rehabilitation in World War I America* (University of Chicago Press, 2011) and coeditor of *Civil Disabilities: Citizenship, Membership, and Belonging* (University of Pennsylvania Press, 2015). Her award-winning scholarship has also appeared in the *Boston Globe, Bulletin of the History of Medicine*, the *Journal of the History of Medicine and Allied Sciences, American Journal of Public Health*, and the *New England Journal of Medicine*. She is currently at work on her next book, *Slouch: The Hidden History of America's Posture Epidemic.*

SHELLEY MCKELLAR, PhD, is the Jason A. Hannah Chair in the History of Medicine at Western University, London, Canada, where she teaches in the Department of History and in the Schulich School of Medicine and Dentistry. She is completing a book on the history of artificial hearts. Her past publications include *Surgical Limits: The Life of Gordon Murray* (University of Toronto Press, 2003) and *Medicine and Technology in Canada* (Canada Science and Technology Museum, 2008), as well as numerous articles. As curator of the Medical Artifact Collection at Western University, she embraces studying and teaching with medical objects.

THOMAS SCHLICH, MD, Dr. habil., is the James McGill Professor of the History of Medicine at the Department Social Studies of Medicine at McGill University. His current research projects include a history of modern surgery, 1800–1914, and the rise of minimally invasive surgery, 1980–2000. Among other works, he has published *Surgery, Science and Industry: A Revolution in Fracture Care, 1950s–1990s* (Palgrave, 2002) and *The Origins of Organ Transplantation: Surgery and Laboratory Science, 1880s–1930s* (University of Rochester Press, 2010).

Index

An italicized page number indicates a figure.

www.ingramcontent.com/pod-product-compliance
Lightning Source LLC
LaVergne TN
LVHW091529200926
848483LV00002B/340